Health and Disease in Human History

The *Journal of Interdisciplinary History* Readers

Health and Disease in Human History
Edited by Robert I. Rotberg

Social Mobility and Modernization
Edited by Robert I. Rotberg

Health and Disease in Human History:
A *Journal of Interdisciplinary History* Reader

Edited by Robert I. Rotberg

The MIT Press
Cambridge, Massachusetts
London, England

Andrew Appleby, "Nutrition and Disease: The Case of London, 1550–1750" *JIH* VI, 1 (Winter 1975); Anne Hardy, "Diagnosis, Death, and Diet in London, 1750–1909" *JIH* XVIII, 3 (Winter 1988); Robert Woods and P. R. Andrew Hinde, "Mortality in Victorian England: Models and Patterns" *JIH* XVIII, 1 (Summer 1987); James C. Riley "Height, Nutrition, and Mortality Risk Reconsidered" XXIV, 3 (Winter 1994); Massimo Livi-Bacci, "Fertility, Nutrition, and Pellagra: Italy During the Vital Revolution" *JIH* XVI, 3 (Winter 1986); Susan B. Hanley, "Urban Sanitation in Preindustrial Japan" *JIH* XVIII, 1 (Summer 1987); Robert McCaa, "Spanish and Nahuatl Views on Smallpox and Demographic Catastrophe in Mexico" *JIH* XXV, 3 (Winter 1995); Dauril Alden and Joseph C. Miller, "Out of Africa: The Slave Trade and the Transmission of Smallpox to Brazil, 1560–1831" *JIH* XVIII, 2 (Autumn 1987); Kenneth F. and Virginia H. Kiple, "Deficiency Diseases in the Caribbean" *JIH* XI, 2 (Autumn 1980); Daniel Blake Smith, "Mortality and Family in the Colonial Chesapeake" *JIH* VIII, 3 (Winter 1978; David Northrup, "African Mortality in the Suppression of the Slave Trade: The Case of the Bight of Biafra" *JIH* IX, 1 (Summer 1978); Myron P. Gutmann and Kenneth Fliess, "The Social Context of Child Mortality in the American Southwest" *JIH* XXVI, 4 (Spring 1996); Irene W. D. Hecht, "Kinship and Migration: The Making of an Oregon Isolate Community" *JIH* VIII, 1 (Summer 1977).

Library of Congress Cataloging-in-Publication Data

Health and disease in human history : a journal of interdisciplinary history reader/ edited by Robert I. Rotberg.
   p. cm.
  Includes bibliographical references.
  ISBN 0-262-18207-6 (hc. : alk. paper)—ISBN 0-262-68122-6 (pbk. : alk. paper)
  1. Disease and history. I. Rotberg, Robert I.

R702.H43 2000
610'.9—dc21

00-035135

Contents

Contributors

Robert I. Rotberg is co-editor of the *Journal of Interdisciplinary History,* President of the World Peace Foundation, Director of Harvard University's Program on Intrastate Conflict, Adjunct Professor at the Kennedy School of Government, and former professor of history and political science at MIT. He is the author or editor of three dozen books on Africa, Asia, and the Caribbean. His most recent book is *Creating Peace in Sri Lanka: Civil War and Reconciliation* (Washington, D.C., 1999).

Dauril Alden is Professor of History, University of Washington. He is the author of *The Making of an Enterprise: The Society of Jesus in Portugal, Its Empire, and Beyond: 1540–1750* (Stanford, 1996) and other books.

Andrew B. Appleby, now deceased, was Associate Professor of History, San Diego State University. He was the author of *Famine in Tudor and Stuart England* (Stanford, 1978).

Kenneth H. Fleiss is Associate Professor of Anthropology, University of Nevada.

Myron P. Gutmann is Professor of History, University of Texas, Austin. He is the author of *Toward the Modern Economy: Early Industry in Europe, 1500–1800* (Philadelphia, 1988) and other books.

Susan Hanley is Professor of Japanese Studies, University of Washington. She is the author of *Everyday Things in Premodern Japan: The Hidden Legacy of Material Culture* (Berkeley, 1997) and other books.

Anne Hardy is Research Fellow, Imperial College, London. She is the author of *The Epidemic Streets: Infectious Disease and the Rise of Preventive Medicine* (Oxford, 1993) and other books.

Irene W. D. Hecht is Senior Associate, American Council on Education, and former President of Wells College. She is the author of *The Department Chair as Academic Leader* (Phoenix, 1998) and other books.

R. Andrew Hinde is Research Fellow, Dept. of Geography, University of Sheffield. He is the author of *Demographic Methods* (London, 1998).

Kenneth F. Kiple is Professor of History, Bowling Green State University. He is the author of *Plague, Pox and Pestilence* (London, 1997) and other books.

Massimo Livi-Bacci is Professor of Demography, University of Florence. He is the author of *The Population of Europe: A History* (Malden, 1999) and other books.

Robert McCaa is Professor of History, University of Minnesota. He is the author of *Marriage and Fertility in Chile: Demographic Turning Points in the Petorca Valley* (Boulder, 1983) and other books.

Joseph C. Miller is Professor of History, University of Virginia. He is the author of *Way of Death: Merchant Capitalism and the Angolan Slave Trade, 1730–1830* (Madison, 1988) and other books.

David Northrup is Professor of History, Boston College. He is the author of *Indentured Labor in the Age of Imperialism, 1834–1922* (Cambridge, 1995) and other books.

James C. Riley is Professor of History, University of Indiana. He is the author of *Sick, Not Dead: The Health of British Workingmen during the Mortality Decline* (Baltimore, 1997) and other books.

Daniel Blake Smith is Associate Professor of History, University of Kentucky. He is the author of *Inside the Great House: Planter Family Life in Eighteenth Century Chesapeake Society* (Ithaca, 1980).

Robert I. Woods is Senior Lecturer, Dept. of Geography, University of Sheffield. He is the author of *An Atlas of Victorian Mortality* (Liverpool, 1997) and other books.

Robert I. Rotberg

Morbidity and Mortality in Human History:

The Struggle to Survive
For more than thirty years, interdisciplinary history has explicitly included the study of how groups and individuals in the past progressed despite disease, nutritional deficiency, poor sanitation, mean and menacing urban streets, fearsome and infectious sea voyages, and the many other morbid and mortal hazards of the last millennium. That populations grew and economies developed is a tribute to many kinds of human advances. But progress, however generously defined, was neither lineal nor consistent. Nor was it equivalent across continents and cultures. This collection of essays suggests the great extent to which exploration, settlement, agricultural growth, colonization, urbanization, and even human stature were influenced by environmental and epidemiological realities, as well as by political and economic responses to those realities.

Methodologically and substantively, these essays depend on a deep understanding of the process of the past—the discipline of history—and an equally full appreciation of the insights and working techniques of other relevant disciplines: anthropology, medicine, nutrition, genetics, psychiatry, statistics, and sanitary engineering.

The thirteen essays in this volume are representative of the dozens of articles and research notes on these and similar subjects that appeared in the *Journal of Interdisciplinary History* during the first three decades of its publication. Indeed, it is not by accident that the original publication dates of these articles range from 1975 to 1996, and exemplify the best work that the *JIH* published during those decades. They also sample several of the many salient issues of mortality and morbidity with which the *JIH* was concerned from its inception and remains concerned: specific diseases and the effect of each on human history; nutrition and economic growth; public health and life and death; the impact of diet and disease on individuals and families as well as the broader sweeps of history; measurements of heights and stature as proxies for generalizations about human progress; and the deployment of medical information and insight to solve historical questions previously presumed to be solely political, social, or economic.

The essays in this volume are representative of the *JIH's* conscious geographical outlook: pioneering work on Britain and the United States certainly appears, but so does paradigmatical research that focuses on the rest of Europe, Africa, Latin America, and Asia, or on two or more geographical and cultural entities at once. To be selected for this volume, the essays, as excellent as they may have been at the time of publication, needed still to be pathbreaking. (Fixed page limits prevented the inclusion of even more of the best of the *JIH* on these and closely allied subjects.)

The late Andrew Appleby's classic examination of the relationship between the lack of nutrition (food scarcity) and the rise of epidemic disease opens this volume both because it was published early in the *JIH*'s development and because it was, and remains, a formative and insightful contribution to the then emerging question of whether malnutrition and poor nutrition lowered resistance to epidemic disease, as traditionally assumed. The received position needed to be reevaluated, particularly to understand the peaks and valleys of English and British population growth. Was improved nutrition protective (as common sense suggested) against disease pathogens? If industrialization lowered workers' standards of living, why did populations increase rapidly? Appleby asked whether there was any decisive relationship between the great epidemic killers of pre-industrial Europe and nutritional deficiencies.

Using a four-century-long price series for bread as a proxy for nutrition among London's poor, and holding constant a number of other important food sources and variables, Appleby suggests that London's poor had few alternative sources of nutrition during grain shortages. After a careful assessment of bills of mortality (which listed causes of death), he finds little correlation between bread prices and plague epidemics. Plague did not break out in London when higher prices prevailed and diets—and presumably resistance—deteriorated. Nor did smallpox. Likewise, he could trace no linkage between high prices, food shortages, and deaths from tuberculosis (or consumption). There may have been a weak relationship between nutritional deficits and typhus.

Mortality classifications were weak and variable. Typhus became less important as a killer as the eighteenth century matured. Convulsions (a mixture of childhood causes of death) killed more and more children as the years advanced, but without a correspondence to long-term falling bread prices. At the same time, despite the increasingly more crowded conditions in London, plague disappeared. Disease, concludes Appleby, should be treated as an "autonomous influence" on population growth.

Anne Hardy also writes about death and diet in Britain, but she begins when Appleby ends, studying the years from 1750 to 1909. She suggests that fewer deaths did not necessarily imply improved nutrition, discusses the unreliability of the statistical surveys employed by her predecessors, and indicates that death rates and causes varied significantly by region within Britain, even within England itself. Ultimately, she warrants only one correlation as strongly explanatory.

Hardy reviews the flaws in the bills of mortality for London, especially their diagnostic weaknesses. Since the bills were compiled by unqualified lay searchers, not medical men, and honesty of reporting was not their strength, she reasons that categories of convulsion and consumption were (as Appleby noted) so imprecise as to be almost useless.

Deaths from convulsions declined from the end of the eighteenth century, when new diagnostic categories like whooping cough, dropsy (tuberculosis meningitis), and croup were introduced. But not until the medical certification of death (a reform from 1839) and the practice of distinguishing between convulsions and diarrhea (which brought about convulsions) as causes of childhood death did the reports and statistics begin to acquire meaning. Indeed, a closer examination of the descriptive term *convulsions* discloses that the category probably included perinatal and crib (sudden infant death syndrome) mortalities.

Re-examining the thesis (advanced elsewhere) that adulterated bread was a prime cause of infant mortality (leading to "convulsions" from the chalk, alum, and bone ashes added to the bread of the poor) in the late eighteenth and early nineteenth centuries in London and Britain, Hardy finds it plausible, based on the better outcomes when potato flour later improved the quality of bread. But she denies the likelihood that ergot of rye was ever a significant cause of infant mortality after 1780. She terms the evidence of ergot in England doubtful, and the connection between ergot and infant convulsions untenable.

With regard to pulmonary tuberculosis, Hardy says that the bills of mortality were exceptionally unreliable. They covered a wider range of complaints than tuberculosis: pneumonia, asthma, chronic bronchitis, some cancers and leukemia, and many more. Any wasting disease was apt to be classified as consumption. Bronchitis was recognized as a separate disease only between 1808 and 1814. Indeed, as deaths from tuberculosis decreased during the nineteenth century, deaths from other lung diseases were rising. This pattern was partially an artifact of the better diagnosis that resulted from the gradual acceptance of Laennec's stethoscope, but it represented no diminution in the number of Londoners dying from diseases of the chest.

The compulsory notification of infectious disease occurred in London only after 1889. Likewise, the contagiousness of various diseases—tuberculosis, for example—did not become recognized until the 1890s. These facts suggest a metaphor for the difficulties that historians face in attempting to associate causes of death with social change. Hardy cautions that the pattern of decline from tuberculosis is too uncertain to permit chronologically precise explanations.

The roles of nutrition and housing as contributory factors in the incidence and prevalence of tuberculosis' rise and fall must remain suspect. For instance, the vaunted associations between increased potato consumption and the reduction of mortality from tuberculosis is doubtful. By the early twentieth century, "when potatoes had long been indisputably a staple starch, more than 90 percent of the British population was infected with tuberculosis" (56). Thus, the contributing causes of mortality from tuberculosis varied with climatic, agricultural, and urban conditions. Nevertheless, concludes Hardy, despite an etiology that demands constant qualification and re-qualification, striking is the discovery that declining mortality from tuberculosis is highly correlated only with rising real wages, especially from 1838 onward.

Robert Woods and P. R. Andrew Hinde examine many of the same issues discussed by Appleby and Hardy; they also review and improve upon the seminal research and writings of Thomas McKeown (*The Modern Rise of Population* [London, 1976]), E. Anthony Wrigley and Roger S. Schofield (*The Population History of England, 1541–1871: A Reconstruction* [Cambridge, Mass., 1981]), and others. They criticize the former for being concerned primarily with national trends at the expense of significant localized environmental variations in levels of mortality and patterns of its causation. They suggest that the latter's life-table models require updating to be useful in the Victorian era. They also take issue with McKeown's strong emphasis on nutritional improvements as the critical explanation for improved life expectations in Britain during the nineteenth and early twentieth centuries.

Although vital statistics were collected and published in England and Wales after 1837, forty-five registration districts show inconsistencies and anomalies. For example, annual sex-specific age at death data are available only for 1855 to 1880 and can be linked to population at risk data only from the 1861 and 1871 censuses. Reliability is problematical: age misreporting is likely, and under-enumeration is a probable factor. The cause-of-death data are also suspect. Before 1869, typhus and typhoid, for example, were combined into one category. Etiology of disease being little understood, other errors and confusion were inevitable (as Hardy also indicated).

Even so, Woods and Hinde say, the vital statistics for England and Wales are rich and potentially fruitful for the 1860s and 1870s. The power of those statistics is even more impressive when compared with similar sources for the rest of Europe and North America. Accurate English life tables date from 1854, that first one relying upon the 1841 census. The next four life tables related average mortality in ten-year intercensal periods to estimates of risk drawn from the 1841 and 1851 censuses.

Woods and Hinde suggest new methods of calculating single-sex life tables for the English family, which, after complicated adjustments, led to thirty-one English model life tables for each sex, and detailed probability-of-dying tables for specific registration districts. This new work enables them to estimate life experiences parallel to the English models of Wrigley and Schofield, but for the full range in mortality experience of 1861.

What Woods and Hinde's re-analysis provides is a new way of estimating age-specific mortality in nineteenth-century Britain. Since certain age groups made more substantial contributions to improvements in life expectations than others, explanations of mortality declines must take age groupings into account. Hence, rises in expectations depended more upon falls in the death rates of children and young adults, not declines in infant mortality. Specifically, as life expectations increased by seven years from 1851 to 1901, deaths of those from one to twenty-four years old fell, whereas the five-year increase in life expectation from 1901 to

1911 was based on mortality reductions for those younger than one year of age.

In addition to demonstrating how an improved understanding of the statistical bases of mortality in England and Wales contributes to re-interpretations of received information, Woods and Hinde also provide elegant cartographical displays of regional variations in England and Wales for 1861, according to life expectation at birth and infant mortality. Their tables display percentages of population in England and Wales in 1861 with respect to levels of life expectation, as well as frequency distributions of causes of death for selected registration districts that show striking variations. These arrays of data lead to the conclusion that infant deaths were caused by water-borne and food-borne diseases. Infant mortality was also higher than expected in Norfolk, Lincolnshire, the East Midlands, and the East Riding of Yorkshire, but lower than expected in the west of Wales and the north and northeast of England.

When Woods and Hinde relate life expectancy and infant mortality to population density (in an attempt to measure the impact of urbanization on mortality), they find that the most crowded cities had the highest levels of infant mortality. But the urban districts vary in such a way that the "simple differences between urban and rural environments are either not entirely captured when measured via population density, or that environmental conditions are rather more complex in their influence on mortality" (83–84). Woods and Hinde also fail to detect any statistically significant relationship between mortality in 1861 and the physician-to-population ratio (much higher in London than in rural England and Wales).

Rather than better nutrition and longer life expectations, Woods and Hinde offer purer water as the most important factor for reducing mortality, particularly in the urban areas. Only when death rates began to fall in the cities of England and Wales did overall expectations of life improve in Victorian England and Wales.

In their later chapter, Kenneth and Virginia Kiple refer to work that demonstrates how stature could reflect the nutritional deprivation of African slaves landed in the Caribbean. James C. Riley, one of the pioneers in using adult height as a proxy for nutritional status, extends this use of anthropometric methodology in another pathbreaking essay in this collection. The *JIH* has published a number of other articles and research notes exploring this important and comparatively new seam of interdisciplinary history.

Measurements of stature provide a method of assessing the distribution of economic and nutritional resources among populations of different eras and geographical locations. Reduced adult height can indicate poorer nutritional status and intimate a higher risk of death. The scientific assumption is that maximum height is achieved when an individual's caloric intake from a protein-rich diet equals, or exceeds, the demands of metabolism, growth, and work. Diets that do not allow individuals, on average, to attain their height potential are by definition insufficient. Declining or otherwise compromised heights can reflect accumulated dietary poverty as well as new or introduced nutritional stress.

Riley studied British males measured in 1866 (and born between 1817 and 1841). The English men in his sample were undersized compared to their modern counterparts, whereas the Scotsmen were taller than their twentieth-century successors. Since this Victorian working-age cohort was measured and weighed, Riley suggests that their nutritional status can be gauged directly, and that their body measurements should permit estimates of their life spans. (Riley's nonrandom sample totaled 3,498 persons. He explains how the sample was drawn and details its strengths and weaknesses, as well as its composition with respect to occupation, class, and so on.)

Contrary to other research populations, the men in Riley's sample displayed no particular variation in nutritional status. Body mass increased with age, as it does in modern populations. Height variations were not pronounced; older men were not shorter than younger men, as is observed and expected in late twentieth-century Britain. Men resident in rural areas were taller and heavier than their urban counterparts; slighter and shorter men migrated to the cities to take up employment in manufacturing. Furthermore, since crude death rates in Britain have declined sharply since 1866 in all regions, Riley can state that English adult males gained height as well as longevity between 1866 and 1980 (the date of a significant modern survey) and Scotsmen gained longevity but lost height. However, by analyzing average body-mass indexes for the men in the Victorian sample and their estimated survival rates, Riley concludes that nutritional deficiency in adulthood played no significant role in the higher mortality of men in the nineteenth century compared to those in the twentieth century. In other words, the nutrition of past populations cannot be judged by height alone; weight matters. Anthropometric historians may have glimpsed only a part of the story.

Elsewhere in Europe, especially in Italy, rising levels of income and better nutrition coincided with a long secular decline in marital fertility. But not in northeastern Italy, which witnessed fertility increases. Why? The literature stresses the limited influence of nutrition on fertility and fecundity. Why did dietary insults play more important roles in northeastern Italy?

In the Veneto, Lombardia, and Emilia, in contrast to neighboring regions of Italy, marital fertility was much higher than it was at the end of the nineteenth century. In northern Italy as a whole (as well as in other sections of the country), fertility had fallen significantly during the same periods. It took fifty years for northeastern Italy's fertility patterns to mirror the low levels of the rest of the nation. Birth control had been practiced in the large urban centers of northeastern Italy, as elsewhere, for several decades. Nuptiality had undergone no meaningful changes. Because infant mortality was rapidly falling, no replacement or insurance effect can explain the fertility increases. Breastfeeding was still universal. Gender balances, as influenced by the out-migration of men, were similar to those elsewhere. Birth registration was complete, too; the fertility results were not statistical artifacts. What was responsible for northern Italy's anomalous fertility pattern?

Contrary to many scholars, Massimo Livi-Bacci maintains that nutrition can have a profound effect on fertility, and that pellagra—a chronic, often fatal disease caused by niacin deficiency—first depressed and then released fecundity in northeastern Italy. Pellagra was most prevalent where diets were dependent on maize, with little or no milk, meat, or vegetables.

Maize became an increasingly popular crop in Italy in the wake of the Napoleonic wars. Maize bread and polenta became the food of the poor. When wheat bread and pasta were expensive, peasants naturally turned to the maize that they grew themselves. The incidence of pellagra increased. In northeastern rural Italy—the heartland of maize consumption (little was exported) and pellagra—the last two decades of the nineteenth century were particularly harsh. The understanding of pellagra as the result of a vitamin deficiency awaited research that was not published until 1912. By then, economic growth and other secular changes had begun vigorously to erode the prevalence of pellagra in northeastern Italy.

Endemic and chronic deficiency diseases ought to depress natural fertility. Diseases like pellagra, which manifests as severe dermatitis, diarrhea, and dementia, could result in reduced libido and reduced frequency of sexual intercourse. The digestive debilitations would certainly have affected fecundity. With pellagra, female mortality is higher than male mortality. But, overall, mortality in the pellagra-affected region of Italy in the second half of the nineteenth century was lower than in other parts of the country.

With the elimination of pellagra, and the nutritional improvements of the late nineteenth century, the barriers to fertility began to fall. Northeastern Italy made up for its lost years, reproducing rapidly until World War I. The secular changes that followed brought the region's demographic patterns in line with those of the rest of the country. By then, pellagra was mostly an unpleasant memory, and marital fertility fell to universal Italian levels.

Potable water and urban sanitary improvements may or may not have been relevant to the fertility story in late nineteenth-century Italy. They were surely critical at that time in Britain, however, as Woods and Hinde discovered. Susan B. Hanley's chapter makes an even stronger case for the importance of waterborne sewage to the growth of cities in preindustrial Japan.

By 1800, 10 percent of Japan's total population was urban; Edo (later Tokyo and once a collection of fishing villages) was one of the largest cities in the world. Kyoto and Osaka were also large. This enormous increase in scale depended on new methods of supplying good water to households and on removing refuse. Edo's population exceeded that of any European city in 1700 and rivaled that of London (which had caught up) in 1800. But because it inhabited a marshy area that was more confined than most European cities, the means of delivering water was a major issue.

Fortunately, the Tokugawa shogun who selected Edo as his capital in 1590 knew that decent water was a limiting factor. One of his key retainers developed a system of tapping spring water and sending it to inner Edo through exposed and covered aqueducts that led to enclosed wooden pipes. This first delivery system was forty-one miles long; it lasted only until the middle of the seventeenth century. Thereafter, river water for drinking, washing, and irrigating rice paddies was delivered to Edo through a fifty-mile-long system. But it, too, soon proved inadequate, and several additional complicated combinations of channels and pipes (metal replacing wood in the nineteenth century) were added to the first two innovations. The engineering skills needed for these accomplishments were great; so were the political arrangements that determined how water could be used, and by whom.

The availability of potable water permitted density of settlement, which created all kinds of urban waste that had to be disposed. Unlike the West, Japan had a practical use for night soil (human excreta) as fertilizer. (Fortunately, it was aged and dried before being applied to fields where consumable crops were grown.) In a country with limited arable land and a growing population to feed, high-quality fertilizer was immensely valuable. Osaka took its night soil away by ship, selling it to farmers along the coast. At first, night soil was bartered for fresh produce; later it was exchanged for silver. Rights to fecal matter and human urine were so important that tenants and landlords were allotted precise shares. The rights to collect human waste were dispersed among guilds and associations, and battles were fought over such rights.

The shogunate had to issue regulations and try to enforce them; toilets were forbidden along rivers and waterways as early as 1648. Seven years later, the people of Edo were commanded to dispose of their solid waste on an island in the bay, not in local rivers. Each ward of the city began to collect its rubbish and transport it to the island, which served as Japan's first dump. Drainage channels followed; even slums channeled run-off waters from streets and roofs into the bay. Judged by these regulatory efforts, and many more, the Tokugawa urban administrations clearly valued cleanliness and proper sanitation.

Hanley concludes that Japanese cities were more hygienic than Western ones from the mid-seventeenth to the mid-nineteenth century. Their urban populations were healthier, and mortality rates lower. Life-expectancy rates were comparable. The plague never reached Japan, and cholera arrived only in the nineteenth century, from the West. But Japan's advances were assisted by the paucity of domestic animals in its cities, as well as its customs regarding hygiene, food, and drink. Carting night soil and urine away, as economic goods, was better than using cesspools, whether covered or uncovered. Even the invention of the water closet in the West helped little; excrement was still flushed into rivers, like the Thames, which also supplied drinking water. New York City was studded with open cesspools into the mid-nineteenth century.

Personal habits seem to have been more advanced, by a century or more, in Japan than in Europe or the Americas. Hanley cites comparative accounts from as early as the seventeenth century that are favorable to the Japanese and that indicate (for a later century) that French and English palaces were "mere latrines" (224). Boiling their water (as in tea) was helpful. So was the Japanese preference for cooking food and not sharing chopsticks, bowls, or teacups. Traditional views of what was pure and impure were also important in reducing epidemics, as were rituals of purification. Even keeping footwear outside houses was protective. Finally, the comparative abundance of water in Japanese cities (as compared to London and other European cities) meant that the people of Japan could bathe more frequently than contemporary Europeans.

Japanese welcomed conformity and government regulation more than Europeans and Americans of the same era did. Not only were the cities divided up into village-sized units for ease of control and administration; they were also supervised from central locations, the better to limit crime and keep abreast of leaking pipes and dirty streets.

That the Japanese were so successful as urban dwellers in the preindustrial period explains why well into the twentieth century they failed to adopt Western advances in sanitary engineering. Even after World War II, Japanese cities shipped night soil to farmers; as late as 1985, only 34 percent of Japanese urban dwellers had access to modern sewer systems. The traditions and methods of modernization that served Japan well as it shifted rapidly from a nation of villages to a nation of cities failed the country during much of the last century.

In Africa and in the Americas, meanwhile, the disease environment was more desperate and destructive than it was in the settled lands of Asia and Europe. The introduction of smallpox into virgin new-world populations is the concern of two articles in this collection: Dauril Alden and Joseph C. Miller write about the transmission of smallpox from Africa to Brazil, and Robert McCaa writes about the impact of smallpox on early-contact Mexico. Both articles question whether or not smallpox alone was responsible for the catastrophic results long attributed to its arrival with foreigners, both conquerors and slaves.

McCaa's problem was to decide whether Mexico's first outbreak of smallpox in 1520 was or was not a catastrophic event at all. Did smallpox kill as many as one-half of the Aztec population, thus occasioning the demographic collapse of indigenous central Mexico and the weakening of Aztec resistance to European conquest? Or was the 1520 epidemic relatively mild and noncatastrophic, as Francis J. Brooks asserted in "Revising the Conquest of Mexico: Smallpox, Sources, and Populations," *JIH,* XXIV (1993), 1–29?

McCaa consulted newly available sources in Spanish and Nahuatl, and reviewed the evidence from standard eyewitness accounts, tax records, and chronicles. He reexamined the six major sources that Brooks consulted. A detailed table sets out all of the relevant sources of information for sixteenth-century Mexican smallpox. Many of the documents attribute the arrival of the pox to a named African slave. Brooks questioned the authenticity of this supposedly eyewitness account, claiming that it was a myth concocted by a Franciscan and copied over and over by subsequent Spanish chroniclers. Brooks was also aware of time lapses— many of the accounts were not recorded until nearly a century after the era of the epidemic.

Taking these historiographical issues into account, McCaa provides a careful reassessment of both the indigenous and the foreign accounts, re-translating and re-thinking questionable words and attributions. He concludes that the indigenous annals and pictographs almost universally describe a widespread epidemic and the destruction of the native elite. Mesoamerica succumbed to Spanish conquest largely because the smallpox killing fields of 1520 removed legitimate local leadership. Likewise, McCaa reports that Brooks used inferior or abridged texts and translations and that the Spanish accounts that Brooks trashed are credible. For McCaa, the contemporary Spanish writings reveal a familiarity with smallpox and smallpox mortality that suggest reliability and lead to "a single conclusion: the smallpox epidemic of 1520 ranked among the three worst demographic crises of the century" (198) For the people of central Mexico, it was a catastrophe. Mortality was enormous, said a contemporary, on a scale "unimaginable to contemporary Europeans" (201).

As Alden and Miller make clear, smallpox was unknown in

the Americas before Europeans landed. It is transmitted via virus-bearing moisture droplets exhaled by the afflicted. Headaches, fevers, chills, and nausea are the initial symptoms, followed by external rashes and attacks on internal organs. Death came to one in four; others were left disfigured. Cures were unknown before the twentieth century, although vaccination was introduced in the nineteenth century.

Hispaniola (modern Haiti and the Dominican Republic) experienced smallpox epidemics as early as 1507, possibly passed from African slaves. The epidemic spread quickly to Puerto Rico and Cuba and then to Mexico. It moved southward rapidly, reaching what is now Argentina in 1558. During the rest of the sixteenth century, the pox primarily killed indigenous Indians in Brazil, thence hopping from one Amerindian area to another. In the next century, slaves began arriving in Brazil from West Africa, the Congo, and Angola in increasing numbers. Frequent fresh outbreaks of smallpox in Brazil throughout that century were attributed to recently landed slaves, many of whom may have been infected in Africa, as well as en route during the notorious middle passage.

Alden and Miller link these many virulent attacks of smallpox in Brazil to cycles of drought and famine in Africa. Hitherto dispersed populations were confined to, and fought over, what the authors call "shrinking living space" (209). These battles for land and resources produced captives who could be sold into slavery and shipped to the African coast for eventual sale in Brazil. Alden and Miller cite several positive associations. They also note that after 1645, climatic improvements in Africa spared Brazil from further major spasms of the pox until the 1660s, when the effects of pestilence were serious. Alden and Miller associate the severity of these morbid episodes to drought and to the outbreak of disease in Angola and the Congo ten years before.

Smallpox was a killer in Brazil throughout the seventeenth century, but the attacks of the 1680s and 1690s were particularly devastating throughout nearly all of the vast colony. The discovery of gold in 1695 led to a demand for increased African slave labor, as well as a collateral increase in the frequency and distribution of smallpox epidemics. At roughly ten-year intervals from 1720, smallpox swept Brazil, killing a great many Africans, Amerindians, and Europeans. The association between aridity, warfare, and contagion in Africa and the subsequent outbreak of disease in

Brazil is as relevant in the eighteenth century as it was in the seventeenth century. It continued even into the nineteenth century, as the transshipment of slaves increased, and the trade shifted from legal to illegal before finally being ended.

Smallpox in Brazil gradually succumbed to preventive vaccination in the nineteenth century. But Alden and Miller also suggest that smallpox was never as deadly in Brazil as it was in Europe, largely because of the dispersal and paucity of population in the colony, and possibly because the tropical epidemiology of smallpox differed in quality from that of its temperate version. Certainly the percentages of the population who died, and the frequency of pandemics, were lower in Brazil then in Europe, plausibly because of the absence of crowded cities. Alden and Miller do not indicate whether Brazil harbored a reservoir of pox, or whether (as they imply) the pox almost always arrived freshly from Africa, where it was endemic.

As imports of slaves into the Americas cascaded during the eighteenth and nineteenth centuries, their total numbers were sustained by forced immigration, not by natural rates of growth. Although slaves in the United States had substantial natural rates of increase, the number of Caribbean slaves decreased. Malnutrition was long presumed to be the most significant contributory cause for the failure of slaves to thrive. Kenneth F. Kiple and Virginia H. Kiple's essay was among the first to prove that slaves in the Caribbean, at least, were malnourished. They single out specific nutritional deficiencies and the diseases that may have been linked to them.

The Kiples' review of the African nutritional heritage finds little animal protein or bovine milk (thanks to the prevalence of tsetse-fly borne parasites), and a limited consumption of green vegetables and fruit. If their survey is accurate, slaves arrived poorly nourished, whatever their terrible middle passage experiences. Indeed, newly imported slaves were shorter on average than American-born slaves. A history of poor nutrition and debilitating illness contracted during the middle passage led in the New World to a susceptibility to pathogenic invasion.

The Kiples reconstruct an ideal (typical) Caribbean slave diet. Even if it were calorically sufficient, it lacked essential minerals and vitamins, as well as fat, thereby exacerbating a deficiency of vitamin A, which is fat soluble. The low fat/high carbohydrate diet of the slaves also led to seriously insufficient intakes of B1, or thiamine. Much of what little their food might have contained was destroyed by cooking, or by rice husking. Even during good times, the Kiples say, Caribbean slave diets were "badly out of balance" (100).

The slaves in the Caribbean suffered from yaws—a skin and bone disease spread by close contact—and neonatal tetanus, neither of which were influenced by nutritional weaknesses. But "sore eyes" and night blindness stemmed from vitamin A deficiency, and beriberi (which included dirt-eating and dropsy) reflected the lack of thiamine. Both complaints were widely prevalent. The death rates of slaves in nineteenth-century Cuba attributed to beriberi were as high as 75 percent on plantations. Infants were particularly hard hit. Those who suffered from a vitamin B deficiency, characterized by stomach pains and skin glossiness, might have found relief during the sugar harvest by drinking the sugarcane juice left over from the sugar-refining process. Planters wrote contemporaneously of the relationship between better diets and freedom from disease.

In the emerging United States, the Chesapeake Bay region also saw a high mortality rate, especially among slaves and other immigrants, but natural increases in population were apparent as early as the beginning of the eighteenth century. Malaria was rife and life expectancies consequently low. These tidewater areas were less healthy than New England, by far. The parish studied in detail by Daniel Blake Smith shows a death rate three times greater than that in early New England towns. Yet, using birth and death registers, and appreciating evidentiary problems with them, Smith finds a slow natural population increase in the Chesapeake area. Before the mid-eighteenth century that increase was barely perceptible, but it rose gradually in the latter half of the century. Elsewhere in Virginia and Maryland, however, rapid natural growth was underway by the 1690s.

Smith's parish grew more slowly than its neighbors, and far more slowly than New England samples, because of a shortage of women (sex ratios were out of balance), higher than comparable death rates, higher than comparable rates on infant mortality, unusual death rates between ages one and four, and lower than comparable life expectancies, The contribution of Smith's essay comes as much from his successful methods for deriving such results from scattered, difficult, and questionable records as from the results themselves. His use of technical, ingenious ways of estimating childhood death rates and adult life expectancies is particularly important. So is his careful comparison of the refractory data from his own Tidewater parish with studies based on data from samples taken elsewhere in colonial America and the Caribbean.

One conclusion is that mortality in colonial times increased as one moved northward toward New England. Since actual as well as average life expectancies were truncated in the Chesapeake, for example, the size of most families was small. Attempts to reconstitute families produce confirming evidence. The controlling demographic fact, Smith says, was the death of parents rather than children. Since most fathers died in their early forties, the Chesapeake area had an overabundance of orphans, and male autonomy arrived at younger ages than elsewhere, accompanied by generous bequests of land and personal property from the deceased. They also married younger. Malaria moved the generations along rather rapidly.

Smith's data reveal that family life in Tidewater Virginia was characterized by an absence of elders. Authority and tradition were weaker than in New England, but opportunity abounded for young men, even more than in England at the time. The area also had more than its expected share of social and political unrest. The implication of Smith's new evidence, teased carefully from sparse and intractable records, is that coastal Virginia was more turbulent and more challenging in the seventeenth and eighteenth centuries than any other region in the colonies.

David Northrup's essay uses the full records of the British navy's West African Squadron to report the heavy loss of lives on slave ships intercepted on the high seas and escorted back to Sierra Leone. Many more slaves died on the African mainland after they were freed. From ascertaining the precise numbers of those who died after their return, Northrup estimates the numbers of West Africans who died as a result of the middle passage, at least during the nineteenth century. He supports other research concluding that as many as 18 percent of the Africans shipped as slaves may have perished during the middle passage in the nineteenth century.

The mortality rates of the slaves varied with the length of time that they were at sea before the warships of the British patrol intercepted them. As common sense would dictate, the longer the voyage—as well as the worse the conditions and the more rotten the food—the greater, in general, was the danger from disease.

But Northrup sometimes found a higher magnitude of loss on short and medium-length voyages. One reason for the anomaly (in addition to the absence of certain voyage length distributions) was food availability, which paradoxically was better on longer voyages. Mortality rates (and the duration of sailings) were also affected by season and by monthly average rainfalls (with their accompanying winds). Since dry-season winds were lighter, voyages with them were longer, and more deadly. Yet, June, a rainy month, was also characterized by high mortality, possibly because of the diseases associated with rougher seas and the closing of ventilators.

Overcrowding, per se, does not appear to have been correlated with higher death rates. Indeed, the data show that the proportion of deaths that occurred during the early weeks of a voyage was greater than that averaged for an entire sailing. Evidently, a slave shipment's place of origin and its conditions during the early part of its voyage were critical. The relationship between ports of embarkation and death rates was direct, locations to the south of the Bight of Biafra being less favored. Northrup found no connection between sex ratios of slaves shipped and mortality, though he did note a positive correlation between the number of children carried and overall death rates.

Child mortality in early twentieth-century rural Texas is the focus of the essay by Myron P. Gutmann and Kenneth P. Fliess in this volume. In particular, they look at the social differences in death rates for children, based on an examination of relevant questions answered in the 1900 and 1910 state censuses, and on county tax assessments. The region showed not only differences in social status, occupation, and socioeconomic condition, but also racial and ethnic differences, and important differences at the subracial and subethnic level. Ancestry was relevant, as was exposure to adverse influences, especially disease.

At the turn of the century, the population of Texas was composed of predominantly white, English-speaking immigrants from other states, or their descendants. Texas also attracted white immigrants from Western Europe, Canada, Asia, and the Americas. One-sixth of the population of the state was of African origin—mainly former slaves, their children, and their grandchildren. About 6 percent of the population was from Germany and Central and Eastern Europe, or had a parent from those areas. Mexicans were the fourth largest group in early Texas, numbering slightly less than the Central and Eastern Europeans. The identification of persons belonging to each of these four categories was based on place of birth and parents' place of birth, as well as by special dictionaries of surnames.

In order to obtain values for childhood mortality, the authors use a model life table that develops an index of the ratio of actual to expected number of births for each woman, or groups of women, in the census sample, allowing them to compare the number born with the number who died. Their results show that rural Texans of African-American and Mexican descent experienced higher levels of child mortality and Germans lower levels than the majority white population ("other white"). But rural Texan African-Americans in the Gutmann–Fleiss sample had better life chances than African-Americans in national samples, and their life chances were improving. Mexican-American children in the rural Texan sample also showed better life expectations than national African-Americans, and their life chances were improving more rapidly than those of any other group.

Gutmann and Fleiss ascribe these sharp differences in life expectations and mortality to county of residence as well as to socioeconomic condition and opportunity. County, in this context, stands as a proxy for population density, levels of poverty, standards of public health and sanitation, access to education, and knowledge about health measures at the family level. How counties fared depended primarily on their population composition, particularly as reflected by the proxy items. The lowest levels of child mortality were experienced by families of farmers and white collar workers. Tenant farmers and skilled workers fared less well; farm and non-farm laboring families experienced the highest rate of loss. Across those categories, African-Americans and Mexican families were afflicted with the most deaths, but the childhood mortality rates for Mexican-Americans decreased generationally. The counties with the highest proportion of Germans had the lowest number of childhood deaths per capita, presumably because of their cultural traditions and habits, as well as their influence on county conditions. As would be expected, taxable wealth strongly influenced the overall results and the county returns.

After accounting for the meaning of these differences and scrutinizing them using multivariate forms of analysis, Gutmann and Fleiss stress the importance of sheer location, in the geographical sense. One favored county had an arid climate, good soils, and clean surface water. A less favored county was lower in elevation, had heavy hard-to-work soils, and more surface water, potentially contaminated. Density of population was also a contributing factor. Overall, access to potable water and well-constructed sanitary facilities seems to have been crucial to the health, and therefore the mortality expectations, of rural Texans. Wealthier Texans with healthier mores had the best prospects, doing far better than the most recent immigrants from more impoverished straits and far better than those who had never enjoyed access to, or expectations of, improved health or medical outcomes.

The final essay in this collection reflects the *JIH's* search for new ways of thinking about existing problems, as well as its search for little appreciated issues that could be examined only by the employment of wholly new methods and approaches. Irene W. D. Hecht links sociohistorical findings to medical data in order to trace the existence of a small, closed population in which gene frequencies are different from those in the general population—a genetic isolate. She then investigates the historical significance of the community that was characterized by being a genetic isolate.

In the 1970s, a lone patient appeared at the Oregon Medical School with a skin condition that was diagnosed as porphyria, a group of hereditary biochemical disorders resulting from the metabolism of porphyrin compounds (which occur when the heme in hemoglobin breaks down). Acute intermittent porphyria, one type of the disease, involves abdominal pain and strange behavior. (King George III's madness was probably this form of porphyria.) Porphyrias are autosomal dominant; offspring will exhibit symptoms if one porphyria gene is received from either parent.

The Oregon patient was of Dutch extraction. A South African study had earlier traced more than 1,000 South Africans with the ailment to a pair of seventeenth-century Dutch immigrants to South Africa. The Oregon patient's relatives, however, showed little penetration of porphyria. Further investigation led to the hypothesis that the patient and his large family of relatives belonged to an isolate, though his community was not isolated geographically in western Oregon. Nor was his family exclusively of one ethnic background; it had undergone much ethnic intermarriage. They were fervent Catholics, as were the earliest white settlers in the Willamette River Valley. Only a medicohistorical collaboration could establish the isolate character of the patient's extended kin system in the Valley.

Hecht reconstructed the families of the Valley community according to the new standard methodology. She used baptism, marriage, and burial records to rebuild all of the relevant families and kin ties. The Oregon census of 1880 and earlier Wisconsin censuses, as well as Dutch migration records, provided valuable information as well. Hecht ultimately could trace the core families of the study to their geographically concentrated German, Belgian, and Dutch roots. She followed them to the Fox River Valley in Wisconsin, and then to Oregon.

One man led the way to Oregon in search of a good location for an agrarian Catholic community. In 1875, three families moved to the Willamette Valley from Wisconsin. Hecht shows how the community grew and prospered, and how it remained faithful to its Catholic core. She explicates and illustrates the strength of kin ties within the group, even as it expanded in size across generations and migrations. The shape of the isolate gradually emerged. But it would not have held together, Hecht says, without two marriage practices—repeat alliances and sibling exchanges—that bound the group into a complex biological network that the participants themselves probably ceased to appreciate or understand. Indeed, those practices probably began even before the first families immigrated. Being concentrated, the resulting gene pool increased the chance of recessive gene pairings.

Hecht concludes that human isolates of historical significance need not be obvious; that is, they need not be geographically specific or easily delineated. They can exist solely on the basis of social practice, and they can operate as isolates amid the activity and normalcy of ordinary society. Nor do they necessarily attract notice, or even realize (after a number of generations) that anything about them is unusual. The science of genetics has something to contribute to the study of social history even if its contribution is neither obvious nor direct.

This volume of essays from the pages of the *JIH* shows how much more complete political, social, and economic histories can be if consideration is given to birth, death, nutrition, disease, and all the complicated ways in which those and other variables interact. It is impossible to consider the Spanish conquest of the Americas without reflecting on the demographic consequences of old world pathogens; it is equally impossible to come to conclusions about the impact of the Atlantic slave trade without a nuanced understanding of disease and mortality before, during, and after the middle passage. Almost every essay in this collection assesses the role of nutrition in susceptibility to disease. Several are conscious of the importance of water and sanitation to mortality, to urbanization, and, ultimately, to the rise and fall of states and civilizations. Methodologically, most of these articles boast meticulous statistics, and several introduce ingenious techniques to solve otherwise intractable problems. One essay even solves a problem that was not known to exist. Together, these contributions represent a continuum of efforts to extend the boundaries of history and to bring new disciplines to bear on problems of the past. In substance and practice, they are a nonrandom, but representative, sample of what the *JIH* has attempted to do from 1970 to 2000.

Andrew B. Appleby

Nutrition and Disease:
The Case of London, 1550–1750

Historians of early modern Europe have often detected a connection between harvest failure and epidemic disease. Helleiner, for example, has written that "subsistence crises invariably engendered epidemic outbreaks" in late medieval Europe. Bowden, speaking of plague in Tudor England, noted that "the striking coincidence of serious plague outbreaks with harvest failures . . . leaves no doubt that these two events were closely related." Contemporaries confirmed the relationship: "first dearth and then plague" was a common saying of the sixteenth and seventeenth centuries, as Meuvret has pointed out.[1] It is easy to reconstruct the process. Following a harvest failure, food prices rose and the poor became progressively malnourished. They ate less and what they ate was worse, as they devoted their limited incomes to grain—which provided the most calories per penny—rather than to a better-balanced but more expensive diet of grains, meat, dairy products, fruits, and vegetables.[2] Malnourishment lowered resistance to disease, allowing a disease already present endemically to grow to epidemic size or providing fertile territory for an epidemic introduced from outside. The

Andrew B. Appleby is Assistant Professor of History at San Diego State University and the author of several articles in the fields of agrarian history and peasant demography.

1   Karl F. Helleiner, "The Population of Europe from the Black Death to the Eve of the Vital Revolution," *The Cambridge Economic History of Europe* (Cambridge, 1967), IV, 69; Peter Bowden, "Agricultural Prices, Farm Profits, and Rents," in Joan Thirsk (ed.), *The Agrarian History of England and Wales*, IV: *1500–1640* (Cambridge, 1967), 633. See also Jaime Vincens Vives, "The Decline of Spain in the Seventeenth Century," in Carlo M. Cipolla (ed.), *The Economic Decline of Empires* (London, 1970), 124: "the persistent state of undernutrition . . . explain[s] the extraordinary virulence of seventeenth-century plagues." Jean Meuvret, "Demographic Crisis in France from the Sixteenth to the Eighteenth Century," in D. V. Glass and D. E. C. Eversley (eds.), *Population in History* (London, 1965), 510. Bartolomé Bennassar, *Recherches sur les grandes épidémies dans le nord de l'Espagne à la fin du XVIᵉ siècle* (Paris, 1969), 32–33, quotes a corregidor of Sepulveda as stating that the plague "has not touched, by God's mercy, well-nourished people."

2   The relative cost of all foodstuffs in early modern Europe is unknown. A study of relative food costs expressed in caloric terms for Paris in the 1780s shows that it cost eleven times as much to buy a certain number of calories in meat as in bread, three times as much in salt fish, six times in eggs, and so forth. Per calorie, bread was much the cheapest food. See R. Philippe, "Une opération pilote: l'étude du ravitaillement de Paris au temps de Lavoisier," in J.-J. Hémardinquer (ed.), *Pour une histoire de l'alimentation* (Paris, 1970), 65.

epidemic in turn was spread rapidly by infected beggars that thronged the roads seeking food. The two—food shortage and disease—went hand in hand, during both the inception and diffusion of the epidemic. This picture is plausible, so plausible as to seem beyond doubt.

Recent studies, however, have questioned one crucial link in this causal chain. The role played by malnutrition in lowering resistance to infectious disease appears less sure than common sense would suggest. Physicians studying starvation in the Warsaw ghetto between 1941 and 1943 and also in Holland in 1945 were struck by the low incidence of such deficiency diseases as scurvy and rickets and also by the relative immunity of these starving people to many infectious diseases.[3] Historians, too, have expressed doubts about the assumed relationship between malnutrition and disease. The late J. D. Chambers argued that infectious disease in pre-industrial England had its own dynamic, largely unaffected by food shortage, and that epidemics slowed, stopped, or reversed population growth in periods of low food prices and, conversely, that demographic expansion often took place during periods of high prices and undoubted shortage simply because epidemics were not frequent or deadly.[4]

The question is important, for if Chambers is correct, we would have at least a partial explanation of why English population stabilized at times—such as 1350 to 1470 and again from 1650 to 1690 and from 1720 to 1750—when grain prices were low and the standard of living of the grain-dependent poor was relatively high. The statement of Sylvia Thrupp that the period "from 1349 to the 1470's, if it was a Golden Age, was the golden age of bacteria" would be confirmed.[5] Disease abounded—and better nutrition in no way protected the poor from periodic epidemics. The absence of any correlation between disease and nutrition would also help to reconcile the evidence that early industrialization led to a lowering of the workers' standard of

3 Ancel Keys et al., *The Biology of Human Starvation* (Minneapolis, 1950; 2v.), II, 1011, writes, in reference to the Warsaw ghetto: "among both children and adults epidemics were very rare and, when they occurred, ran a benign course." (Typhus fever should be excepted from this observation.) See also *ibid.*, I, xv, 20, 448–453; II, 1009–1040; Emil Apfelbaum, *Maladie de Famine* (Warsaw, 1946); Leonard Tushnet, *The Uses of Adversity* (New York, 1966); Frederick Hocking, *Starvation* (Sydney, 1969). For the view that malnutrition increases the virulence of infectious disease, see N. S. Scrimshaw, C. E. Taylor, and J. E. Gordon, *Interactions of Nutrition and Infection* (Geneva, 1968).
4 Chambers, *Population, Economy and Society in Pre-Industrial England* (Oxford, 1972), esp. chs. 1, 4.
5 Quoted in *ibid.*, 22, 81–82.

living with the seemingly conflicting data that show a rapid rise in population and, for the first time, an excess of births over deaths in many of the larger cities, including London.[6] It should perhaps be added here that no one denies that malnutrition lowers a human's resistance to certain diseases, such as tuberculosis, or that certain diseases arise directly from dietary deficiencies, such as pellagra or scurvy. What has been questioned is the interplay between the great epidemic killers of pre-industrial Europe—plague, smallpox, typhus, influenza, to name four—and nutritional deficiencies.

The purpose here is to explore the relationship—if any—between malnutrition and certain specific diseases in London for the period 1550–1750, in the hope of adding to the available evidence. We will pay particular attention to plague from 1550 to 1680 and to other diseases from 1630 to 1750, a period when the authorities systematically identified ailments other than plague for the first time. The beginning date for the plague study is determined by the data on nutrition, which begin only in 1545. The ending date of 1680 marks the disappearance of plague from London. Separate mortality figures for typhus, "fever," and smallpox were not given until 1629, which explains the starting date for these comparisons. Consumption figures are available from 1657. The study was not carried past 1728 for typhus and fever because they were lumped together after that date. The final cutoff of 1750 for the remaining diseases is somewhat arbitrary; we chose to limit this essay to pre-industrial England.

The two basic sources used in this study are London bread prices and London bills of mortality. Perhaps a word about these and the methodology used is in order.

The bread prices were the maximum permissible retail prices, in pence, that could be charged for a four-pound wheaten loaf, as set by the assize of bread.[7] The price series is virtually complete and runs from 1545 to 1925. Our primary interest, however, is not in prices but in malnutrition. The problem is to relate these bread prices to possible caloric, protein, or vitamin deficiencies among the London

---

6   The literature on the standard of living during the industrial revolution is extensive; see E. J. Hobsbawm and R. M. Hartwell, "The Standard of Living during the Industrial Revolution: A Discussion," *Economic History Review*, XVI (1963), 120–146. For urban births, see Chambers, *Population*, 103.
7   The London bread prices have been published in B. R. Mitchell and Phyllis Deane, *Abstract of British Historical Statistics* (Cambridge, 1962), 497–498.

poor. We know that bread was the core of the poor man's diet.[8] Very likely bread purchases were his single most important outlay, exceeding what he spent on clothing or housing. But we do not know precisely how dependent the poor were on wheat bread, as differentiated from other breads or grains. Nor do we know to what extent the poor shifted from wheat to another, cheaper grain in times of dearth, or what other, non-grain substitutes might have been added to their diet. Despite these shortcomings in our knowledge, it is possible to show that London wheat bread prices accurately reflect the general level of nutrition. If these prices rose, the nutrition of the poor deteriorated, especially in periods of prolonged high prices. And it is in these prolonged shortages that one would expect to find a greater incidence of disease, if indeed malnourishment made men more vulnerable to infection.

Let us consider the problem of alternative foods that might have substituted for wheat bread when wheat prices were high. During a dearth, the poor no doubt ate more low-priced grains—oats, barley, and rye, if they were available—and less wheat, which always tended to be more expensive per measure.[9] This tactic stretched their available money but would not have fended off malnutrition during a long, severe dearth. Some years ago, Hoskins argued that the price of other grains (and all other foods) tended to follow the price of wheat. Recently, this contention has been questioned by Harrison, who has shown that there were frequent divergences in grain price movements.[10] But this does not mean that when the price of wheat went up, the poor simply switched to another, more modestly priced grain. All too often, in times of extreme wheat shortage all other grains rose swiftly in

8 Judging from the controls and regulations that all authorities throughout Western Europe set to cover virtually every transaction. No other commodity was so thoroughly regulated. See Jack C. Drummond and Anne Wilbraham, *The Englishman's Food, A History of Five Centuries of English Diet* (London, 1958), 41.

9 See Bowden, "Agricultural Prices," 601–602, 612. In 1641, Henry Best was selling oats at 14s. the quarter, barley at 22s. the quarter, rye at 27s. 6d. the quarter and white wheat at 35s. the quarter. See J. Thirsk and J. P. Cooper (eds.), *Seventeenth-Century Economic Documents* (Oxford, 1972), 356.

10 W. G. Hoskins, "Harvest Fluctuations and English Economic History, 1480–1619," *Agricultural History Review*, XII (1964), 40; C. J. Harrison, "Grain Price Analysis and Harvest Qualities, 1465–1634," *ibid.*, XIX (1971), 138–143. According to our calculations, Harrison constructed his 31-year moving averages by adding the prices for the 15 preceding years, the year in question, and the following 15 years, making a correct total of 31 years. He then apparently divided by 30, instead of 31, which gave him a constant error of 3–4 percent. Anyone wishing to use Harrison's averages should first check his calculations.

price, as a glance at Harrison's grain price graphs reveals. In general, a shortage of one grain meant the shortage of another, particularly when prices remained high for longer than one year.

The crises of 1555–56 and 1596–97 are cases in point.[11] These two periods beyond doubt saw the worst harvest failures of the sixteenth century. In each year of these two crises, the prices of all grains were very high; sometimes wheat rose more than the other grains; sometimes their increase surpassed that of wheat. In 1555, wheat did not quite reach dearth levels but the average of all grains did, thanks to the incredible price of barley. (Here, "dearth" is specifically defined as 50 percent or more above the thirty-one-year moving average price of the grain in question.) The next year there was a dearth of wheat and oats. Barley prices moderated somewhat but remained higher than in any year prior to 1555. In 1596–97, the same pattern can be quickly discerned; 1596 was a terrible year, with wheat, barley, oats, and rye all reaching unprecedented levels. The next year was slightly improved but again all grains were well above their normal price. Perhaps it bears repeating: In bad years, particularly in a run of bad years, the poor could not turn from one grain to another and find it at a reasonable price, even assuming that it was available.

So much for grains. What about other alternatives, such as beans, peas, or dairy products? The poor stretched their bread grain with beans and peas and apparently consumed some milk, cheese, and butter in normal years. Both beans and peas were very dear during the two crises we have chosen as examples.[12] Prices for dairy products are not available for 1555–56, but in 1596–97 they reached a new high, although the increase was not startling from a percentage standpoint. Cattle and sheep prices remained about average during the two crises but the poor man could not afford to replace his usual grain purchases with meat. Indeed, the relative price stability of cattle and sheep suggests that they were of minor importance in the diet of the poor. Had they been of any consequence, buying pressure would have forced prices higher. In this connection, it is interesting to note that wheat prices were less volatile than prices of the cheaper grains.[13] In a

11 The following price data are drawn from Peter Bowden, "Statistical Appendix," in Thirsk, *Agrarian History*, 814–870. The quality designation for "dearth" is that used by Hoskins and Harrison in their articles. See also Bowden, "Agricultural Prices," 626.
12 Bowden, "Statistical Appendix," 818–820.
13 See Harrison, "Grain Price Analysis," 139–141.

bad year, the price of wheat had to rise only slightly to put it out of the reach of the poor because initially it was expensive. Oats or barley, on the other hand, started at a lower quantity price and would have had to move up proportionally more before becoming too dear.

Less is known about other foodstuffs eaten by the poor. Salt fish evidently played an increasing role in their diet during the sixteenth century, although it was not available in quantities sufficient to substitute for bread in times of harvest failure. The same might be said of fruits and vegetables. The poor in the late sixteenth century were eating more vegetables than before and a further increase in fruit and vegetable consumption was reported after the Restoration.[14] But it is doubtful that either fruits or vegetables were much of a factor in the average diet. The orchards and gardens near London could not have sufficiently expanded their output in the short term to offset the shortage of other foods.

In sum, it seems highly unlikely that the poor had any cheap alternative foodstuffs in time of grain shortage. Probably the poor man tightened his belt and cut down on all purchases except basic grains stretched with peas, beans, and other fillers. As William Harrison said, the poor were reduced to living on "horsse corne, beanes, peason, otes, tares & lintels" when the grain harvest failed.[15] If this was true, they faced a decline in both the quantity (in caloric terms) and quality (in terms of nutritional value) of their food. Naturally, the degree of malnutrition would have varied with the length and severity of the shortage, becoming progressively greater the longer prices remained high and the higher they went.

The other major source for this study, the London bills of mortality, also contain certain strengths and weaknesses. Occasional bills survive for the sixteenth century but usually show only plague deaths in years of plague epidemics. Beginning in 1629, however, the bills regularly show yearly total mortality for 130 London and adjoining parishes from a variety of causes, being arranged under various disease or accident headings.[16] The headings occasionally were changed, to

---

14 Drummond and Wilbraham, *Englishman's Food*, 29–30, 38–39, 55; Thirsk and Cooper, *Economic Documents*, 80.
15 Quoted in Drummond and Wilbraham, *Englishman's Food*, 88.
16 The origin of the bills is discussed in Thomas R. Forbes, *Chronicle from Aldgate* (New Haven, 1971), 46–50. T. Birch (ed.), *A Collection of the Yearly Bills of Mortality, from 1657 to 1758 inclusive . . .* (London, 1759). Some earlier bills are included in this volume but not the occasional bill for the sixteenth century. The number of parishes varied, some being added from time to time as London grew.

reflect shifting patterns of disease or changing concerns of the authorities. Because they show only mortality and not morbidity, the bills are useful only for tracing fatal diseases. A widespread epidemic of influenza might have left all London prostrate but if it resulted in no deaths, it would have left no trace on the bills.

More important, the bills pose a problem of reliability. The cause of each death in each parish was reported to the parish clerk by the parish "searcher," often an old woman whose only qualification was her willingness to undertake an unpleasant task for a few pennies in pay. She would visit the house of the deceased, view the body, and perhaps discuss the cause of death with relatives or whomever might offer an opinion as to why the person had died. Because of this rather haphazard method of determining cause of death, certain allowances should be made for error. Do these errors invalidate the bills as a source of medical information? This seems to depend upon the disease under consideration. Certain diseases are easy to identify—smallpox, for instance[17]—and mistakes in diagnosis would have been statistically insignificant. Plague was much feared and its symptoms were well known, particularly in a city like London where it was endemic for many years. However, plague was occasionally misdiagnosed; the jump in typhus deaths during a plague epidemic, for example, suggests that some plague cases were misidentified as typhus, through ignorance or fear of the magistrates.[18] But here allowances can be made. Smallpox, plague, and typhus, can be confidently traced through the bills of mortality.

More difficult to assess would be deaths from "Ague and Feaver" or "Consumption and Tissick," to cite just two catchall headings used in the bills. Myriad ailments could be masquerading under the first and just about any lung disorder could come under the second. The identity of a great killer of children, "convulsions," is obscure, although the name apparently described the symptoms. In spite of these problems, the data in the London bills are probably more complete and accurate than any available elsewhere in England at that time.

Finally, it should be mentioned that London offers one great advantage to our study. The transmission of disease is complex,

17 Charles Creighton, *A History of Epidemics in Britain* (Cambridge, 1891), II, 534: "there is hardly anything more distinctive or more loathsome."
18 See Birch, *Bills of Mortality*, 11. The authorities would isolate a house to prevent the disease from spreading. Needless to say, many householders were anxious to avoid the inconvenience of being cooped up for a long period.

involving the twin poles of exposure to the disease and receptivity when once exposed. We are interested here only in receptivity—the resistance of the host—so that it would be advantageous to reduce exposure to a constant. London offers a closer approximation to this constant than would a rural area where exposure would have fluctuated enormously. This is not to say that everyone in an urban area such as London was exposed at all times to every possible contagious ailment. But from a statistical standpoint, it is as close as we can come to such a perfect constant, enabling us at least partly to isolate receptivity to disease.

The correspondence between plague and London bread prices is set out in Fig. 1. It should be noted that bread prices in this and subsequent figures and tables have been dated not by the harvest year but by the following year, when the prices actually would have prevailed. Thus, the harvest year of 1562 runs from the end of September, 1562, to the end of September, 1563. In a year of shortage, such as 1562–63, most of the privation would have fallen in 1563, rather than immediately following the harvest in 1562. Accordingly, we have dated the year 1563 to facilitate comparisons with disease. As the reader will see, the high prices of 1563 thus coincide with the plague epidemic of that year, rather than being off by one year.

We can find little correlation between high bread prices and plague epidemics in London. Between 1550 and 1670 five epidemics ravaged the city—in 1563, 1593, 1603, 1625, and 1665. A lesser epidemic struck in 1636.[19] Of these epidemics, only one fell in a year of real shortage: 1563, when the price of bread soared 65 percent above normal. In the plague year of 1625, prices were 20 percent above normal. Apart from these, prices in epidemic years were average or below average.[20]

What might be termed the "reverse" correlation is even less apparent. Years of dearth did not lead to plague epidemics, even though the disease smoldered endemically in the city. Periods of

19 For dates of plague epidemics, see J. F. D. Shrewsbury, *A History of Bubonic Plague in the British Isles* (Cambridge, 1970), 189–194, 221–231, 266–270, 315–336, 372–377, 445–481. The bills of mortality do not cover the first epidemic mentioned here, that of 1563.

20 "Normal" is here defined as the 15-year moving average price of bread, i.e., prices for seven years back, seven forward, and the year in question, added together and then divided by 15. There are too many gaps in the material to use a 31-year moving average as did Hoskins, "Harvest Fluctuations," 43.

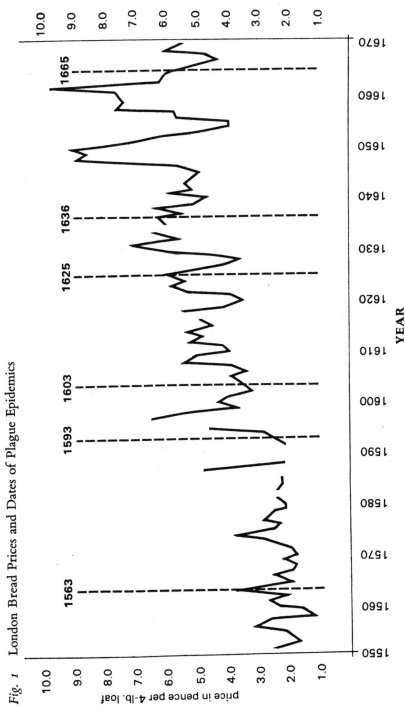

Fig. 1 London Bread Prices and Dates of Plague Epidemics

terrible shortage in the 1550s, the late 1590s (when real wages fell to their lowest point), the late 1640s, and the early 1660s did not trigger epidemics, although the poor must have suffered severe malnutrition. During all of these food crises, except possibly during the dearth of the 1550s,[21] plague was endemic to the city. If deteriorating dietary levels meant falling resistance, and if resistance in turn was a factor, plague epidemics would have broken out. But none did. In the grave food crisis of the late 1640s, plague diminished in intensity as the price of bread rose. The first of five bad years, 1647, saw considerable disease in the city, but as the subsistence crisis worsened, the numbers dying of plague declined dramatically, as Table 1 shows:

Table 1 Plague Deaths and Bread Prices
—Short-Term Divergence

YEAR	PLAGUE DEATHS	BREAD PRICES IN PENCE PER 4-LB. LOAF
1644	1,492	5.1
1645	1,871	4.8
1646	2,436	5.3
1647	3,597	6.8
1648	611	9.0
1649	67	8.6
1650	15	9.0
1651	23	7.4
1652	16	6.4
1653	6	4.8

In short, the London evidence accords with the statement of the French demographer and medical doctor, J.-N. Biraben, that "famine does not seem to increase the virulence of plague by diminishing, for example, an individual's resistance. The plague is a sufficiently grave disease that all those who contract it, even the well-nourished, have little chance of recovery."[22]

21 W. G. Hoskins, "Epidemics in English History," *The Listener* (Dec. 31, 1964), 1044: "Between 1500 and 1665 ... London was free from plague not more than a dozen years." E. H. Phelps Brown and Sheila V. Hopkins, "Seven Centuries of the Prices of Consumables, Compared with Builders' Wage Rates," in E. M. Carus-Wilson (ed.), *Essays in Economic History* (London, 1962), II, 189. Shrewsbury, *History of Bubonic Plague*, 189.
22 *Annales de Démographie Historique, 1968* (Paris, 1968), 15. Statistically, the correlation coefficient between the independent variable, London bread prices, and the dependent

Turning from plague to other diseases, we find a somewhat confused picture in the period 1630–1750. Bread prices did not continue to rise as they had throughout the sixteenth century. Extreme short-term fluctuations continued, however, and must have brought great distress to the poor, even though the secular price trend was no longer disadvantageous. The periods that would have known the greatest malnutrition—and therefore a heightened incidence of disease if a connection exists between the two—were in the years 1647 through 1651, 1658 through 1663, 1693 through 1699 and 1709 through 1710. Isolated bad years, such as 1631, would not have been as great a threat to health as these periods of prolonged high prices.

If we look in detail at Fig. 2, which charts the deaths from "spotted fever," that is, typhus, against the bread prices, we find no rise in deaths during the terrible late 1640s. There was a greater incidence of disease in the dearth of the late 1650s and early 1660s, but deaths were low in the dreadful year of 1662 (the 1661 harvest year), when prices reached their high point for the century, 59 percent above normal.[23] The death totals attributed to typhus in 1636 and 1665 should be viewed with suspicion; probably they were plague deaths mistakenly attributed. It is possible that the two killers were present at the same time. If so, there was no connection with the price of bread, which had fallen well below its average.

Later in the seventeenth century a correlation between bread prices and typhus mortality becomes more apparent.[24] The years 1674, 1694, 1698, and 1710 saw both high prices and high mortality. It is difficult to see why a difference exists between the first part of the period and the last, that is, why no price-mortality correlation is discernible until about 1660. It seems unlikely that the disease changed its character and suddenly began to affect only malnourished individuals. During the sixteenth century the disease had been recognized as a close companion of famine; it was one of the so-called "famine

variable, plague deaths, for all 50 years from 1629 through 1681 when both figures are available is −.059. This is statistically insignificant at the 5 percent confidence level. All prices were adjusted one year forward, as in the graphs, to correspond to the year when most of the harvest results would be felt. We would like to thank the Economic Resources Laboratory and the Computer Center, both of San Diego State University, for their help with these computations.

23   See footnote 20 above.

24   For the 89 years from 1629 through 1728 when both price and typhus mortality data are available, the correlation coefficient is .144. This is statistically insignificant at the 5 percent confidence level.

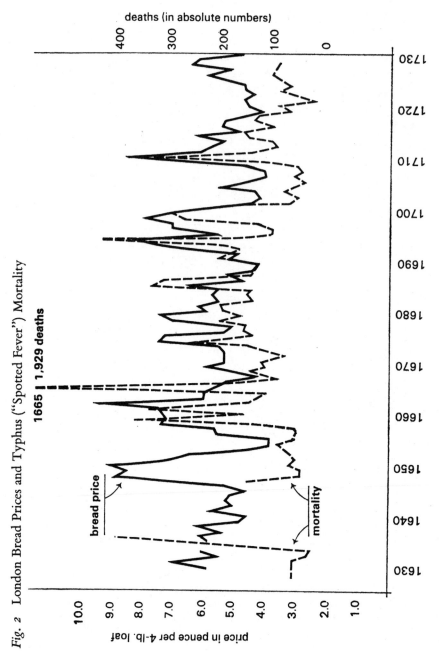

Fig. 2 London Bread Prices and Typhus ("Spotted Fever") Mortality

fevers."[25] Possibly the answer lies in the years during the 1630s and 1640s for which we have no mortality figures. Typhus has two characteristics that bear on the question: The disease confers immunity on its survivors, and children sicken but seldom die from it.[26] If there was a widespread epidemic a few years prior to the dearth of 1647–51, the pool of infectables might not have grown to the size necessary for another epidemic. This would have been particularly true if large numbers of children had been immunized by the earlier epidemic. If this conjectural explanation has any validity, it suggests that normally there was a correlation between nutritional levels and the spread or virulence of typhus, but that the lack of sufficient numbers of susceptible persons made this connection inoperable in the dearth of the late 1640s.

Typhus mortality seems to have tapered off after 1700 and the keeping of separate death figures was discontinued for the disease after 1728. The decline in the per capita incidence of the disease occurred earlier, for the number of typhus deaths remained surprisingly constant from 1630 to 1728, at a time when the city grew substantially. Quantitatively typhus was not an important killer at any time, except in the suspect year, 1665.

Smallpox mortality (Fig. 3) seems to have had no correlation with bread prices.[27] High prices and heightened mortality sometimes coincided, as in 1674 and 1710, but these appear to have been random. The course of smallpox deaths was a jagged, sawtooth affair, with minor epidemics occurring regularly about once every three years. If, for some reason, deaths were fewer than usual for several years, a larger epidemic invariably followed. This seems to explain the heightened death tolls in 1674 and 1710. Like typhus, smallpox conferred immunity on those fortunate enough to survive, but, unlike typhus, children

25 Typhus was the one epidemic disease usually present in the ghettos of occupied Poland. See Isaiah Trunk, *Judenrat* (New York, 1972), 143–172. Famine may be associated with typhus because famine discourages cleanliness, which in turn encourages body lice, the carriers of typhus. Famine can also promote crowding (for example, when beggars thronged into a city seeking charity) which helps to spread the disease. Resistance to typhus may not depend upon on the nutrition of the host.
26 On typhus, see John C. Snyder, "The Typhus Fevers," in T. M. Rivers and F. L. Horsfall, Jr. (eds.), *Viral and Rickettsial Infections of Man* (London, 1959), 799–827; J. W. D. Megaw, "Typhus Fevers and other Rickettsial Fevers," in Lord Horder (ed.), *The British Encyclopedia of Medical Practice* (London, 1952; 2d ed.), XII, 390–414.
27 For the 111 years from 1629 through 1750 when both price and smallpox mortality data are available, the correlation coefficient is −.145. This is statistically insignificant at the 5 percent confidence level.

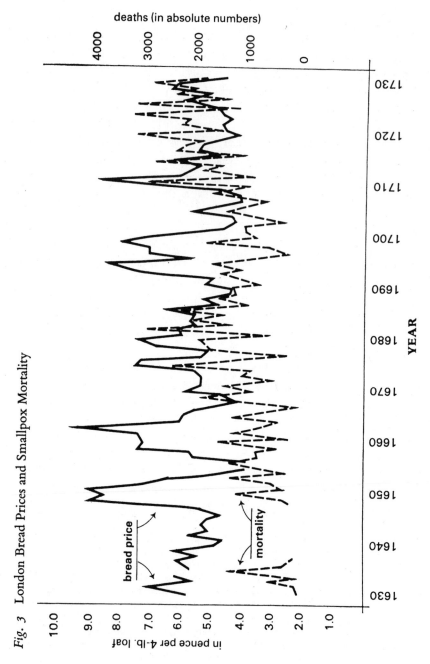

Fig. 3 London Bread Prices and Smallpox Mortality

had no special resistance to it. Since almost everyone in London was exposed in childhood to smallpox, only children provided a source of unexposed victims.[28] At regular intervals an epidemic attacked those children who had not previously been exposed. As the graphs indicate, smallpox mortality was quantitatively important, running almost ten times that of typhus. The searchers had no difficulty differentiating between smallpox and plague, for in neither 1636 nor 1665 were smallpox deaths elevated, as typhus deaths had been.

"Ague and fever" was another major killer of the time. Probably both influenza and malaria would have fallen into this category. Aside from these two, it is impossible to say exactly what diseases seventeenth- and eighteenth-century physicians included under that heading, and it is extremely unlikely that the searchers had any specific idea of what diseases to include or exclude. Whatever collection of ailments the terms encompassed, "ague and fever" killed more people in the average year than smallpox. As with typhus, the correlation between "ague and fever" mortality and bread prices is nonexistent in the 1640s and early 1650s,[29] but thereafter some correlation can be found, although it is far from consistent. As Fig. 4 reveals, there is a divergence of the two after 1710. The mortality from ague and fever rose slowly throughout the period, paralleling the increase in the city's population.[30]

In the 1650s and 1660s, "consumption and tissick" was the greatest killer in London, carrying off between three and four thousand persons per year. "Tissick" apparently is an antiquated spelling of phtisic, another name for pulmonary consumption, or tuberculosis. Fig. 5 sets out the correlation between consumption and bread prices from 1650 to 1750. Consumption and other pulmonary ailments, such as emphysema, are generally acknowledged to be extremely sensitive to nutrition. A correlation between deaths and bread prices would be

28 See C. W. Dixon, *Smallpox* (London, 1962).
29 Chambers thought it noteworthy that the "seven ill years" in the 1690s were relatively healthy years (*Population*, 91–94). In London, the generally low level of mortality from the great epidemic diseases in the 1640s seems equally surprising. The prolonged bad years from 1647 through 1651 provoked no heightened mortality from typhus, smallpox, or fever, although the degree of malnutrition probably was greater than at any other time in the seventeenth century.
30 The correlation coefficient for all 89 years from 1629 through 1728 for which figures are available is − .020. This is statistically insignificant at the 5 percent confidence level. E. A. Wrigley, "A Simple Model of London's Importance in Changing English Society and Economy 1650–1750," *Past & Present*, 37 (1967), 45, offers the following round figures for London's population: 200,000 in 1600; 400,000 in 1650; 575,000 in 1700; 675,000 in 1750.

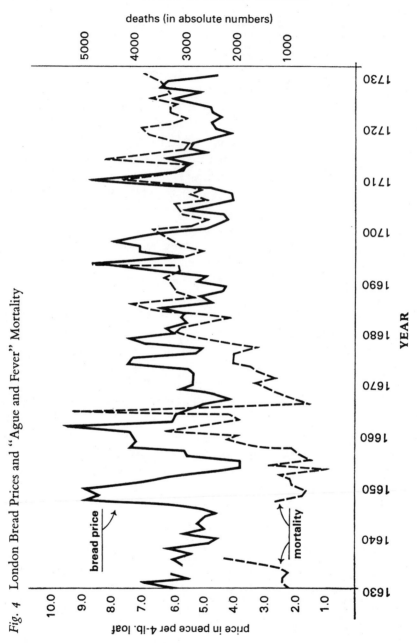

Fig. 4 London Bread Prices and "Ague and Fever" Mortality

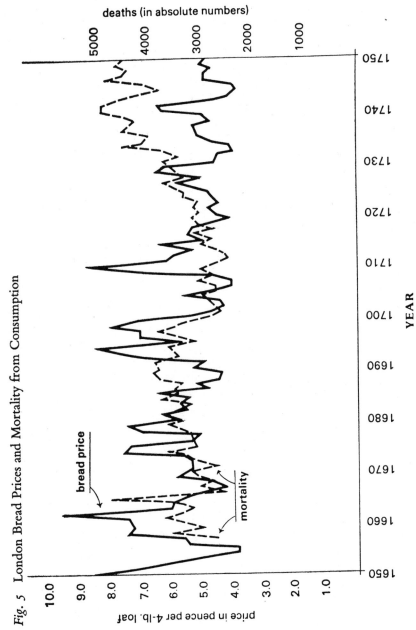

Fig. 5 London Bread Prices and Mortality from Consumption

expected, particularly following a prolonged dearth, such as that of the 1690s. But here again, any correlation is questionable.[31] The graph of consumption shows deaths rising gradually until about 1692, then falling for about thirty years before once again ascending, this time to new heights. What may have prompted the decline in consumption mortality in the first three decades of the eighteenth century? Prices were both more volatile and also absolutely higher than later in the 1730s and 1740s when consumption deaths again increased. Possibly weather played a role; winters may have been milder in the years of low mortality. Further research needs to be done to isolate each environmental factor. But all in all, it is hard to see any connection between consumption and bread price levels in this one historical instance.

It would be a mistake to push our evidence too far. The identification and classification of disease was far from sure. The 1665 mortality figures shown for typhus, fever, and consumption all suggest that plague deaths were falsely attributed to each of these.[32] Such mistakes hardly inspire confidence in the evidence. On the other hand, the various diseases follow approximately the pattern one would expect, aside from any correlation with bread prices. The pattern for smallpox, for example, was the logical one for a disease that virtually all Londoners were exposed to early in life—small epidemics, recurring every few years, and striking only the previously unexposed children. The picture of consumption mortality, too, is as expected: only small variations from year to year in the death toll from this endemic, wasting disease.

We have suggested that disease mortality levels corresponded to bread prices in two instances: typhus and "ague and fever." Certainly neither correspondence can be said statistically to be established, but only in these two was there *any* correspondence.[33] As we noted before, typhus was an insignificant disease from a demographic standpoint. "Ague and fever" was much more important but it too was dwarfed

31 Tushnet, *Uses of Adversity*, 54, 60. The correlation coefficient between bread prices and consumption mortality was −.066 for the 94 years from 1657 through 1750. This is statistically insignificant at the 5 percent confidence level.

32 The deaths attributed to consumption may, of course, have been caused by pneumonic plague. Both diseases involve the coughing of blood, although the course of pneumonic plague is much more rapid than that of consumption.

33 See notes 24 and 30, above. The statistical correlation of fever mortality to bread prices was actually slightly negative. Any positive correlation appears only on the graph.

by the myriad of other diseases which show no correspondence to bread price levels. The greatest killer in the eighteenth century was "convulsions," a childhood disease (or group of diseases) that killed a progressively greater number of children each year, at a rate unaffected by long-term falling bread prices.

Environmental factors appear to have been less important than one might expect in the course of London mortality. The bread price level was not determining, although these prices were a suitable index of nutritional levels. Another environmental factor that should have played a considerable role was the density of population, or the crowding factor. As London grew, mortality from epidemic disease should have increased disproportionally, because the chances of exposure were greater. But this, too, seems doubtful. Plague disappeared,[34] and typhus declined in importance.

The relative unimportance of environmental factors in London suggests that it was possible for disease to have been extremely virulent in the fifteenth century, despite relatively low population density and relatively good diet, and quite mild during the early industrial revolution, despite increased population density and perhaps deteriorating nutrition. Largely independent of environmental factors, the course of disease may have to be treated as an autonomous influence on population growth.[35]

34 For reasons that remain unclear.
35 In another place, we have argued the complement to this view: that starvation, unassisted by disease, could determine population change. See "Disease or Famine? Mortality in Cumberland and Westmorland, 1580–1640," *Economic History Review*, XXVI (1973), 403–432.

YEAR	PLAGUE	TYPHUS	SMALLPOX	FEVER	CONSUMPTION
1629	0	32	72	956	—
1630	1,317	58	40	1,091	—
1631	274	58	58	1,115	—
1632	8	38	531	1,108	—
1633	0	24	72	953	—
1634	1	125	1,354	1,279	—
1635	0	245	293	1,622	—
1636	10,400	397	127	2,306	—
1637	3,082	—	—	—	—
1638	—	—	—	—	—
1639	—	—	—	—	—
1640	1,450	—	—	—	—
1641	3,067	—	—	—	—
1642	1,824	—	—	—	—
1643	996	—	—	—	—
1644	1,492	—	—	—	—
1645	1,871	—	—	—	—
1646	2,436	—	—	—	—
1647	3,597	145	139	1,260	—
1648	611	47	400	884	—
1649	67	43	1,190	751	—
1650	15	65	184	970	—
1651	23	54	525	1,038	—
1652	16	60	1,279	1,212	—
1653	6	75	139	282	—
1654	16	89	812	1,371	—
1655	9	56	1,294	689	—
1656	6	52	823	875	—
1657	4	56	835	997	2,757
1658	14	123	409	1,800	3,610
1659	36	368	1,523	2,303	2,982
1660	14	146	354	2,148	3,414
1661	20	335	1,246	3,490	3,788
1662	12	148	768	2,601	3,485
1663	9	128	411	2,107	3,260
1664	6	116	1,233	2,258	3,645
1665	68,596	1,929	655	5,257	4,808

a The absence of figures indicates the absence of data. Zero mortality is shown as zero. The headings have been modernized. In the bills of mortality, the headings change from time to time. For example, what we have labelled typhus was called "purples and spotted fever" in 1629, "spotted feaver and purples" in 1657, "spotted fever" in 1670, "spotted fever and purples" in 1673, then again "spotted fever" in 1675, only to merge with "ague and fever" in 1729 in a grouping including fever, "malignant fever, spotted fever and purples" in 1729.

1666	1,998	141	38	741	2,592
1667	35	96	1,196	916	3,087
1668	14	148	1,987	1,247	2,856
1669	3	114	951	1,499	3,162
1670	0	121	1,465	1,729	3,272
1671	5	77	696	1,343	2,710
1672	5	112	1,116	1,615	3,165
1673	5	144	853	1,804	3,320
1674	3	285	2,507	2,164	3,785
1675	1	143	997	2,154	3,148
1676	2	156	359	2,112	3,223
1677	2	155	1,678	1,749	3,272
1678	5	204	1,798	2,376	3,448
1679	2	160	1,967	2,763	3,675
1680	0	193	689	3,324	3,427
1681	0	199	2,982	3,174	3,784
1682	0	140	1,408	2,696	3,464
1683	0	148	2,096	2,250	3,241
1684	0	139	1,560	2,836	3,862
1685	0	333	2,496	3,832	3,502
1686	0	314	1,062	4,185	3,569
1687	0	144	1,551	2,847	3,473
1688	0	139	1,318	3,196	3,867
1689	—	129	1,389	3,313	3,981
1690	—	203	778	3,350	3,783
1691	—	193	1,241	3,490	3,928
1692	—	161	1,592	3,205	3,512
1693	—	199	1,164	3,211	3,547
1694	—	423	1,683	5,036	3,702
1695	—	105	784	3,019	3,181
1696	—	102	196	2,775	3,471
1697	—	137	634	3,111	3,820
1698	—	274	1,813	3,343	3,582
1699	—	306	890	3,505	3,351
1700	—	189	1,031	3,676	2,819
1701	—	68	1,095	2,902	2,678
1702	—	53	311	2,682	2,730
1703	—	74	898	3,162	2,831
1704	—	61	1,501	3,243	3,013
1705	—	41	1,095	3,290	2,784
1706	—	54	721	2,662	2,716
1707	—	42	1,078	2,947	3,049
1708	—	62	1,687	2,738	2,796
1709	—	118	1,024	3,140	3,040
1710	—	343	3,138	4,397	2,706
1711	—	142	915	3,461	2,520

YEAR	PLAGUE	TYPHUS	SMALLPOX	FEVER	CONSUMPTION
1712	—	96	1,943	3,131	2,551
1713	—	102	1,614	3,039	2,745
1714	—	150	2,810	4,631	3,029
1715	—	161	1,057	3,588	2,842
1716	—	100	2,427	3,078	3,189
1717	—	137	2,211	2,940	2,764
1718	—	132	1,884	3,475	3,106
1719	—	124	3,229	3,803	3,206
1720	—	66	1,440	3,910	3,054
1721	—	84	2,375	3,331	3,188
1722	—	22	2,167	3,088	3,107
1723	—	51	3,271	3,321	3,352
1724	—	84	1,227	3,262	3,371
1725	—	59	3,188	3,277	3,240
1726	—	84	1,569	4,666	3,764
1727	—	102	2,379	4,728	3,340
1728	—	94	2,105	4,716	3,491
1729	—	—	2,849	5,235	3,544
1730	—	—	1,914	4,011	3,728
1731	—	—	2,640	3,225	3,425
1732	—	—	1,197	2,939	3,719
1733	—	—	1,370	3,831	4,601
1734	—	—	2,688	3,116	4,139
1735	—	—	1,594	2,544	4,064
1736	—	—	3,014	3,361	4,554
1737	—	—	2,084	4,580	4,441
1738	—	—	1,590	3,890	4,326
1739	—	—	1,690	3,334	4,429
1740	—	—	2,725	4,003	4,919
1741	—	—	1,977	7,528	4,981
1742	—	—	1,429	5,108	4,716
1743	—	—	2,029	3,837	4,353
1744	—	—	1,633	2,670	3,865
1745	—	—	1,206	2,690	4,015
1746	—	—	3,236	4,167	4,887
1747	—	—	1,380	4,779	4,560
1748	—	—	1,789	3,981	4,487
1749	—	—	2,625	4,458	4,623
1750	—	—	1,229	4,294	4,543

Anne Hardy

Diagnosis, Death, and Diet: The Case of London, 1750–1909

There are two basic approaches to historical study: the general and the particular. Most historians are more gifted at one, yet can appreciate and be stimulated by the other; the best history successfully combines the two perspectives. In interdisciplinary history above all, the two approaches meet in a complex and delicate relationship. The modern emphasis on statistical methods has added a further dimension of both vision and error to the historian's craft. The history of mortality is one area where the use of statistical methods seems irresistible, and where the pitfalls of so doing are numerous.

When McKeown published his classic *Modern Rise of Population* in 1976, the novelty of the statistical survey technique, authoritatively applied by a medically qualified historian, gave great stimulus to historical mortality studies. The social history of medicine was a relatively new field, and the flaws in the technique were not immediately apparent. In the last decade, medical history has developed rapidly, and although the importance of McKeown's work remains unchallenged, the validity of statistical surveys in furthering our understanding of historical mortality must be seriously questioned. In a recent article, Matossian used the statistical survey technique in an attempt to emphasize the importance of diet in mortality by showing a causal relationship between fungus contaminated cereals and declining mortality in eighteenth- and nineteenth-century London. Matossian's essay is an excellent example of the misuse of eighteenth- and nineteenth-century statistics. The time has clearly come to draw attention to the shortcomings of these statistics, so that English mortality studies may be placed on a sounder footing.[1]

Anne Hardy is Research Fellow at Imperial College, London.

The author is grateful to Irvine Loudon and Lise Wilkinson for their comments on an earlier draft of this article.

1 Thomas McKeown, *The Modern Rise of Population* (London, 1976). For recent work critical of McKeown, see Robert Woods and John Woodward (eds.), *Urban Disease and*

In simple statistical terms there may be some basis for Matossian's argument, but attention to the interpretation of contemporary medical terminology and to the realities of English climate and diet raises serious qualifications to the thesis with respect to mortality from specific causes. Neither the London bills of mortality, nor the Registrar-General's statistical series, the sources for all statistical discussion of London's mortality in this period, were models of diagnostic accuracy. The London bills of mortality, it is well known, were not compiled by qualified medical men, but by unqualified "searchers," whose diagnostic skills were undoubtedly limited, whose honesty was sometimes doubtful, and whose charity to the families of the dead was probably considerable. The early pioneers of public health and medical statistics, from John Graunt in the seventeenth century to Thomas Bateman in the early nineteenth, were unanimous in their advice that the bills of mortality were liable to great diagnostic inaccuracy. Medical men themselves were not unaware of vagueness in many of their own diagnostic categories, and attempts were made to refine terminology throughout the period. Such medical reinterpretations were probably slow to filter through to the searchers. Although all of their information should be treated with some caution, certain categories of disease, including convulsions and consumption, the principal props of Matossian's argument, should be regarded with great skepticism.[2]

CONVULSIONS   The decline in deaths from convulsions in the period after 1750 should not be measured simply against selected death rates from the period 1750 to 1754, but against the broad spectrum. Total infant mortality (under five and under two) apparently fell in the later eighteenth century, but remained disconcertingly stable in the nineteenth. The relationship between the

Mortality (London, 1985); Mary Kilbourne Matossian, "Death in London, 1750–1909," *Journal of Interdisciplinary History,* XVI (1985), 183–197. McKeown himself used only post-registration data because of the diagnostic unreliability of the bills of mortality, and he drew attention to the less serious shortcomings of mortality statistics since 1839.

2   William Heberden, *Observations on the Increase and Decrease of Different Diseases* (London, 1801), 44; Thomas Bateman, *Reports on the Diseases of London,* (London, 1819), 6–8, 22, 47–48. The subject of the general reliability of the bills of mortality was thoroughly investigated by William Ogle in 1892. Ogle saw no reason to depart from the traditional medical view of the searchers. Ogle, "An Inquiry into the Trustworthiness of the Old Bills of Mortality," *Journal of the Statistical Society,* LV (1892), 442–443.

falling number of deaths from convulsions and the overall decline in infant mortality may be significant, but in far wider terms than Matossian allows.[3]

Throughout the period, convulsions was a handy term for describing a multiplicity of ills; its application may also, at one level, reflect nosological fashion. When the bills of mortality began to specify cause of death in 1629, the list of children's diseases included both convulsions, and "Chrisomes and Infants." From 1629 until 1726, when it finally disappeared, deaths attributed to the latter declined while those from convulsions rose. Both Heberden the Younger and Marshall after him considered that this change in incidence was one of name only. As Heberden remarked, there was little doubt that "some children's diseases, formerly called chrysoms and infants, are now accumulated under the general head of convulsions." Since chrisoms deaths largely related to deaths in the first month of life, the term convulsions may, in the first part of the eighteenth century at least, have covered general neonatal mortality.[4]

When deaths from convulsions began to decline at the end of the eighteenth century, it was after the incorporation of new diagnostic categories: cough and whooping cough (1740), dropsy in the brain (1790), and croup (1793). "Dropsy in the brain" certainly reduced the total number of convulsions deaths. The term was used for tuberculous meningitis, a not uncommon cause of death, which was often described as convulsions or hydrocephalus. Marshall noted this development particularly:

> *Coughs, Croup, and Dropsy in the Brain,* all indicate a determination, since 1790, to fill up the void of Mortality which the diminution under the head of *Convulsions* seems disposed to occasion. *Dropsy in the Brain,* in particular, appears to deserve attention: how far this Disease may have been confounded with Convulsions, or otherways, prior to 1790, is a point I must leave to the Medical Professor to determine.[5]

3   Matossian, "Death in London," 186; Heberden, "On the Mortality of London," *Medical Transactions of the College of Physicians,* IV (1813), 112–113; Thomas R. Edmonds, "The Mortality of Infants in England," *Lancet* (Jan. 1836), 690–694; Anthony S. Wohl, *Endangered Lives* (London, 1983), 10–11.
4   Heberden, *Observations,* 42–3; John Marshall, *Mortality of the Metropolis* (London, 1832), v.
5   *Ibid.*

Wohl, discussing the importance of premature births and perinatal and neo-natal mortality for the nineteenth century, suggests "fatal convulsions" as one category to describe these deaths. He is undoubtedly correct, but the link between convulsions and diarrhea should not be dismissed. Fatal diarrhea in infants often terminates in convulsions, and contemporaries probably viewed the two as related. In Cullen's nosology, used by Marshall, convulsions were placed among the causes of infant deaths, but were described as belonging to the nervous diseases, of the order *spasmi*, most of which were clearly bowel disorders. Once convulsions and diarrhea were distinguished in the Registrar-General's classification after 1839, and with the medical certification of death, a greater degree of precision separated deaths which had previously been generally denominated convulsions.[6]

The July to September peak in convulsions deaths, evident after 1839, also suggests that there be caution in accepting the term convulsions as meaning the same thing throughout the period 1750 to 1909. Later analysis of Heberden's data revealed that, between 1797 and 1799, convulsions were most fatal in the four *coldest* months of the year. They were least fatal, by a small margin, in the warmest months. This pattern again strongly suggests a wider interpretation of convulsions that included perinatal, and perhaps also respiratory, "crib," and other cold weather infant deaths. After 1839, however, the likelihood increases that registered convulsions mortality, like that of diarrhea, relates to improper feeding. During the summer and autumn months many women were out at work, and babies were cared for by others. Dry-nursing was not always carried out responsibly, and the risks to infants were high. The risks of weaning were in any case high, for it was principally carried out through the introduction of cereal foods, and the risks of digestive upset and of celiac disease were considerable. But the summer months were in themselves unhealthy for the London poor, whose unventilated homes, heated by the sun and the family's domestic fire, rapidly became stifling. Infants were especially vulnerable to heat disorders and dehydration, for parents were generally over-anxious about their warmth. The summer peak of convulsions after 1839 may disguise no more

6 Wohl, *Lives,* 15–16; Francis B. Smith, *The People's Health* (London, 1979), 85.

than a variety of non-specific bowel and heat-induced disorders in young infants.[7]

Although summer bowel complaints probably reflect a range of food and general hygiene problems, the role of bread and cereals in infant mortality throughout the year should be considered, in view of Matossian's thesis. Adulterated bread was certainly considered a cause of infant mortality in the late eighteenth century. With the addition of chalk, alum, and bone-ashes to London bread, it would be surprising if vulnerable infants were not in one sense poisoned by being weaned on pap made with this bread. The substitution of potato flour for these additives in the late eighteenth and in the nineteenth centuries made for a healthier "wheaten" loaf. But if adulterated bread may be considered a possible element in deaths from convulsions, it is most unlikely that ergot of rye had a role to play in this mortality. By the 1780s, when deaths from convulsions began to decline, rye had for some time ceased to play any considerable role in the diet of London, and indeed of southern England. Rye flours continued to be used in some parts of the English counties throughout the nineteenth century, but there is no evidence of major local variations in convulsion mortality coinciding with rye areas.[8]

Regional consumption of rye apart, the evidence for the presence of ergot in England is doubtful. The grounds for linking ergot with infant convulsions are even more debatable. Convulsive ergotism is a familial affection. Had convulsive ergotism been responsible for infant convulsion deaths in England on the scale which Matossian claims, the adult population would not have been unaffected, and there would certainly have been positive contemporary documentation. No such documentation exists.

7 William Guy, "Temperature and its Relation to Mortality," *Journal of the Statistical Society*, XLIV (1881), 253; John Sykes, "The Certification and Classification of the Causes of Death," *Public Health*, II (1889), 37. It was estimated that 90% of the children put out to dry-nurse by wet-nurses died after a few weeks. Bateman, *Reports*, 88, 240, 247; Medical Officer's Annual Report (MOAR) (Newington, 1860), 25.
8 Tobias Smollett, *Humphrey Clinker* (London, 1771; repr. 1967), 152. As late as 1893 it was thought that both potato and maize flour were often used in considerable quantities in bread making: Alfred Hill, "The Influence of Food Adulteration on Health," *Public Health*, V (1893), 355; Matossian, "Mold Poisoning: An Unrecognised English Health Problem, 1500–1800," *Medical History*, XXV (1981), 79; Edward J. Collins, "Dietary Change and Cereal Consumption in Britain in the Nineteenth Century," *Agricultural History Review*, XXIII (1975), 97–115.

Further, the regularity of the curve of infant convulsions deaths is at odds with the nature of egotism. Ergot is above all an epidemic infection: its presence in rye demands very particular weather conditions, which may not occur every year. In fact, rye becomes dangerous only in exceptional years. Quite apart from the disappearance of rye from the southern English diet in the eighteenth century, the suggestion that ergotism was responsible for an annual toll of infant deaths is untenable.[9]

CONSUMPTION   The analysis of the pattern of deaths from consumption in eighteenth- and nineteenth-century London is both simpler and more complex than that of convulsions. On the one hand we are dealing with a recognizable disease, rather than with a symptom; on the other hand, the etiology of the disease is very complex. Nor was the historical recognition of pulmonary tuberculosis straightforward, and the bills of mortality are exceptionally unreliable with respect to this disease. The term "phthisis," and hence also "consumption," in its Greek derivation means simply "wasting," and it was in this sense that it was used, during the eighteenth and much of the nineteenth centuries, to cover a wider range of diseases than pulmonary consumption alone. In later eighteenth-century veterinary texts, it can be found as a synonym for pneumonia. In the early nineteenth century five types of phthisis were identified, deriving from Cullen's listing of five causes of phthisis: haemoptysis, suppuration of the lungs resulting from pneumonia, catarrh, asthma, and, the commonest, tubercule. Even by the end of the nineteenth century, old habits lingered. In 1892, for instance, the example of phthisis was used to demonstrate the unreliability of the Registrar-General's statistics: Wales showed a very high phthisis mortality partly because the proportion of uncertified deaths was high, but also because "every death from wasting disease is apt to be certified as 'consumption'." But pulmonary tuberculosis was not the only disease

9 George Barger, *Ergot and Ergotism* (London, 1931), 2–5, 27, 98; Frank J. Bove, *The Story of Ergot* (New York, 1970), 8; David van Zwanenburg, "A Singular Calamity," *Medical History*, XVII (1973), 206; Thomas D. Wyllie and Lawrence G. Morehouse (eds.), *Mycotoxic Fungi, Mycotoxins, Mycotoxicoses* (New York, 1978), III, 148. For a graphic account of the effects of convulsive ergotism in adults, see John G. Fuller, *The Day of St. Anthony's Fire* (London, 1968).

to cause wasting; deaths from internal cancers and leukemia were probably often registered as "phthisis."[10]

If phthisis was used to describe deaths from a variety of causes other than pulmonary tuberculosis, statistics of phthisis mortality should, above all, be studied in conjunction with those for bronchitis. In the eighteenth century, especially, deaths registered as the result of consumption disguised mortality from chronic bronchitis, which was also listed as "cough" and "asthma." The identification of bronchitis as a separate disease took place only between 1808 and 1814. Before this, deaths which were primarily due to bronchitis, but were immediately due to other complaints, were classified under the last: consumption, pneumonia, dropsy, or pleurisy. Given the blanket application of phthisis, and the similarity of bronchitis symptoms—cough, generally with thick and copious expectoration, sometimes with haemoptysis—to those of pulmonary tuberculosis, it is a fair assumption that, before the work of Buxton and Badham, most deaths that were subsequently registered as bronchitis were classified as phthisis. Haemoptysis was usually equated with phthisis, but it is also very common in bronchiectasis, which results from chronic bronchitis.[11]

The evidence of Willan on this point is significant. He tested the accuracy of the bills of mortality with respect to pulmonary complaints against cases in his own dispensary practice in the years 1795 and 1796. His results confirmed one third of London's total mortality to be due to *respiratory disease*. This finding has been taken as evidence for the diagnostic reliability of the bills, but in fact it was misleading. Willan was referring to respiratory deaths in general, and not phthisis in particular:

10   For the etiology of tuberculosis, see William Topley and Graham S. Wilson, *Principles of Bacteriology, Virology and Immunity* (London, 1984; 7th ed.), III, 33–61. On the misuse of the term consumptive, see Bateman, *Reports*, 22–23; Heberden, *Observations*, 44; Charles Vial de Sainbel (trans. anon.), *The Works* (London, 1795), 67, 105; *Edinburgh Medical and Physical Directory* (Edinburgh, 1807), II; anonymous review of Alfred Haviland, *The Geographical Distribution of Disease in Great Britain* in *Public Health*, V (1893), 14. See also, John Landers, "Mortality, Weather and Prices in London 1675–1825: A Study in Short-Term Fluctuations," *Journal of Historical Geography*, XII (1986), 349–350.

11   See Victor C. Medvei, "Isaac Buxton (1773–1825)," *British Medical Journal* (1957), I, 279–280; Robert L. Richards, "Charles Badham M.D., F. R. S. (1780–1845)," *Journal of the History of Medicine*, XI (1956), 54–65.

The article of pulmonary consumption includes cases of ulcerations of the lungs, and alteration of their texture, in consequence of pneumonic Inflammation and repeated Catarrhs. I apprehend not more than a fourth part of the whole number of cases put down could be referred to proper phthisis, arising from the slow and successive suppurations of tubercules in strumous constitutions.[12]

Both in Willan's own account and in the bills of mortality, phthisis included a wide range of respiratory disease other than pulmonary consumption, principally, on Willan's description, chronic bronchitis. Indeed Willan suggests that not more than 25 percent of pulmonary consumption, and probably rather less, were from true phthisis.

The link which Matossian detects between cold and phthisis deaths in the years before about 1830, and the disappearance of the connection after that, confirms the suspicion that this pattern actually reflects the addition to pulmonary tuberculosis death numbers of deaths due to bronchitis. The correlation of low winter temperatures and severe fogs with high mortality from bronchitis in particular was well recognized, certainly·by the mid-nineteenth century. Although deaths from tuberculosis were gradually decreasing, contemporaries were aware that deaths from other lung diseases were rising—"so that the sum of the two shows no progressive decrease." The Royal Commission on Tuberculosis, reporting in 1898, admitted that:

The true significance of the alteration of the rates of mortality as time has gone on is to an important extent obscured by the increasing accuracy of diagnosis, by changes in nomenclature, and by the different extent to which deaths have been medically certified.[13]

12 Robert Willan, *Reports on the Diseases in London* (London, 1801), 84–85. For the misinterpretation of Willan, see John Brownlee, "Investigation into the Epidemiology of Phthisis in Great Britain and Ireland," *Medical Research Council Reports*, XVIII (1918), 41–42. Brownlee construed "pulmonary complaints" as "consumption," and used Willan as evidence for the accuracy of the bills. In this interpretation, he was clearly mistaken. Willan's findings were substantially confirmed by Buxton a few years later. See Isaac Buxton, *An Essay on the Use of a Regulated Temperature in Winter–Cough and Consumption* (London, 1810), 10–23.

13 Matossian, "Death in London," 194; *Twenty–Seventh Annual Report of the Registrar-General*, British Parliamentary Papers (BPP), XIX (1866), 71–72; *Forty-Second Annual Report of the Registrar-General*, BPP, XXVII (1881), 30; *Royal Commission on Tuberculosis*, BPP, LXIX (1898), 338.

It was only in the early decades of the nineteenth century, with the adoption of percussion followed by the gradual acceptance of Laennec's stethoscope, that the medical diagnosis of tuberculosis began to become more precise. The number of bronchitis deaths, however, was probably swollen by the addition of deaths really due to consumption.[14]

Tuberculosis was a socially sensitive disease in the nineteenth century. The popularly accepted view was that it was, in some form, hereditary. Efforts were often made to disguise its presence, or otherwise to explain deaths from it. In these endeavors, families were frequently assisted by their medical attendants. It was common to ascribe phthisis deaths to bronchitis or pneumonia, the condition most prominent at the time of death. This practice became more frequent around 1840, when the institution of registration and the medical certification of deaths introduced a barely acceptable form of bureaucatic intrusion into English life.[15]

From the mid-1850s, the mechanisms of preventive medicine further breached traditional English domestic privacy. Whereas the visits of the searchers had been tolerated, the intervention of preventive officers was resented and avoided if possible. In well-to-do households, it was generally impossible for the preventive authorities to ascertain the presence of smallpox; after the introduction of the compulsory notification of infectious diseases in 1889, there were bitter complaints of the infringement of privacy. The delay in making pulmonary tuberculosis notifiable stemmed partly from its reputation as a hereditary disease. Concealment from official eyes and official records was probably a priority in an unknown percentage of cases; and it appears likely that concealment became important, perhaps increasingly so, only after the bills of mortality were replaced by certification and registration.[16]

14 Robert Young Keers, *Pulmonary Tuberculosis: A Journey down the Centuries* (London, 1978), 35–51.

15 Arthur Ransome, "The Etiology and Prevention of Phthisis," *Lancet* (Mar. 1890), 531. For the hereditary idea and family concealment of tuberculosis, see James Niven, "Inquiry into the Conditions in which the Infection of Consumption is Operative," *Public Health*, III (1891), 463; Dennis Vinrace, *The War Against Consumption* (London, 1901), 20; René and Jean Dubos, *The White Plague* (Harmondsworth, 1956), 6. For similar attitudes and problems in France, see Pierre Guillaume, *Du deséspoir au salut; les tuberculeux au 19e et 20e siècles* (Paris, 1986).

16 On the concealment of smallpox, see *Lancet*, I (1871), 284; on the protection of

The difficulties which historians face in working on a disease like consumption are considerable. The detailed local investigations by medical officers of health and the central medical department, which provide most of our information on the communicable diseases for this period, are virtually absent for tuberculosis before the infectiousness of the disease was accepted in the early 1890s. Even then, specific, rather than general, epidemiological studies are rare. Medical officers seeking to study the disease met with formidable obstacles: patients gave false addresses or moved house to escape inquiry and publicity. Compulsory notification of consumption was not achieved before 1912, partly because of fears that official recognition would deprive patients of the means of livelihood.[17]

Mortality figures remain our best guide to the incidence of pulmonary tuberculosis in a given area, but they should never be used without qualification, and they should always be considered in their local context. Local climate, demography, diet, social and sanitary conditions, occupational and institutional structure, all have a bearing on the interpretation of historical tuberculosis mortality. In wealthy urban areas, for example, registered mortality is more likely to reflect the incidence of the disease on the upper-class residential population: servants who fell terminally ill returned to their homes, often in the country, to die. Poor urban areas with many common lodging houses, on the other hand, often attracted a tubercular population whose infection had been acquired elsewhere: the lodging house was the last resort before the workhouse. The presence of hospitals could also swell local death rates from the disease, whether obviously as in Chelsea, the location of the Brompton Hospital, or unobtrusively as in St. Marylebone, where private hospitals and nursing homes became increasingly numerous in the Victorian period.[18]

---

privacy, see *Newington Vestry Annual Report* (1891), 79; Ransome, "The Prevention of Consumption by Disinfection," *Public Health*, IV (1892), 322; MOAR (Whitechapel, 1878), I, 13. The 1836 Registration Act marked the beginning of bureaucratic interest in domestic affairs. The introduction of public health officers in 1856 and the Notification Act of 1889 intensified the possible degree of interference.

17 Niven, "Inquiry," 463; John T. Hammack, "The Relation between Density of Population and Mortality from Consumption," *Transactions of the National Association for the Promotion of Social Science*, II (1859), 567.

18 MOAR (St. Giles, 1863), 11; MOAR (Westminster, 1898), 47; Arthur Newsholme, *Fifty Years in Public Health* (London, 1935), 244–260.

The pattern of decline of mortality from respiratory tuberculosis before about 1840 is too uncertain to allow for chronologically precise explanations of its cause. Later nineteenth-century contemporaries were convinced that the disease was on the decline, just as their forebears, at the turn of the eighteenth century, had been convinced it was increasing. Consumption remained a major killer throughout the nineteenth century: in the 1890s the disease was still recognized to be a serious problem, responsible for some 70,000 deaths a year nationally. Overall, however, the reduction in tuberculosis mortality by over one third in the late nineteenth century is too large to be accounted for solely by greater accuracy in diagnosis and the disguising of tuberculous deaths.[19]

Although the debate over the respective roles of nutrition and housing as contributory factors in causing respiratory tuberculosis continues, caution should be exercised in attempting to resolve the problem of the disease's decline with blanket explanations. The lesson to be learned from local studies is that a wide variety of factors influenced regional tuberculosis mortality. In the case of London, the apparent sharp fall in tuberculosis deaths in the 1830s is suspect because of the change in methods of death registration, and the extreme unreliability of the bills of mortality in those years. Although it is probable that tuberculosis deaths were decreasing at this time, the available statistics cannot assess reliably the extent or chronology of the decline over the period 1750 to 1909. The very sharp fall between 1831 and 1838, with a further fall in 1841, after which registration procedures were tightened up, and the continuing but much more gentle decline thereafter, strongly suggests the operation of a redistribution factor.[20]

The same statistical uncertainty bedevils attempts to estimate nutritional patterns in this period. Although it may be puzzling that deaths from pulmonary tuberculosis apparently began to decline in the "hungry half century," there is little real evidence

19 Bateman, Reports, 21; George B. Longstaff, "On the Recent Decline in the English Death Rate," Journal of the Statistical Society, XLV (1884), 224; Ransome, "Etiology," 531.
20 On housing versus nutrition in tuberculosis, see, for example, Jay Winter, The Great War and the British People (London, 1986), reviewed by Linda Bryder in Welsh History Review, XIII (1986), 245–248. On regional variations in tuberculosis, see Gillian Cronje, "Tuberculosis and Mortality in England and Wales, 1851–1910," in Woods and Woodward (eds.), Urban Disease, 79–101. Ogle, "Inquiry," 451, is particularly stern on the reliability of the bills after 1832.

to link this decline with increased potato consumption. Until the 1820s at least, potato consumption represented a decline in living standards in popular estimation, and was probably resorted to only in times of stress; bread consumption, if it fell, did so only fractionally in the first half of the nineteenth century. In any case, the role of the potato in reducing susceptibility to tuberculosis infection must remain doubtful. By the early twentieth century, when potatoes had long been indisputably a staple starch, more than 90 percent of the British population was infected with tuberculosis.[21]

It is also unlikely that the problems created by modern agricultural techniques existed in the past, or that the conditions promoting the development of *fusaria* were constantly present in the granaries. *Fusaria* are essentially field fungi—that is, they become established and grow before harvest, and once harvest is complete they are replaced by storage fungi. By the time the grain has been milled, the field flora have practically disappeared, or been removed with the bran, and the storage flora are well developed. Two types of *fusarium* only do not conform to this pattern: *f. tricinctum,* which contains T-2 toxin, occurs in grain overwintered in the fields, and has been responsible for alimentary toxic aleukia in a limited area of the Soviet Union; and *f. graminearum,* which is an advanced decay fungus, appears after deterioration and increased water activity in stored grain. As with all molds, temperature is crucial to the development of these fungi, both in the field and in storage. Although there is no doubt that they did occur in previous centuries (it was not English practice to overwinter grain in the field, however), and did cause localized outbreaks of mold poisoning from time to time, it is only since the introduction of modern mechanical techniques for harvesting, prestorage, bulk drying, and storage in silos of enormous size that mold has become a major problem in temperate climates. In the undoubtedly well-ventilated granaries of eighteenth- and nine-

21 John Burnett, *Plenty and Want* (London, 1966), 7, 11, 12, 41–42. Burnett observes that Salaman's estimates of potato consumption (used by Matossian, "Death in London," 193) were drawn from doubtful sources. Burnett, *Plenty,* 7n. For tuberculosis infection in Britain, see Sheridan Delepine, *Final Report of the Departmental Committee on Tuberculosis,* BPP (London, 1913), II, 27, cited in Bryder, "The Problem of Tuberculosis in England and Wales, 1900–1950," unpub. D.Phil. diss. (Oxford Univ., 1985), 15. See also Edward R. Long, "The Decline of Tuberculosis," *Bulletin of the History of Medicine,* VIII (1940), 826.

teenth-century northern Europe, *fusaria* can have been only an intermittent problem.[22]

There were also variations in the local pattern of tuberculosis mortality and in the pattern of the disease's overall decline. By the 1880s, it had become clear that the decline in mortality from pulmonary tuberculosis since 1850 was greatest (between 15 and 28 percent) in the age group five to thirty-five, with the most progress made by those between fifteen and twenty-five. Death rates were also falling faster among women.

These facts, the well-known occupational influences, and the regional variations in mortality described by Cronje, should be taken into account in attempting any general explanation of the falling death rate from consumption. Consumption was more fatal in the big cities and their hinterlands—for example, in London and the metropolitan counties, and in the northern textile towns. Rural death rates were generally lower than urban ones; but death rates for females were high in Suffolk and Cumberland, and for males in Sussex. Did women in Suffolk and Cumberland and men in Sussex eat more bread and fewer potatoes than their spouses? Cronje is surely correct in stating that the causes of prevailing tuberculosis mortality must have been as variable as local conditions in the regions.[23]

The etiology of tuberculosis is undoubtedly complex. Although the influence of regional, local, and personal factors is clear, it is intellectually difficult to reconcile all these different elements with a sustained long-term fall in mortality, such as is

22 Claude Moreau (trans. and ed. Maurice O. Moss), *Moulds, Toxins and Food* (New York, 1979), 12–13, 220–223. Alimentary toxic aleukia (ATA) has only been recognized in the Soviet Union between latitudes 50–60° north and longitudes 40–140° east, in an area of badly drained clay soil where the winter temperature is of the order −10 to −15°C, and the summer temperature 15–25°. The grain becomes toxic only in spring, with the active growth of the fungus, and the optimum temperature for production of T-2 toxin is 1.5 to 4°C. Koomi Kanai and Eiko Kondo, "Decreased Resistance to Mycobacterial Infection in Mice Fed a Trichothecene Compound (T-2 Toxin)," *Journal of Japanese Medical Science and Biology*, XXXVII (1984), 97–104 (cited by Matossian, "Death in London," 195), state that T-2 toxin is present in "several of the genus *fusaria*," but they do not specify which. Moreau, in his authoritative text, *Moulds, Toxins and Food*, lists 20 species of *fusaria* and their associated toxins. The only species of *fusaria* here stated to contain T-2 toxin is *f. tricinctum (Cda) Sn. and H.,* that identified with ATA.

23 Longstaff, "Recent Decline," 225–226. Among occupations associated with a high incidence of pulmonary tuberculosis were printing, boot and shoe-making, tailoring, tin mining, and slate quarrying. See also Cronje, "Tuberculosis," 94, 97.

apparent since 1838. There is a temptation to seek a single significant underlying cause for this remarkable mortality decline.
Viewing these elements against the general eighteenth- and nineteenth-century background, and taking into account the age-specific nature of decreasing phthisis mortality between 1850 and
1880 and widespread primary infection in the early twentieth
century, one may point to rising living standards as a fundamental
cause of decline. But one might equally convincingly point to
increased personal optimism as another.

Psychological stress is a recognized trigger of post-primary
tuberculosis; if, after 1800, poverty was no longer perceived as
inevitable, the effects of optimism would first be registered among
the naturally most optimistic age-group—those under thirty-five.
Such an explanation is at least as likely as the contention that
rising potato consumption reduced the immunosuppressant effect
of moldy cereals (unproven in man), and so increased resistance
to *mycobacterium tuberculosis*. Continuing high levels of tuberculosis
in urban areas where poverty remained dire and living standards
low (and potato consumption was undoubtedly high by the mid
to later nineteenth century), and where the high risk infection
factors of overcrowding and poor ventilation were particularly
great, are arguments against the latter thesis in its present elementary format. Evidence that declining tuberculosis mortality is
highly correlated with rising real wages remains the single most
dependable factor in an etiology fraught with variables.[24]

Although few would disagree that, in terms of curative medicine,
medical intervention made a positive contribution to the mortality
decline which London experienced in the nineteenth century, it
would be rash on this basis to dismiss the evidence of medical
observers, and to rely simply on the interpretation of unqualified
statistical evidence to resolve the question of why English mor-

24 Topley and Wilson, *Principles,* 33–61; *ibid.* (6th ed.), II, 1728–1729; Franklin H. Top
and Paul F. Wherle, *Communicable and Infectious Diseases* (St. Louis, 1981; 9th ed.), 679. E.
Anthony Wrigley and Roger S. Schofield, *The Population History of England, 1541–1871:
A Reconstruction* (Cambridge, Mass., 1981), 411–412. The experiments of Kanai and Kondo
with laboratory mice cannot be held to be very valid in relation to human, pre-twentieth-
century European experience. This has been implicitly argued above, but without information as to the duration of the immunosuppressant function of T-2 toxin in man, effective
dosages etc., the relation between *fusarium* and tuberculosis mortality must remain spec-
ulative.

tality declined in this period. The diagnostic unreliability of several major "cause of death" categories invalidates this type of statistical survey for the eighteenth and much of the nineteenth centuries. If Matossian believes that the available statistics permit London's mortality trends to be explained with "scientific precision," she is misguided. The suggestion that improved diet was the significant factor in modern mortality decline is not a new one, and is one that has been much debated since McKeown's *Modern Rise of Population*. Here again, oversimplified explanations should be treated with care: man did not live by bread alone, and nutritional history, like the history of disease, cannot be determined within a framework of preconceived ideas and in that vacuum in which the determination to be "scientific" so often places historians. Our knowledge of the relationship between diet and mortality, and of the historical behavior of different diseases, can be advanced only by detailed local studies which take account not only of a wide range of local circumstances, but also of statistical pitfalls, the etiology of specific diseases, and contemporary medical observations.[25]

25 It is possible that, overall, medical intervention contributed substantially to mortality. This argument is present in Smith, *People's Health*. For positive evidence on this score, see Irvine Loudon, "Death in Childbed from the Eighteenth Century to 1935," *Medical History*, XXX (1986), 1–41. For discussion of diet and mortality, see, for example, "Hunger and History," a special issue, *Journal of Interdisciplinary History*, XIV (1983), 199–534.

Robert Woods and P.R. Andrew Hinde

Mortality in Victorian England: Models and Patterns

Much of our knowledge and understanding of the secular decline in mortality that began in Europe and North America in the nineteenth century is based on the work of McKeown and his fellow researchers. McKeown's analysis starts with eighteenth-century England; it moves forward in time and then outward to encompass Europe. In his model the cause of death components of variations in mortality levels are isolated before the reasons for changes in the balance of these components are inferred.[1]

McKeown's principal arguments may be summarized as follows. There are four possible ways in which a secular decline in mortality could occur. First, living standards, diet, and housing conditions can improve substantially. Second, sanitary conditions and public health in general can be improved by administrative intervention by national or local governments. Third, particular diseases may decline in importance for reasons which are independent of human intervention. Fourth, the application of medical science may directly reduce the level of morbidity and mortality. For late nineteenth-century England, the beneficial effects of the

Robert Woods is Senior Lecturer in the Department of Geography, University of Sheffield, and is co-editor of *Urban Disease and Mortality in Nineteenth-Century England* (London, 1984). P. R. Andrew Hinde is Junior Research Fellow in the Department of Geography, University of Sheffield.

The authors thank the Nuffield Foundation and the Wellcome Trust for financial support and E. Anthony Wrigley and John Woodward for their comments.

1   The most substantial summary is to be found in Thomas McKeown, *The Modern Rise of Population* (London, 1976). See also, *idem,* "Fertility, Mortality and Causes of Death: An Examination of Issues Related to the Modern Rise of Population," *Population Studies,* XXXII (1978), 235–242; *idem,* "Food, Infection, and Population," *Journal of Interdisciplinary History,* XIV (1983), 227–247. See also, *idem* and R. G. Record, "Reasons for the Decline of Mortality in England and Wales during the Nineteenth Century," *Population Studies,* XVI (1962), 94–122; McKeown, Record, and R. D. Turner, "An Interpretation of the Decline in Mortality in England and Wales during the Twentieth Century," *Population Studies,* XXIX (1975), 391–422.

fourth possibility were largely discounted, but the other three were given considerable prominence by McKeown. Half of the mortality decline was linked to improvements in living standards, especially diet; a quarter with the sanitary revolution; and a further quarter with autonomous changes in certain diseases, scarlet fever for instance.[2]

Those who have sought to criticize this interpretation have emphasized the value of McKeown's list of possibilities and even the priority that he gives them. But they have questioned the allocation of relative weights, arguing, for example, that the direct evidence for general improvements in diet in the Victorian era is not as strong as it needs to be or that the indirect influence of medical science and the medical profession was, if not substantial, at least not negligible. The dangers of using the McKeown interpretation as a general world model have also been stressed.[3]

There are, in addition, several other difficulties. The McKeown interpretation relies both on an imperfect set of data, especially as it relates to the reporting of cause of death, and on limited temporal and spatial perspectives on the pattern of variation in mortality. These data problems are discussed below. Wrigley and Schofield's estimates of life expectation at birth (e_0) for England suggest that the limited improvements that did occur between 1750 and 1850 merely redressed the five to seven year decline of the seventeenth century. Substantial national improvements in mortality were clear only from the 1850s and 1860s onwards when e_0 stayed above forty. The rise in e_0 was accelerated after 1900 by the decline in infant mortality ($_1q_0$), which had remained high during the last half of the nineteenth century. During this half century (1851 to 1901) e_0 increased by approximately seven years in England and Wales. Although this is not inconsiderable, a further five years were added by 1911. Since

2   See also, Woods and John Woodward (eds.), *Urban Disease and Mortality in Nineteenth-Century England* (New York, 1984), 29–33.
3   On diet see, Derek J. Oddy, "The Health of the People," in Theo Barker and Michael Drake (eds.), *Population and Society in Britain, 1850–1980* (London, 1982), 121–139; Oddy, "Urban Famine in Nineteenth-Century Britain: the Effect of the Lancashire Cotton Famine on Working Class Diet and Health," *Economic History Review*, XXXVI (1983), 68–86. On the indirect influence of the medical profession, Woodward, "Medicine and the City," in Woods and Woodward, *Urban Disease*, 65–78; Samuel H. Preston, "The Changing Relation between Mortality and Level of Economic Development," *Population Studies*, XXIX (1975), 231–248.

McKeown deals with the periods 1848–1854 to 1901 and post-1901 separately, the significance of sudden changes in infant mortality after 1901 for longer term trends in life expectation may be blurred. McKeown is concerned only with national trends and presents, thereby, an impression of uniformity in his interpretation that belies the significant environmental variations which appear to have existed in both the level of mortality and the structure of cause-of-death patterns.[4]

Our approach to these issues develops an alternative yet complementary perspective by focusing in detail on the pattern and structure of mortality in the nineteenth century. We are particularly concerned with two aspects: variations in age-specific mortality together with regional or local differences in mortality. Although McKeown was to some extent concerned with the former, he took virtually no account of the latter. Yet the range of life chances experienced by Victorians was considerable. More specifically, we are concerned with two sets of problems: first, the estimation of model life tables which will assist the study of changes in the age-specific structure of mortality; and, second, the influence of environment on variations in the level of mortality. Although our solutions to these problems may not represent a reinterpretation of McKeown's position, they will at least add to the debate by providing a more sophisticated description of the underlying mortality conditions.[5]

We begin by considering the availability and quality of civil registration data, especially mortality statistics, in Victorian England and Wales. We proceed to a review of the official English Life Tables (ELTs) and the construction of English model life table systems (differentiated here and throughout from official ELTs). The last two sections consider regional variations in mortality

4 E. Anthony Wrigley and Roger S. Schofield, *The Population History of England, 1541–1871: A Reconstruction* (Cambridge, Mass., 1981), 230, Table 7.15. The best estimates of e_0 for England and Wales in the nineteenth century are 1801, 37; 1811, 38; 1821, 38; 1831, 40; 1841, 40; 1851, 41; 1861, 41; 1871, 42; 1881, 44; 1891, 46; 1901, 48; 1911, 53. See Woods, "The Effects of Population Redistribution on the Level of Mortality in Nineteenth-Century England and Wales," *Journal of Economic History*, XLV (1985), 645–651. The rise in e_0 between 1750 and 1850 from about 35 to 40 occurred despite the effects of urbanization and the redistribution of population from low mortality rural to high mortality urban areas.

5 McKeown and Record, "Reasons for the Decline," 100. See also Woods and Woodward, *Urban Disease*, 39.

patterns and the influence of environmental factors, as well as the maldistribution of members of the medical profession in the nineteenth century.

VITAL STATISTICS   Civil registration began in England and Wales in July 1837. The country was divided into forty-five registration counties and over 600 registration districts, each one of which had a superintendent registrar who was responsible for the compilation of information on births, marriages, and deaths. Of the three, mortality registration was, even from the 1830s, the most comprehensive, since both age at death and cause of death were recorded on a sex-specific basis. The registrar general, based in London, was responsible for the preparation of an annual report, which normally provided a commentary on the course of vital events together with a series of tables reporting annual vital statistics. Special reports on, for example, occupational mortality, were frequently appended, but the degree of detail reported was also liable to vary from year to year. Supplements were also prepared for the twenty-fifth (1862), thirty-fifth (1872), forty-fifth (1882), fifty-fifth (1892), sixty-fifth (1902), and seventy-fifth (1912) annual reports. They gave summaries of the vital statistics for the decades 1851–1860, 1861–1870, 1871–1880, 1881–1890, 1891–1900, and 1901–1910. In 1911 the districts were abandoned as civil registration units in favour of the new local government areas.

Registration districts should therefore provide a convenient scale for the analysis of mortality patterns between 1838 and 1910, but, apart from the decennial supplements, age at death data were only published in the eighteenth (1855) to the forty-seventh (1884) annual reports. Thereafter registration counties were employed and, for the forty-fourth (1881) to the forty-seventh (1884) reports, male and female ages at death were not published separately. Annual sex-specific age at death data are only available for the period 1855 to 1880 and can only be related to population at risk data from the 1861 and 1871 censuses.[6]

6   There is no comprehensive guide to the publications of vital statistics by the registrar general between 1837 and 1911. Most, but not all, of the reports, abstracts of statistics, supplements, and incidental items on specific issues are to be found in Parliamentary Papers (PP). John M. Eyler, *Victorian Social Medicine: The Ideas and Methods of William Farr* (Baltimore, 1979), provides an interesting insight on the work of the General Register Office and on William Farr, one of its most influential members.

Our analysis of mortality variations rests, therefore, on statistics drawn from the twenty-fourth (1861), twenty-fifth (1862), and twenty-sixth (1863) annual reports of the Registrar General of Births, Deaths and Marriages, together with the 1861 census of population, and is complemented by cause of death data from the *Supplement to the Thirty-Fifth (1872) Annual Report* for 1861 to 1870. It focuses on the registration districts and ignores those periods for which only decennial or county data are available. Decades and counties are not used for similar reasons: the former cover too long a time span and the latter too large an area; both obscure some of those very environmental variations that we seek to uncover.

The reliability of these data is difficult, if not impossible, to judge. There is no reason to believe that death reporting was particularly inaccurate, but there are grounds for suspecting some bias in the age at death and age structure data, and especially the data on cause of death. The former have been examined in some detail by Lee and Lam for England and Wales as a whole. They concentrate on the age structure of the female population from the 1821 and the 1841 to 1931 censuses, but they also analyze the male structures for 1861 to 1871. Their results suggest, for example, the need to adjust the number of 0–4 year olds given in the 1861 and 1871 censuses by 1.0162 for males and 1.0488 for females. They refer particularly to the high degree of age misreporting in the 1841 census.[7]

Unfortunately, the methods employed are not amenable to use with registration district data since the differences in age-structures that occur between two censuses are likely to be affected by age-specific net migration. Even Lee and Lam focused their analysis on the female population to avoid, among other things,

7 Ronald D. Lee and David Lam, "Age Distribution Adjustments for English Censuses, 1821 to 1931," *Population Studies*, XXXVII (1983), 445–464. There have been attempts to estimate the extent of birth under-registration, but these have relied on the assumption that death registration was relatively accurate. See David V. Glass, "A Note on the Under-Registration of Births in Britain in the Nineteenth Century," *Population Studies*, V (1951), 70–88; Michael S. Teitelbaum, "Birth Under-Registration in the Constituent Counties of England and Wales, 1841–1910," *Population Studies*, XXVIII (1974), 329–343. The recent study by Dov Friedlander et al., "Socio-Economic Characteristics and Life Expectancies in Nineteenth-Century England: A District Analysis," *Population Studies*, XXXIX (1985), 137–151, ignores the problem in its indirect estimation of e_0 for registration districts by decades.

the problems associated with the presumed higher migration of men. Age-structure distortions and the variable level of under-enumeration remain intractable problems when using registration district data. The reporting of cause of death must also be treated with caution since the etiology of many of the most important infectious diseases was little understood by members of the medical profession in the mid-nineteenth century. For instance, typhus and typhoid were combined in the registrar general's statistics up until 1869. These statistics also employ a nosography that is very broad, containing as it does one category for other diseases, which is normally also the largest single category.

Despite these drawbacks, the vital statistics for England and Wales are particularly rich and potentially fruitful, especially for the 1860s and 1870s and when compared with those statistics available in other European countries and in North America.[8]

LIFE TABLES   Although the publication of official English Life Tables (ELTs) began in 1843, an accurate national life table only became available in 1854 with the appearance of Farr's ELT 3. Both of the first two English Life Tables rely on age structure data from the 1841 census which, as we have already seen, was particularly suspect. However, ELT 3 was based on age at death figures for 1838 to 1854 together with population at risk estimated from the 1841 and 1851 censuses. ELTs 4 to 7 all adopted a similar principle by relating average mortality in ten-year inter-censal periods to at risk estimates drawn from two censuses. ELT 8 provides the pattern for modern English Life Tables by employing mortality data for 1910 to 1912 and for the 1911 census. The probability of dying ($_nq_x$) functions for ELTs 3 to 8 are given in Table 1, together with life expectations at five ages, for males and females separately. In each case, the original full life tables have been abridged in the conventional way.[9]

8   On the United States, see, for example, Eileen M. Crimmins and Gretchen A. Condran, "Mortality Variation in U.S. Cities in 1900: A Two-Level Explanation by Cause of Death and Underlying Factors," *Social Science History*, VII (1983), 31–59; Condran and Crimmins, "Mortality Differentials between Rural and Urban Areas of States in the Northeastern United States, 1890–1900," *Journal of Historical Geography*, VI (1980), 179–202. On longer-term trends in Philadelphia, Condran and Rose A. Cheney, "Mortality Trends in Philadelphia: Age- and Cause-specific Death Rates, 1870–1930," *Demography*, XIX (1982), 97–123. On urban France, Preston and Etienne van de Walle, "Urban French Mortality in the Nineteenth Century," *Population Studies*, XXXII (1978), 275–297.
9   The first eight English Life Tables are to be found as follows: ELT 1, PP 1843/xxi; ELT

Table 1   The Probability of Dying ($_nq_x$) for English Life Tables 3 to 8

AGE GROUPS	ENGLISH LIFE TABLES					
	3	4	5	6	7	8
MALES	1838–54	1871–80	1881–90	1891–1900	1901–10	1910–12
0	0.1636	0.1586	0.1610	0.1719	0.1443	0.1204
1–4	0.1368	0.1276	0.1043	0.0940	0.0721	0.0606
5–9	0.0468	0.0342	0.0240	0.0218	0.0166	0.0168
10–14	0.0248	0.0177	0.0100	0.0122	0.0101	0.0096
15–19	0.0310	0.0235	0.0188	0.0188	0.0153	0.0139
20–24	0.0425	0.0337	0.0263	0.0250	0.0206	0.0186
25–29	0.0467	0.0412	0.0354	0.0298	0.0242	0.0212
30–34	0.0515	0.0495	0.0443	0.0372	0.0312	0.0263
35–39	0.0581	0.0597	0.0543	0.0497	0.0398	0.0343
40–44	0.0675	0.0723	0.0669	0.0632	0.0508	0.0448
45–49	0.0808	0.0869	0.0829	0.0799	0.0674	0.0603
50–54	0.1015	0.1096	0.1056	0.1037	0.0913	0.0827
55–59	0.1298	0.1405	0.1395	0.1394	0.1262	0.1170
60–64	0.1733	0.1859	0.1906	0.1885	0.1742	0.1648
65–69	0.2414	0.2527	0.2600	0.2579	0.2388	0.2319
70–74	0.3374	0.3472	0.3551	0.3569	0.3393	0.3292
75–79	0.4575	0.4664	0.4800	0.4811	0.4630	0.4562
80–84	0.5895	0.6019	0.6267	0.6194	0.5900	0.5934
85+	1.0000	1.0000	1.0000	1.0000	1.0000	1.0000
e_0	39.91	41.35	43.66	44.13	48.53	51.50
e_1	46.65	48.05	50.97	52.22	55.68	57.51
e_5	49.71	50.87	52.75	53.50	55.90	57.14
e_{10}	47.05	47.60	49.00	49.63	51.81	53.08
e_{85}	3.73	3.56	3.29	3.45	3.53	3.72
FEMALES						
0	0.1347	0.1287	0.1311	0.1407	0.1174	0.0977
1–4	0.1326	0.1247	0.0986	0.0898	0.0689	0.0615
5–9	0.0463	0.0318	0.0218	0.0216	0.0173	0.0166
10–14	0.0263	0.0182	0.0093	0.0128	0.0106	0.0099
15–19	0.0327	0.0235	0.0194	0.0182	0.0143	0.0132
20–24	0.0442	0.0326	0.0262	0.0221	0.0173	0.0155
25–29	0.0490	0.0386	0.0341	0.0270	0.0208	0.0181
30–34	0.0536	0.0449	0.0415	0.0335	0.0265	0.0224
35–39	0.0588	0.0520	0.0478	0.0427	0.0334	0.0285
40–44	0.0649	0.0603	0.0546	0.0518	0.0414	0.0361
45–49	0.0728	0.0701	0.0657	0.0628	0.0529	0.0471
50–54	0.0844	0.0834	0.0849	0.0814	0.0705	0.0639
55–59	0.1139	0.1144	0.1137	0.1127	0.1001	0.0902
60–64	0.1557	0.1578	0.1577	0.1580	0.1374	0.1274
65–69	0.2191	0.2215	0.2238	0.2238	0.1942	0.1856
70–74	0.3095	0.3126	0.3175.	0.3185	0.2983	0.2782
75–79	0.4261	0.4283	0.4391	0.4396	0.4116	0.3989
80–84	0.5572	0.5628	0.5798	0.5771	0.5436	0.5398
85+	1.0000	1.0000	1.0000	1.0000	1.0000	1.0000
e_0	41.85	44.62	47.18	47.77	52.38	55.35
e_1	47.31	50.14	53.24	54.53	58.31	60.31
e_5	50.33	53.08	54.92	55.79	58.53	59.94
e_{10}	47.67	49.78	51.10	51.97	54.53	55.91
e_{85}	3.98	3.88	3.71	3.80	3.94	4.19

ELT 3 also provides the basis for Wrigley and Schofield's attempt to construct a series of model life tables that would capture the pattern of age-specific mortality particular to England. They needed a family of life tables spanning a range of mortality levels in order to carry out aggregative back projection on the population of England prior to 1871. Looking first at the four families of models constructed by Coale and Demeny and comparing each with ELT 3, they observed that, although the North model provided the closest correspondence, the fit, particularly for females between ages twenty and fifty-five, was not close. To use ELT 3 unmodified as the basis for a family of specifically English life tables was considered undesirable because of the serious problem of age misreporting, especially among the elderly, in the 1841 census. Wrigley and Schofield's solution to this problem was to splice rates of $_nq_x$ from Coale and Demeny's North model above age fifty onto those from ELT 3. The appropriate North model rates were found to be at level 9.45 and were obtained by linear interpolation between levels 9 and 10 of the English life table. As for level 10 of the English family, the other levels were calculated by applying the ratios of $_nq_x$ between any two levels in the North tables to that English table. They present their new English family for both sexes combined for values of e_0 ranging from 23.54 to 45.66 (levels 3 to 12).[10]

Wrigley and Schofield's method produces a set of life tables which probably well reflects the English mortality experience. In order for the method to be of use in the analysis of mortality during the Victorian period, however, it needs to be extended to encompass a range of values of e_0 more appropriate to the late nineteenth century. Moreover, it is desirable to present the family in a form which is easier to use. In the following paragraphs we suggest ways in which these modifications could be made and compare the results with those from an alternative and entirely empirical method of constructing model life tables.[11]

---

2 females, in a letter to the registrar general by Farr on "The Finance of Life Assurance" (1853) and males in PP 1859/xii; ELT 3, in Farr, *English Life Table. Tables of Lifetimes, Annuities, and Premiums* (London, 1864); ELT 4, PP 1884/xx; ELT 5, PP 1895/xxiii, pt 1; ELT 6, PP 1905/xviii (also compares ELTs 3, 6); ELTs 7 and 8, PP 1914/xiv.

10 Wrigley and Schofield, *Population History of England*, 708–714; Ansley J. Coale and Paul Demeny, *Regional Model Life Tables and Stable Populations* (New York, 1983; 2nd ed.).

11 The most recent set of United Nations model life tables is presented in family patterns

We first followed Wrigley and Schofield's method, and calculated single-sex life tables for levels 7 to 17 of the English family in which e_0 for males ranges from 32.34 to 56.39 and for females from 34.27 to 59.30, thereby encompassing most of the Victorian experience of mortality. The eleven life tables for each sex so generated were then treated analogously to the set of 326 used by Coale and Demeny. Regression equations were estimated for the relationships between $_nq_x$s and e_{10} ($_1q_0$, $_4q_1$, $_5q_5$, . . . , $_5q_{75}$ against e_{10}). Coale and Demeny's original models used 80+ as the final open-ended age category. Here we prefer to use the more conventional 85+ category and are thus obliged to estimate $_5q_{80}$. Like Wrigley and Schofield, we have based our estimate on the work of Gabriel and Ronen, who relate $_5q_{80}$ to $_5q_{75}$.[12]

Finally, we need to estimate e_{85}, but here we are assisted by Coale and Demeny's extended model system which gives e_{100}. We therefore obtained an equation relating e_{85} to l_{85} by a simple regression of the values of e_{85} given in levels 7 to 17 of their extended North model tables on the corresponding l_{85} values. The final stage of the exercise involved the calculation of $_nq_x$s for levels of e_0. In a fashion similar to Coale and Demeny, this calculation was accomplished by choosing values of e_{10}, the independent variable, by an iterative procedure so that $_nq_x$s corresponding to e_0 levels one year apart from 30 to 60 could be found for males and females separately. This complicated exercise yields thirty-one English model life tables for each sex: $_nq_x$s for e_0s equal to 30, 35, 40, 45, 50, 55, and 60 are shown in Table 2.[13]

The vital statistics and the census age structure data described above also provide the means of estimating sex-specific life tables for each of the registration districts in England and Wales in 1861

but organized so that e_0 is set at 35, 36, 37, 38, . . . 75 for males and females independently. This ordering differs from the Coale and Demeny system, where male and female e_0s are tied, and from Wrigley and Schofield, where they are combined. See United Nations, *Model Life Tables for Developing Countries* (New York, 1982).

12 K. R. Gabriel and Ilana Ronen, "Estimates of Mortality from Infant Mortality Rates," *Population Studies,* XII (1958), 164–169.

13 The extended system is reported in the second edition of Coale and Demeny, *Regional Model Life Tables.* Table 1 above gives e_{85} so that all the abridged life table functions can be estimated. Additional $_nq_x$s may be found by interpolation between adjacent e_0 levels. In life table notation, $_nq_x$ is the probability of dying between age x and age $x + n$ (infant mortality is $_1q_0$); l_x is the number of persons alive and aged x (l_0 is the radix of a life table, the assumed number of births per year); and e_x is life expectation in years aged x (e_0 is life expectation at birth).

Table 2 The Probability of Dying ($_nq_x$) for English Model Life Tables based on the Wrigley and Schofield Method

AGE GROUPS	e_0						
MALES	30	35	40	45	50	55	60
0	0.2327	0.1942	0.1611	0.1321	0.1064	0.0836	0.0636
1–4	0.2022	0.1642	0.1309	0.1018	0.0769	0.0557	0.0391
5–9	0.0692	0.0566	0.0456	0.0361	0.0278	0.0207	0.0149
10–14	0.0360	0.0298	0.0243	0.0196	0.0154	0.0118	0.0087
15–19	0.0428	0.0363	0.0307	0.0258	0.0214	0.0174	0.0137
20–24	0.0584	0.0496	0.0421	0.0355	0.0295	0.0241	0.0191
25–29	0.0644	0.0546	0.0462	0.0389	0.0322	0.0262	0.0207
30–34	0.0710	0.0602	0.0510	0.0429	0.0356	0.0290	0.0229
35–39	0.0804	0.0681	0.0576	0.0483	0.0400	0.0325	0.0255
40–44	0.0931	0.0789	0.0668	0.0562	0.0467	0.0380	0.0300
45–49	0.1104	0.0939	0.0799	0.0677	0.0566	0.0465	0.0370
50–54	0.1346	0.1163	0.1009	0.0872	0.0748	0.0632	0.0519
55–59	0.1808	0.1568	0.1364	0.1185	0.1021	0.0868	0.0718
60–64	0.2383	0.2093	0.1849	0.1634	0.1435	0.1245	0.1054
65–69	0.3458	0.3073	0.2753	0.2467	0.2203	0.1946	0.1681
70–74	0.4573	0.4095	0.3697	0.3344	0.3014	0.2690	0.2352
75–79	0.6065	0.5514	0.5060	0.4653	0.4271	0.3888	0.3478
80–84	0.7266	0.6794	0.6405	0.6056	0.5728	0.5401	0.5049
85+	1.0000	1.0000	1.0000	1.0000	1.0000	1.0000	1.0000
e_{85}	2.83	2.92	3.05	3.24	3.49	3.82	4.29
FEMALES							
0	0.2053	0.1722	0.1437	0.1189	0.0970	0.0811	0.0598
1–4	0.2153	0.1761	0.1425	0.1124	0.0865	0.0692	0.0442
5–9	0.0750	0.0614	0.0497	0.0393	0.0303	0.0240	0.0157
10–14	0.0416	0.0344	0.0282	0.0227	0.0179	0.0145	0.0100
15–19	0.0502	0.0420	0.0349	0.0287	0.0233	0.0193	0.0141
20–24	0.0666	0.0561	0.0471	0.0393	0.0323	0.0273	0.0205
25–29	0.0740	0.0621	0.0572	0.0436	0.0358	0.0302	0.0226
30–34	0.0815	0.0684	0.0572	0.0475	0.0389	0.0326	0.0242
35–39	0.0889	0.0747	0.0626	0.0520	0.0426	0.0358	0.0267
40–44	0.0957	0.0813	0.0689	0.0584	0.0488	0.0419	0.0324
45–49	0.1054	0.0902	0.0771	0.0660	0.0559	0.0485	0.0385
50–54	0.1181	0.1024	0.0888	0.0775	0.0670	0.0592	0.0486
55–59	0.1546	0.1339	0.1162	0.1013	0.0875	0.0773	0.0634
60–64	0.2158	0.1885	0.1651	0.1455	0.1273	0.1138	0.0952
65–69	0.3072	0.2711	0.2402	0.2145	0.1905	0.1725	0.1476
70–74	0.4336	0.3872	0.3474	0.3148	0.2838	0.2606	0.2282
75–79	0.5742	0.5215	0.4763	0.4398	0.4046	0.3779	0.3403
80–84	0.6989	0.6538	0.6150	0.5838	0.5535	0.5306	0.4985
85+	1.0000	1.0000	1.0000	1.0000	1.0000	1.0000	1.0000
e_{85}	2.89	3.07	3.19	3.35	3.56	3.83	4.16

and 1871. Here we have only utilized the 1861 census by relating to it the mean annual age at death data for 1861 to 1863. We have also found it necessary to combine a small number of the registration districts to permit comparison with demographic structures for other periods and, in this instance, to treat London as a single unit. The case of London poses a particular problem since, although we know the number of deaths that occurred in public institutions, especially in workhouses and hospitals, we have no way of relating those deaths to the normal districts of residence of the deceased. Since many of London's inner districts provide such facilities for the outer suburbs, the registration district based pattern of mortality is liable to severe distortions. We are left with 590 units covering England and Wales, most of which are single registration districts.[14]

The registration district specific life tables provide the possibility of estimating a new set of tables parallel to Wrigley and Schofield's English models but based on the range of mortality experience in 1861. The method used to estimate this set of empirical models was analogous to that outlined above. The $_nq_x$ functions were regressed against e_{10} using the two sets of 590 life tables separately, but e_{10} and e_{85} were both related to e_0 in this case. The model $_nq_x$ was found by substituting $e_0 = 30$ to 60 in the regression equations with e_{10}, and the resulting e_{10} estimates in the equations to find $_nq_x$s for the standard age groups. The $_nq_x$ functions corresponding to e_0s equal to 30, 35, 40, 45, 50, 55, and 60 for males and females were estimated in a fashion compatible with Table 2. These empirical models and our version of Wrigley and Schofield's English models are illustrated in Figure 1 for males, where the l_x functions from ELTs 3, 5, 7, and 8 are compared.

Figure 1 makes clear (as would a similar figure for females) that our empirical model and the Wrigley and Schofield English

14 In 1861–1863 nearly 15% of deaths in London occurred in public institutions. Of those deaths 56% were in workhouses and a further 29% were in general hospitals. Any districts having both workhouses and general hospitals were therefore likely to show excessive death rates. In the St. George-Hanover Square, Westminster, Whitechapel, and St. Olave-Southwalk districts deaths in public institutions exceeded 20%; in Hampstead they were only 6% and in Lewisham 3%. On poverty, fertility, and infant mortality in London, see Woods and Woodward, Urban Disease, 25; Woods, "Social Class Variations in the Decline of Marital Fertility in Late Nineteenth-Century London," Geografiska Annaler B, LXVI (1984), 29–38.

Fig. 1 The l_x Functions of Two Forms of Model Life Table Systems, Males.

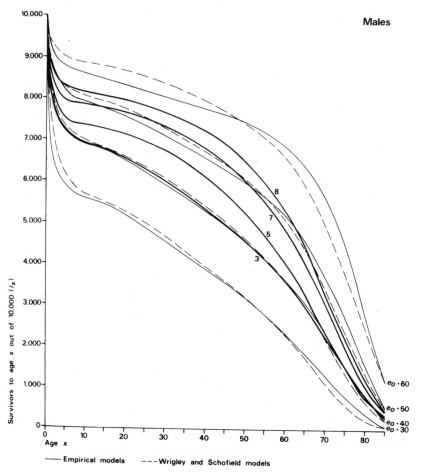

models relate well to each other when e_0 is 30 to 50. But as e_0 approaches 60, divergence becomes more accentuated. Comparison with ELTs 3, 5, 7, and 8 also shows that the models are likely to perform least well when e_0 is in the 50s, but that between 30 and 50 the models will prove to be reasonably reliable. We would expect our empirical model to be least reliable at the extremes of observation since its estimation relies solely on data for 1861, but the models based on the Wrigley and Schofield method should remain reliable so long as the North system fits closely to the English experience. In general, estimated model English life tables, but particularly the system based on Wrigley and Schofield's method, appear to work well over the e_0 range 30–60, and especially 30–50.

Our purpose in estimating these English model life tables is twofold. First, we are concerned to emphasize the importance of changes in age-specific mortality in the late nineteenth century. Figure 1 helps to illustrate the important point that certain age groups made more substantial contributions to the rise in life expectations than others and thus that our understanding of mortality decline must focus on those particular ages. The movement of e_0 from 40 to 50 is related especially to the fall in mortality among children and young adults, but not among infants, adults, and the elderly. Once e_0 exceeds 50, further substantial improvements are only possible with a fall in infant mortality. In England and Wales, the seven-year increase in e_0 between 1851 and 1901 is closely linked with particular changes in the age structure of mortality between 1 and 24, whereas the five-year rise in e_0 between 1901 and 1911 is associated with additional changes in mortality among those under one year of age. This point is demonstrated most effectively if one scans across the rows for age groups 1–4 to 10–14 in Table 2.[15]

Second, model life table systems offer a means of checking demographic data for internal inconsistencies and of enabling calculations to be made on estimates of local mortality and fertility in circumstances where vital statistics or census data are incomplete.[16]

15 For a detailed examination of the fortunes of each age group in Victorian England, see F. Barry Smith, *The People's Health, 1830–1910* (London, 1979). Preston and van de Walle, "Urban French Mortality," 280, also emphasize the cohort-specific nature of the mortality decline in urban France, as does Michael R. Haines, "Mortality in Nineteenth-Century America: Estimates from New York and Pennsylvania," *Demography,* XIV (1977), 311–332, for childhood mortality in New York, 1850–1865 to 1900–1902. The point is also illustrated in Woods and Woodward, *Urban Disease,* 39.

16 See Woods and Christopher W. Smith, "The Decline of Marital Fertility in the Late Nineteenth Century: The Case of England and Wales," *Population Studies,* XXXVII (1983), 216–224, on the estimation of social-class specific fertility measures which are dependent upon availability of reliable model life tables. Hinde and Woods, "Variations in Historical Natural Fertility Patterns and the Measurement of Fertility Control," *Journal of Biosocial Science,* XVI (1984), 309–321, gives further examples. On the use of model life tables with U.S. data, see Haines, "The Use of Model Life Tables to Estimate Mortality for the United States in the Late Nineteenth Century," *Demography,* XVI (1979), 289–312.

REGIONAL VARIATIONS   Whereas life tables provide a most convenient means of representing the structure of age-specific mortality, life expectation at birth (e_0) and infant mortality ($_1q_0$) give simple summary indices of the levels of mortality which avoid the distortion inherent in local variations in the age structure of the population at risk of dying. Life expectation and infant mortality are shown in Figures 2 and 3 respectively for both sexes combined in 1861. Both reveal a considerable range in the mortality experience. When e_0 for England and Wales as a whole was in the low 40s, many rural districts in the south and especially the southwest of England and Wales had e_0s above 50 in the early 1860s; in other districts, particularly in the urban industrial areas of Lancashire, Yorkshire, and the northeast, e_0 was less than 35. Similarly, $_1q_0$ was about 0.130 nationally, but was below 0.100 in

Fig. 2   Life Expectation at Birth (e_0), England and Wales, 1861 (shown by registration districts with both sexes combined).

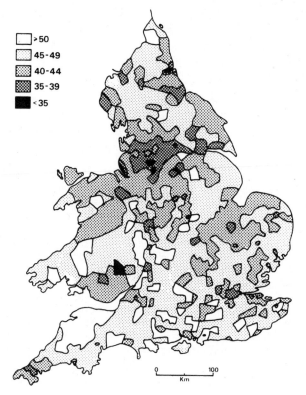

> 50
45-49
40-44
35-39
< 35

0   100
Km

Fig. 3 Infant Mortality ($_1q_0$), England and Wales, 1861 (shown by registration districts with both sexes combined).

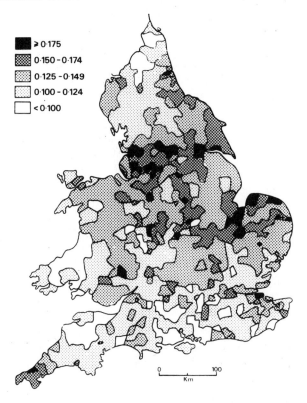

the south, southwest, and extreme north and in excess of 0.175 in most urban industrial centers, along the east coast, and in the Fenlands. Table 3 illustrates the extent of the variability in mortality by expressing the percentage of the total national population living in districts with varying life expectations and infant mortalities in 1861. Whereas about 90 percent of the population lived in districts with e_0s above 35 but less than 50, 80 percent experienced infant mortality at levels between 0.100 and 0.175. Substantial percentage reductions in $_1q_0$ (and thus e_0) could be achieved merely by relocation between districts.[17]

Table 3 also serves to illustrate the inherent problems associated with treating England and Wales as a single unit, for the

17 Woods, "Effects of Population Redistribution."

Table 3 Percentage of Population in England and Wales in 1861 Living in Registration Districts with Various Levels of Life Expectation at Birth (e_0) and Infant Mortality ($_1q_0$).

e_0	PERCENTAGE	$_1q_0$	PERCENTAGE
50 and over	4.14 (4.81)	0.175 and over	14.66 (17.04)
45–49	25.41 (29.53)	0.150–0.174	38.01 (27.96)
40–44	28.04 (32.59)	0.125–0.149	25.20 (29.29)
35–39	36.62 (26.34)	0.100–0.124	18.37 (21.35)
Less than 35	5.80 (6.74)	Less than 0.100	3.75 (4.36)

NOTE: The percentages in brackets exclude the influence of London.

origins of the secular decline of mortality lie not only in the reduction of childhood mortality, but also in the convergence of mortality levels between urban and rural areas by 1911. McKeown's interpretation, as we have already remarked, does not emphasize this important point. In consequence, it probably reduces the significance that should be attached to changes in the specifically urban environment. We return to this issue, but first we consider in detail the patterns shown in Figures 2 and 3.[18]

It might be thought that those districts with extremely low or high mortality would have had different cause-specific patterns; but closer analysis reveals not only that differences were less obvious than one would assume, but also that the analysis itself is fraught with problems. Table 4 shows frequency distributions of causes of death for six Devon registration districts compared with six drawn from south Lancashire for 1861 to 1870. The Devon districts all had e_0s in excess of 50 in the 1860s. Those in south Lancashire had particularly high mortality, with e_0 less than 35 in several cases. Scarlet fever, diarrhea and dysentery, and lung diseases seem to have been more important in the urban environment, whereas heart disease was more prominent in Devon. The death of women during childbirth was more significant in Lan-

18 By 1911 e_0 was 53 in England and Wales, but 52 in London, 51 in large towns, 53 in small towns, and 55 in rural areas. In 1861 e_0 had been, respectively, 41, 37, 35, 40, and 45. See Woods, "The Spatial Dynamics of the Demographic Transition in the West," in *idem* and Philip Ress (eds.), *Population Structures and Models* (London, 1986), 21–44, for the derivation of these estimates. This convergence effect is also noticeable in France. See Preston and van de Walle, "Urban French Mortality," 278.

cashire. Yet the most significant category is "other causes," which accounts for 15 percent of all deaths in the Lancashire districts and 24 percent in Devon. Table 4 also repeats the exercise for infant deaths with males and females combined; 44 percent of infant deaths fall into the "other causes" category in Devon and 30 percent in Lancashire. In Devon 16 percent of all deaths occurred among infants with the corresponding number being 25 percent in Lancashire. In the former 29 percent of "other causes" deaths were among infants; the number was 48 percent in the latter. Further, in terms of infant mortality, the most notable difference between Devon and Lancashire lay in the prominence of the diarrhea and dysentery category in Lancashire.[19]

Table 4 Frequency Distributions of Causes of Death for Six Registration Districts in Devon and Lancashire, 1861–1870 (Total Deaths and Infant Deaths).

	MALES		FEMALES		INFANT DEATHS	
CAUSES OF DEATH	DEVON	LANCASHIRE	DEVON	LANCASHIRE	DEVON	LANCASHIRE
1. Smallpox	0.13	0.56	0.06	0.49	0.03	0.47
2. Measles	1.45	2.32	1.41	2.41	1.73	1.99
3. Scarlet fever	2.38	5.22	1.97	5.21	0.72	1.23
4. Diphtheria	0.77	0.51	0.86	0.56	0.36	0.30
5. Whooping cough	1.54	2.37	2.35	3.17	4.26	4.06
6. Typhus	3.34	4.33	3.69	4.40	0.52	0.46
7. Diarrhea and dysentery	1.38	6.41	1.17	6.54	2.93	15.11
8. Cholera	0.43	0.28	0.36	0.21	0.39	0.14
9. Other zymotic diseases	2.46	2.45	2.18	2.31	1.53	1.50
10. Cancer	1.69	0.62	3.13	1.69	0.00	0.01
11. Scrofula and tabes	1.62	1.75	1.33	1.53	2.60	2.54
12. Phthisis	9.78	10.11	12.26	11.26	1.20	0.59
13. Hydrocephalus	1.60	1.86	1.23	1.45	2.86	2.40
Diseases of:						
14. Brain	11.91	12.91	10.02	11.55	15.72	20.82
15. Heart and dropsy	7.65	4.23	10.31	5.34	0.81	0.29
16. Lungs	16.01	18.29	13.34	17.15	16.80	15.63
17. Stomach and liver	4.73	3.71	4.93	4.08	2.51	1.89
18. Kidneys	1.98	1.37	0.84	0.77	0.13	0.04
19. Generative organs	0.02	0.02	0.48	0.34	0.00	0.01
20. Joints	0.25	0.42	0.35	0.34	0.00	0.04
21. Skin	0.31	0.21	0.22	0.20	0.55	0.27
22. Childbirth	—	—	1.39	2.03	—	—
23. Suicide	0.46	0.41	0.09	0.15	—	—
24. Other violent deaths	4.14	4.08	1.53	1.55	0.72	0.61
25. Other causes	24.30	15.56	24.50	15.26	43.63	29.60

19 The 6 Devon districts were Okehampton, Crediton, South Molton, Torrington,

Several points emerge from Table 4 and the percentages cited above, but three need to be stressed. First, the comparison of cause-specific mortality patterns between areas experiencing extreme mortality conditions is thwarted by the existence of the large residual category "other causes." Second, infant mortality is relatively more important in the urban area and part of the reason for the excess of infant deaths must be attributed to water- and food-borne diseases. Third, there are sufficient similarities between the cause of death patterns of these contrasting populations to imply differences in the levels of morbidity and even the case fatality rates in circumstances where e_0 differs by at least fifteen years.[20]

A second approach to examining the patterns shown in Figures 2 and 3 involves an analysis of the relationship between life expectancy at birth and infant mortality. One would expect to find a particularly strong association between e_0 and $_1q_0$ since infant deaths, as we have seen, represented from 15 to 25 percent of all deaths. It should therefore be possible to predict $_1q_0$ from e_0. Figure 4 shows the relationship among the 590 districts in 1861. Clearly the inverse relationship is significant and strong, but, when one proceeds a stage further and considers the regression residuals, a striking pattern of regional clustering emerges. Infant mortality is higher than would be predicted given a knowledge of life expectancy at birth in Norfolk, Lincolnshire, the East Midlands, and the East Riding of Yorkshire, but is lower in the west of Wales and the extreme northeast and north of England (Figure 5). In the remainder of England and Wales $_1q_0$ is either effectively predicted by e_0 or the residuals are scattered in an isolated and random fashion. This pattern also gives encouragement to our construction of national model life table systems

Bideford, and Holsworthy (average e_0 and $_1q_0$ in 1861, 52.04 and 0.088). The 6 Lancashire districts were Salford, Manchester, Oldham, Bury, Rochdale, and Haslington (average e_0 and $_1q_0$ in 1861, 35.13 and 0.180).

20 Little seems to be known about variations in case fatality rates, but, in two populations subject to similar disease patterns, the one living in an urban environment may experience the higher case fatality rate and thus higher mortality. Although certain diseases were more prevalent in urban areas (the effect of population density on measles, for instance), the effect of high case fatality rates would have exacerbated the situation. In those populations with the very worst mortality levels both morbidity and case fatality rates may have been higher.

Fig. 4 The Relationship between Infant Mortality ($_1q_0$) and Life Expectation at Birth (e_0), England and Wales, 1861 (based on registration district data with both sexes combined).

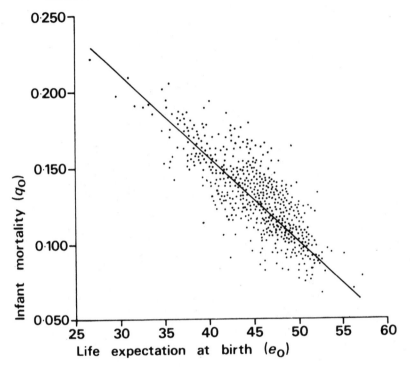

since, for most of the populous districts, $_1q_0$ and e_0 were closely related.[21]

It is not at all obvious why there should have been such differences between the east and the west, but an analysis of causes of death may help to resolve the matter. Table 5 is compatible with Table 4. It employs the same method on data drawn from six registration districts round the Wash, on the east coast of England, and from six districts along Cardigan Bay in Wales. Those in the east all had high positive residuals in Figure 5 and those in the west high negative ones. In the east 23 percent of all

21 In 590 districts the relationship between $_1q_0$ (Y) and e_0 (X) in 1861 was $Y = 0.3528 - 0.0049X$ ($r^2 = 64.90\%$, significant at 99.99%).

Fig. 5 Residuals from the Regression of $_1q_0$ on e_0 (see Fig. 4).

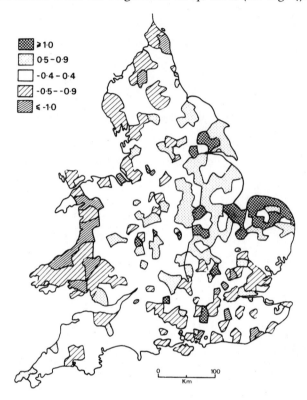

deaths occurred among infants, with 13 percent being the number in the west; in the former 47 percent of "other causes" deaths were among infants and in the latter the number was 18 percent. Apart from the importance of this "other causes" category, there do appear to be certain differences between the cause of death patterns which led to the west experiencing infant mortality levels as low as Devon and the east as high as parts of Lancashire, although both east and west have approximately similar e_0s. As for Lancashire, the percentage distribution of causes of death for infants in the east emphasizes diarrhea and dysentery, and diseases of the brain and lungs. Mortality among adults in the west appears to differ from that in Devon as a result of the greater importance of phthisis (pulmonary tuberculosis), among other causes. To oversimplify, e_0 in the east fell below the level one would expect of a rural area because water and food-borne diseases increased

Table 5 Frequency Distributions of Causes of Death for Six Registration Districts in the East of England and West of Wales, 1861–1870 (Total Deaths and Infant Deaths)

CAUSES OF DEATH	MALES		FEMALES		INFANT DEATHS	
	EAST	WEST	EAST	WEST	EAST	WEST
1. Smallpox	0.46	0.30	0.32	0.31	0.41	0.36
2. Measles	1.41	0.57	1.29	0.43	1.02	0.43
3. Scarlet fever	2.78	2.41	2.91	2.59	0.77	1.58
4. Diphtheria	2.10	1.79	2.34	2.19	0.41	0.76
5. Whooping cough	1.95	1.17	2.49	1.97	4.66	4.32
6. Typhus	3.44	3.60	3.74	3.40	0.45	0.50
7. Diarrhea and dysentery	3.01	0.53	2.91	0.42	5.68	0.65
8. Cholera	0.15	0.16	0.17	0.17	0.17	0.04
9. Other zymotic diseases	2.29	2.60	2.40	2.32	1.36	1.62
10. Cancer	1.38	1.47	2.79	1.78	0.00	0.00
11. Scrofula and tabes	1.45	1.32	1.23	0.93	1.72	0.61
12. Phthisis	8.90	18.16	11.23	17.36	0.67	0.72
13. Hydrocephalus	1.11	0.49	0.88	0.35	1.28	0.40
Diseases of:						
14. Brain	10.93	11.89	9.91	10.79	13.82	36.26
15. Heart and dropsy	5.90	4.46	6.79	6.07	1.16	0.00
16. Lungs	12.48	8.24	10.68	6.46	10.73	4.25
17. Stomach and liver	3.76	3.31	3.96	2.61	1.25	0.94
18. Kidneys	2.09	1.12	0.81	0.29	0.08	0.00
19. Generative organs	0.02	0.00	0.63	0.13	0.00	0.00
20. Joints	0.33	0.06	0.19	0.01	0.05	0.00
21. Skin	0.62	0.18	0.30	0.07	0.31	0.25
22. Childbirth	—	—	1.48	1.70	—	—
23. Suicide	0.45	0.13	0.16	0.05	—	—
24. Other violent deaths	4.21	3.86	1.53	0.81	0.80	0.18
25. Other causes	28.45	32.18	28.77	36.79	53.20	46.13

infant mortality to an extent comparable with many urban districts; in the west tuberculosis among adults similarly depressed e_0 where conditions were otherwise favorable to very low infant mortality.[22]

Beyond these observations, we are left to speculate as to the underlying causes of the disease patterns that created differences in the balance between infant and adult mortality in the east and the west.[23]

22 The 6 districts in the east were Wisbech, Walsingham, Docking, Freebridge Lynn, Spalding, and Holbeach (average e_0 and $_1q_0$ in 1861, 43.47 and 0.173). The 6 districts in the west were Cardigan, Newcastle-in-Emlyn, Aberayron, Aberystwyth, Machynlleth, and Dolghelly (average e_0 and $_1q_0$ in 1861, 45.28 and 0.097).

23 Unlike our earlier speculations regarding variations in case fatality rates, we now

ENVIRONMENTAL CONDITIONS   One of the most abiding impressions to be gained from conditions in nineteenth-century Britain both from Victorians and subsequent observers relates to the poor life chances experienced in urban areas, and especially in large cities, compared with that in small towns and rural areas. Probably the most simple method of examining this particular form of environmental influence is to relate life expectancy and infant mortality to population density. This examination may be performed relatively easily as Figures 6 and 7 show. The associations are significant in both cases, although there is considerable vari-

Fig. 6   The Relationship between Life Expectation at Birth (e_0) and Log. Population Density in Persons per Square Kilometer, England and Wales, 1861 (based on registration district data with both sexes combined).

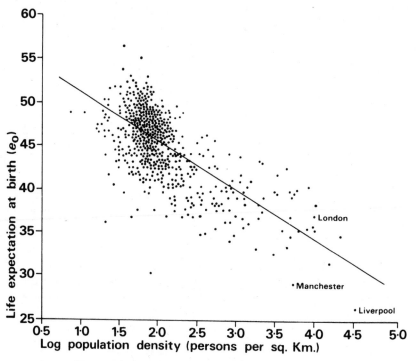

appear to be dealing with an instance in which the pattern of infectious diseases differed between rural environments.

Fig. 7   The Relationship between Infant Mortality ($_1q_0$) and Log. Population Density in Persons per Square Kilometer, England and Wales, 1861 (based on registration district data with both sexes combined).

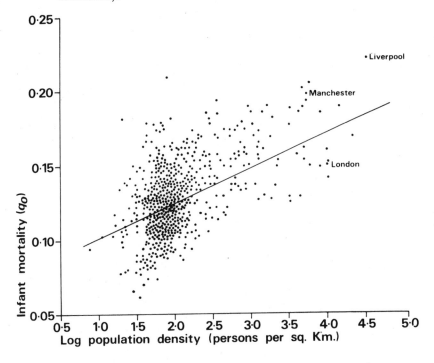

ation about the regression line. In the low population density rural areas e_0 does tend to be higher than in the high density urban areas, but there are clearly also rural areas in which e_0 is lower than one would expect from a knowledge of their population densities. Our comparison of east and west in Table 5 illustrates some of the possible reasons for finding relatively poorer life chances in certain low density areas. There is also variation among the urban districts most, but not all, of which have an e_0 less than 41. Similar comments could be made regarding the association between $_1q_0$ and population density. There is a statistically significant association, but the degree of variation suggests that simple differences between urban and rural environments are either not entirely captured when measured via population density, or that environmental conditions are rather more complex in their influence on mortality. Neither of these findings is surprising, but they do caution us against overhasty and oversimplified explanations.[24]

It has been argued by McKeown that medical science and the medical profession in general had a relatively limited influence on mortality in the nineteenth century. This being so, one would not expect a population well served by doctors to be any more healthy or to have any better life expectation than one with only limited access to members of the medical profession. Figure 6 shows that the well-supplied areas comprise parts of London and surrounding districts together with small southern towns, resorts, and spas. In London in 1861 there were 805 persons per doctor, but 304 in the St. George-Hanover Square district and 4,379 in Bethnal Green. Doctors were thinly distributed, especially in Lancashire and south Staffordshire, and in the most remote rural areas, particularly in Wales and in the rural hinterlands of well-supplied market towns.[25]

There appears to be no statistically significant link between mortality (either e_0 or $_1q_0$) and the population:doctor ratio shown in Figure 8. But it is difficult to believe that morbidity and mortality could not have been ameliorated in, for example, the Lancashire cotton towns, if there had been more doctors to inform employers and local councils of the dangers to public and personal health, or in the East End of London, where few doctors worked and even fewer lived.[26]

24 In 590 districts the relationship between e_0 (Y) and population density in persons per square kilometer (X) was $Y = 56.4460 - 5.5433 \log X$ ($r^2 = 46.59\%$, significant at 99.99%) and between $_1q_0$ (Y) and X it was $Y = 0.0762 + 0.0272 \log X$ ($r^2 = 30.44\%$, significant at 99.99%) in 1861. See Farr, *Vital Statistics* (London, 1885), 172–176, for analogous calculations for 1841–1850 and 1851–1860 using death rates. See also, Friedlander et al., "Socio-Economic Characteristics."

25 The figures for population: doctor ratios are taken from the 1861 population census and relate to the total population and the number of physicians, surgeons, and apothecaries in that year. See Woodward, "Medicine and the City," 69–70; M. Jeanne Peterson, *The Medical Profession in Mid-Victorian London* (Berkeley, 1978); Ivan Waddington, *The Medical Profession in the Industrial Revolution* (Dublin, 1984). Some 45% of the 768 physicians lived in just 3 districts (Kensington, St. George-Hanover Square, and Marylebone). In most of the East End districts there were 1,500 persons per doctor, but most of the doctors were surgeons or apothecaries.

26 The relationships of e_0 and $_1q_0$ to persons per doctor yield r^2s of 0.55% and 1.15%, respectively. Neither are significant. Marilyn E. Pooley and Colin G. Pooley, "Health, Society and Environment in Victorian Manchester," in Woods and Woodward, *Urban Disease*, 148–175, deals with the case of Manchester in some detail. See also, Cheney,

Fig. 8 The Ratio of Population to "Doctors," England and Wales, 1861

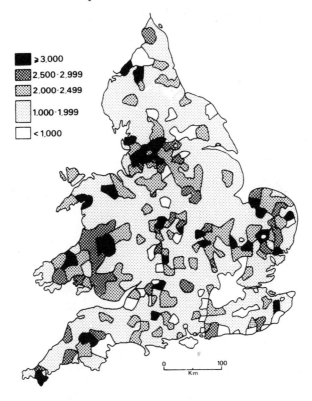

Our analysis of Victorian mortality has stressed shortcomings in McKeown's interpretation of mortality decline by presenting a more detailed demographic account of the patterns. We have focused particularly on those aspects that are critical for a general understanding of the mortality transition. First, we have emphasized the age-specific aspects of mortality decline by constructing sets of English life tables based, respectively, on modifications to the North family and on the experience of English and Welsh registration districts in 1861. These models (Table 2 and Figure 1) and the official English Life Tables (Table 1) demonstrate the

"Seasonal Aspects of Infant and Childhood Mortality: Philadelphia, 1865–1920," *Journal of Interdisciplinary History*, XIV (1984), 561–585, on the indirect influence of members of the medical profession via the Philadelphia Board of Health and the application of preventive medicine which eventually affected childhood and infant mortality. Also, Condran and Cheney, "Mortality Trends in Philadelphia," 119.

cohort-specific nature of mortality reduction, with children, young adults, adults, infants, and the elderly experiencing improved life chances in a sequential fashion. Second, we have stressed the existence of variations between mortality conditions in different environments, especially the urban and the rural, and have indicated the potential significance of differences in case-fatality rates. The cross-sectional analyses of mortality conditions in 1861 emphasize these points. England and Wales must not be treated as an undifferentiated whole since to do so will only mislead explanations of demographic change. Urban conditions, especially in the large towns, must improve before national levels of life expectation can be raised. Cause of death statistics not only highlight inherent problems of interpretation, but also suggest certain specific patterns of infectious diseases operating in particular rural environments.

What are the implications of our work for the McKeown interpretation? McKeown's list of the four possible ways in which mortality could have declined has not been affected. Indeed it seems likely that we should accept that each played a role. But the importance that McKeown attached to each item does require review.[27]

It is still difficult to evaluate the role of the medical profession in the nineteenth century and in this regard our evidence has also proved negative. Medical men were unevenly distributed in relation to the general population and in consequence their influence was severely limited in certain areas, especially in the large provincial centers. McKeown's evidence regarding scarlet fever need not be disputed since it corresponds well with the observed decline in childhood mortality.[28]

McKeown places particular emphasis on improvements in nutrition during the nineteenth and twentieth centuries as the major cause of population growth. He argues that in England and Wales these nutritional improvements are associated with the reduction in the impact of tuberculosis. Our analysis has shown the overwhelming significance of urban-rural differences and thus the necessity for urban life chances to improve before the national level of mortality can change radically. Urban living conditions

27 Condran and Cheney, "Mortality Trends in Philadelphia," 119 for instance.
28 McKeown, *Modern Rise of Population*, 99; *idem* and Record, "Reasons for the Decline of Mortality," 117.

improved in the late nineteenth century and began to catch up with rural conditions. From 1900, with the fall in infant mortality, all areas experienced accelerated increase in life expectation. If improvements in nutrition are to be credited with having a major influence on these changes, it must be shown that there were substantial differences between urban and rural diets and that the nutritional level of the urban population accelerated particularly rapidly from the mid-nineteenth century. There is very little evidence to support this argument. It is most likely that the urban environment itself changed as a result of improvements in public health and especially in the quality of water supply. This single factor of improvements in public health was of the greatest importance in narrowing the distribution of mortality experiences between environments and thus of raising the national level of life expectation. Our stress on environmental variations leads us to reemphasize that part of McKeown's original list dealing with the sanitary revolution. Under this broad heading we would include related aspects that stem from advances in the effectiveness of local administration, such as the control of housing quality.[29]

We conclude that McKeown overstates the case for mortality decline caused by improvements in nutrition. Life expectation increased in England and Wales between 1850 and 1900 because conditions in the large cities were ameliorated mainly because of improvements in water supply and sanitation in conjunction with the increased efficiency of local administration. After 1900 the decline in mortality was accelerated by the dramatic fall in infant mortality, which again occurred most rapidly in the large urban centers. The worst effects of nineteenth-century urbanization were counteracted in the last decades of the Victorian era and this improvement alone was sufficient to begin the secular decline in national mortality rates.

Our final comments relate to two further points. First, the method adopted by McKeown (when the impossible has been

29 On tuberculosis, see Gillian Cronjé, "Tuberculosis and Mortality Decline in England and Wales, 1851–1910," in Woods and Woodward, *Urban Disease*, 79–101. Work on American and French mortality differentials seems to support this view. See, for example, Preston and van de Walle, "Urban French Mortality," 290–291; Condran and Cheney, "Mortality Trends in Philadelphia," 120; Robert Higgs and David Booth, "Mortality Differentials within Large American Cities in 1890," *Human Ecology*, VII (1979), 353–370; Higgs, "Cycles and Trends of Mortality in Eighteen Large American Cities, 1871–1900," *Explorations in Economic History*, XVI (1979), 381–408.

eliminated, whatever remains, however, improbable, must be the truth) should be avoided in historical analysis: it rejects the need for strong positive evidence in order for the improbable to become acceptable. It is particularly unfortunate that this logic led Mc-Keown to stress the importance of nutrition so forcefully. More recent research has demonstrated that the relationships between nutrition, morbidity, mortality, and fertility are very complicated. Extremely poor diets will exacerbate morbidity, increase mortality, and depress fertility; but improvements only in moderately poor nutrition will not on their own lead to dramatic changes in mortality. Second, the demographic analysis presented here stresses both the diversity of mortality patterns between environments (the composition effect) and changing age-related conditions (the cohort effect). It highlights new clues which should change our view of what was possible in the nineteenth century, especially in large towns and cities.[30]

30 See the contributions to *Hunger and History: The Impact of Changing Food Production and Consumption Patterns on Society*, a special issue of the *Journal of Interdisciplinary History*, XIV (1983), 199–534, for a comprehensive survey of the debates and evidence relating to the effects of variations in nutrition on demographic and social history.

James C. Riley

Height, Nutrition, and Mortality Risk Reconsidered

ered Recent excursions in anthropometric history have sought to reconstruct the nutritional status of prior populations by measuring height at ages when growth has been, or is nearly, completed. The idea that height may serve as a proxy for nutritional status is based on inferences from anthropometric research showing that human stature and bulk—height and weight—reflect prior nutritional experience in the sense that they provide a record of how much individuals have eaten, net of other demands on food energy. Of the two measures, height is more useful as an indicator of nutritional status during growth, and weight standardized for height is a more valuable indicator of recent nutritional status after the completion of growth. Since few historical sources detail both heights and weights of past populations, anthropometric research has focused on measurements of stature. The argument has regularly been made that children and adults who are short, compared to members of the same genetic group at other points in time, have had a poorer nutritional status, regardless of their weight or girth.

Population-level measurements of height sometimes show dramatic changes over time. In most European societies, people have gotten taller. Their gains in stature have often roughly coincided with gains in income, material comfort, life expectancy, and other measures of well-being. But the evidence about heights, interpreted in this way, has not related a story of uniform change. In the United States, the average height of young adults dimin-

James C. Riley is Professor of History, Indiana University. He is the author of *Sickness, Recovery, and Death: A History of Ill Health* (Iowa City, 1989); *The Eighteenth-Century Campaign to Avoid Disease* (New York, 1987).

The author thanks Michael Richardson and his colleagues in Special Collections, University Library, University of Bristol for bringing the Beddoe collection to my attention and helping me make use of it. Greg Farrar, Seneka Johnson, Jeff Leising, Scott Locke, David Mutchnik, and Dayatra Smith entered and proofed data. George Alter, Sheila Cooper, Timothy Cuff, Robert Fogel, John Komlos, Elyce Rotella, George Stolnitz, and Martha Zuppan made helpful comments on earlier drafts. Data entry was funded by Public Health Service Grant S07 RR 7031N.

ished during the nineteenth century, a finding that led Fogel to suggest that there was a broad deterioration in the well-being of Americans during the middle decades of the century, a period of rapid economic growth. In the Austrian Empire and throughout Western Europe, heights declined among people born from the 1750s to the 1780s, and remained low among those born from the 1780s through the 1830s before increasing once again. By the 1780s, Komlos argues, 30 to 40 percent of Europeans were chronically malnourished, and their circumstances did not improve until after the 1830s, even though it is known, from other sources, that mortality declined sharply during that period. Fogel, too, maintains that poor nutrition was widespread, arguing: "for many European nations prior to the middle of the nineteenth century, the national production of food was at such low levels that the lower classes were bound to have been malnourished"; and that "chronic malnutrition was widespread in Europe during the eighteenth and nineteenth centuries." In Britain, heights of people nearing the end of their growth diminished among birth cohorts from the 1830s until the 1870s, in the middle stages of Britain's industrial modernization. From the decline in heights during this time, Floud, Wachter, and Gregory conclude that the middle rather than the early years of industrialization eroded nutritional status.[1]

These findings challenge conclusions about economic performance in Europe and the United States which were reached using more conventional sources, by suggesting that nutritional status,

---

1 Robert W. Fogel, "Nutrition and the Decline of Mortality since 1700: Some Preliminary Findings," in Stanley L. Engerman and Robert E. Gallman (eds.), *Long-Term Factors in American Economic Growth* (Chicago, 1986), 439–555; Robert W. Fogel, "The Conquest of High Mortality and Hunger in Europe and America: Timing and Mechanisms," in Patrice Higonnet, David S. Landes, and Henry Rosovsky (eds.), *Favorites of Fortune: Technology, Growth, and Economic Development since the Industrial Revolution* (Cambridge, Mass., 1991), 40, 47; John Komlos, *Nutrition and Economic Development in the Eighteenth-Century Habsburg Monarchy: An Anthropometric Study* (Princeton, 1989), 73; Roderick Floud, Kenneth Wachter, and Annabel Gregory, *Height, Health and History: Nutritional Status in the United Kingdom, 1750–1980* (Cambridge, 1990), 136–137, 151, 259, 264, 270. However, using evidence about convicts transported to Australia, Nicholas and Steckel challenge Floud, Wachter, and Gregory's conclusions, arguing that nutrition deteriorated early in the industrial revolution, up to c. 1820. Stephen Nicholas and Richard N. Steckel, "Tall but Poor: Nutrition, Health, and Living Standards in Pre-Famine Ireland," National Bureau of Economic Research Historical Paper 39 (Cambridge, Mass., 1992).

as measured by the stature of young adults, could deteriorate during periods of putative economic expansion. Measurements of stature appear to capture a way to assess shortcomings in the output and distribution of economic, and specifically nutritional, resources. Anthropometric historians have expanded upon this implication by suggesting that the poorer nutritional status can be associated also with survivorship prospects. Poorer nutritional status, as revealed by lower adult height, is taken to signal a higher risk of death. Moreover, in the view of some of these scholars, heights provide a way to make comparisons about health status across countries and time. This article examines a fresh body of manuscript information about the anthropometric status of a large group of British males measured during the 1860s. The evidence is used as an opportunity to review and to challenge some of the assumptions most often made in anthropometric histories.[2]

Anthropometric research is based on the recognition of a triangular relationship among food intake, demands for energy, and growth. Calories consumed by an individual provide the energy needed for metabolic processes, work, recreation, disease resistance, and growth. Since metabolic processes make a prior claim, the other claimants may suffer when caloric intake is insufficient to sustain all of these activities at their maximum levels. Shortfalls in final height, compared to the height potential of a population, are taken to reflect prior nutritional stress, and stress is equated with malnutrition.

According to nutritionists, the proportion of potential height that an individual achieves is determined by net nutrition and by the composition of the individual's diet. Maximum height would be achieved by an individual whose caloric intake regularly equaled or exceeded the demands of metabolism, growth, work, and other claimants, and whose diet included large quantities of protein-rich foods, especially meat and dairy products, which promote growth. Although it is widely recognized that certain foods are rich in protein—for example, some 38.4 percent of the

2 Floud, Wachter, and Gregory, *Height, Health, and History,* xvii–xviii; Fogel, "Biomedical Approaches to the Estimation and Interpretation of Secular Trends in Equity, Morbidity, Mortality, and Labor Productivity in Europe, 1750–1980," unpub. paper (Chicago, 1987), 79.

energy in beef is protein—protein needs amount to only 10–15 percent of the energy supply, and less than 10 percent among adults whose energy intake is high. Thus, it is useful to distinguish the composition of diets that promote growth, which should be rich in protein, from diets that satisfy present-day nutritional recommendations, in which protein needs may be high or low. Many foods other than meat and dairy products also supply generous allowances of protein energy; for example, wheat flour furnishes about 13.2 percent of its energy in protein. Protein needs can be met by diets poor in meat and dairy products, but they can be surpassed, and growth in infancy and childhood promoted, by diets particularly rich in such high quality protein foods.[3]

Diets are often divided into groups of the "good" and the "bad." In anthropometric histories, good diets are those that result in rising heights, or in heights that are stable at a high level. For example, eighteen-year-old entrants to Harvard University from private schools (that is, schools charging tuition, indicating the high socioeconomic status of their pupils) averaged 180.59 cm in the 1930s, and did not gain in height between then and the 1950s, whereas their public school counterparts did gain significantly in height.[4] The implication is that the diet of wealthy Americans in the 1910s and 1920s, when university students of the 1930s were growing up, allowed their height potential to be achieved, whereas diets in other socioeconomic groups did not, for some decades yet, allow them to reach their potential. Bad diets are those that result in low heights, compared to the stature achieved by counterparts in other cohorts, or in declining heights.

Lower heights can be reached along two bad-diet paths. On one, they are achieved because caloric intake fails to match the demands of metabolism, growth, work, and other claimants, especially at moments in the life cycle of particular importance for growth. On the other, they are achieved by a change in dietary composition, and most efficiently by a shift away from protein-rich foods. Shortfalls in height may actually reflect prior dietary composition rather than nutritional stress.

3 Reginald Passmore and Martin A. Eastwood, *Human Nutrition and Dietetics* (Edinburgh, 1986; 8th. ed.), 12, 14–27, 47–50, 211, 518.
4 Harry Bakwin and Sylvia M. McLaughlin, "Increase in Stature—Is the End in Sight?," *Lancet* (5 Dec. 1964), 1195–1196.

In a study of the adult population of Norway during the period 1963–1975, Waaler found that mortality risks decline as height rises, except possibly for the very tall. He summarized those findings in a series of curves, each portraying variations in survival risk by age, with one series dividing people by their heights and another series by a standard measurement combining height and weight. Waaler's curves of the distribution of mortality risk by age and height among men and women show, especially at lower adult ages, that taller Norwegians had a lower mortality risk. Waaler also found low heights to be associated with certain diseases, especially obstructive lung disease, tuberculosis, and some neoplasms.[5]

Anthropometric historians have often cited Waaler's findings as grounds for using evidence about stature to estimate mortality risk and to associate mortality risk with nutritional status. But it is important to notice Waaler's assumptions and cautions. As for assumptions, Waaler's model suggests that nutritional status during childhood, the net effect of which is reflected in the height achieved around age twenty to twenty-four, at the end of growth, influences survival throughout life rather than merely in the growth years. Waaler did not offer estimates of the association between poor nutritional status in childhood, as measured by body size, and survivorship in childhood. It is easy to suggest ways in which poor nutrition during infancy and childhood would lead to elevated rates of mortality among infants and children. But it is more difficult to explain how poor nutrition in infancy or childhood would affect the survival prospects of individuals between twenty and fifty years later. One explanation for the association lies in methodology. Waaler adopted a simple model that, for each age group, considered only two factors, height (or height-for-weight) and survival. The model omits other factors, such as income and socioeconomic status, known to be associated with both height and survival. Bivariate models often yield exaggerated claims about the predictive power of the one explanatory variable they contain. In this case there are good theoretical grounds for supposing that a multivariate model would sharply

5 Hans Th. Waaler, "Height, Weight, and Mortality: The Norwegian Experience," *Acta Medica Scandinavica,* Supp. 679 (1984), 14.

reduce the putative power of height, or height-for-weight, to predict survival.[6]

As for cautions, Waaler concluded that survival prospects *within a population* rise with height. That conclusion is different from the view that, when comparing populations across space or time, taller populations have the advantage in survivorship. Waaler argued that taller individuals lived longer, and diets that promote greater growth reduced mortality.

In the late nineteenth century, most nutritionists, drawing a spurious association between energy needs and protein needs, recommended diets rich in protein energy, such as provided by fish, meat, milk, beans, and peas. In recent decades, however, nutritional advice has shifted toward promoting diets containing strictly limited quantities of meats and dairy products, especially those high in saturated fats and cholesterol, because, among adults, diets rich in those components are associated with cardiovascular disease. According to present-day advice, a "good" diet that promotes maximum growth in childhood becomes a "bad" diet in adulthood by promoting a higher risk of cardiovascular disease. Some nutritionists also argue that children should restrict their intake of saturated fats and cholesterol, which implies that maximum heights should be achieved only through a carefully selected diet rich in protein, but not rich in the two other elements present in meat and dairy products.[7]

The manuscript sources discussed here provide no direct information about nutritional status, but the issue of good nutrition is central to the interpretation of anthropometric evidence. The population under study, British males measured in 1866, can be divided into two groups: Englishmen and Scotsmen. The Englishmen were much shorter than their modern counterparts, which

6 Research in this area has produced inconclusive results. D. J. P. Barker and associates argue that childhood influences, including height and weight, help explain the origins of diseases suffered in adulthood. But J. Elford and associates find the associations weak or ambiguous. See the research review in "Heart Disease: In the Beginning," *Lancet,* 339 (6 June 1992), 1386–1388. Aviva Must, Paul F. Jacques, Gerard E. Dallal, Carl J. Bajema, and William H. Dietz, "Long-term Morbidity and Mortality of Overweight Adolescents: A Follow-up of the Harvard Growth Study of 1922 to 1935," *New England Journal of Medicine,* CCCXXVII (1992), 1350–1355, suggests close associations between obesity in adolescence and later health problems, but does not appear to take other pertinent variables into account.

7 Karl Y. Guggenheim, *Nutrition and Nutritional Disease: The Evolution of Concepts* (Lexington, Mass., 1981), 151–152.

implies that they, like other nineteenth-century populations, did not achieve their potential height. The Scotsmen were slightly taller than their modern counterparts, which implies that they came closer to achieving their potential height in the nineteenth century than have their counterparts in the more recent past. The men in question were measured *and* weighed, which makes it possible to use both height and height-for-weight to gauge nutritional status. The leading question is what the body measurements of these men suggest about their survivorship prospects.[8]

SOURCES AND EVIDENCE   Around 1865 Beddoe, a physician and amateur physical anthropologist, set out to explore the racial characteristics of people living in the British Isles. To judge from the questions that he asked and the evidence that he published, Beddoe believed that distinctive racial groups existed in Britain and that their distinctiveness would show up in height, weight, and the color of hair, eyes, and complexion. The results were inconclusive, although Beddoe and other physical anthropologists continued to believe that they were discovering the physical attributes of race, and introduced additional attributes, such as head size. Beddoe's curiosity about height and weight, which seems to have derived from earlier work by Broca, was not often followed up by later race scientists. Although Beddoe gathered data about height and weight with another purpose in mind, those data serve here as one of the earliest known measurements of stature and bulk in a large group of people.[9]

In search of information about height, weight, and coloring, Beddoe enlisted the assistance of numerous friends, acquaintances, and contacts across Britain, providing them with handwritten forms requesting measurement of groups of men "taken indiscriminately as to size" and, if possible, also a report on eye and hair color, and complexion. In this way, Beddoe gathered a large

8 Some information about weights in historical populations is also supplied by Komlos, "The Height and Weight of West Point Cadets: Dietary Change in Antebellum America," *Journal of Economic History,* XLVII (1987), 905, 911; Timothy Cuff, "The Body Mass Index of West Point Cadets in the Nineteenth Century," unpub. paper (Pittsburgh, 1989).
9 University Library, University of Bristol, Special Collections, John Beddoe Collection DM2, in several cartons of anthropological notes (hereinafter Beddoe collection). Broca extracted heights from conscription lists in an effort to identify racial types and locales. See Francis Schiller, *Paul Broca: Founder of French Anthropology, Explorer of the Brain* (Berkeley, 1979), 139.

body of information that formed the basis for a monograph in which he divided the individuals about whom he had received reports into groups based on place of birth; averaged their heights and weights, converting those to equivalents without clothing or footwear; and where possible discussed coloring of hair, eyes, and complexion. In extended footnotes, Beddoe reported what he believed he had learned about the physical traits of racial groups, discussing such topics as "the Northamptonshire breed." Although he received some information about men of lower and higher ages than the limits he stated, twenty-three and fifty, Beddoe did not publish those data. Since the manuscript reports from and correspondence with his collaborators have been preserved in the archives of the University of Bristol, individual-level information was extracted from the original records, including height, weight, age, occupation, place of residence at measurement, and place of birth. These characteristics form the basis of this investigation.[10]

Beddoe made a large number of decisions about how to collect and interpret information, and many of those decisions influence the evaluation and interpretation given here. Altogether, Beddoe published information about 8,583 men born in England, Ireland, Scotland, and Wales. The body of data to be discussed here, referred to as the Beddoe group, deals with 3,498 men— the entire part of the full set that met the standards of data accuracy and selection that I applied. The largest number of records omitted deal with men listed in reports in which the collaborator gave weights only to the nearest stone (14 lbs. or 6.35 kg) or score (20 lbs. or 9.07 kg). Rounded figures suggest inaccuracy in reporting and measurement. Some collaborators acknowledged this possible inaccuracy by writing Beddoe that they had been unable to obtain precise values. Beddoe gathered information about the weights of clothing and shoes worn by subjects, and the height added by footwear. He distinguished subjects who were measured wearing footwear from those that were not. This information, along with other such distinctions, gave Beddoe a way to adjust

---

10 The phrase "taken indiscriminately as to size" and others like it appeared repeatedly on the forms that Beddoe provided. John Beddoe, *On the Stature and Bulk of Man in the British Isles* (London, 1870), 73, 75. A Paradox3 version of the file is available from the author on request, as is also a more detailed description of the decisions that Beddoe made about collecting and interpreting data.

values for clothed subjects to the unclothed values that he wanted to consider.[11]

Like other records used in anthropometric research, Beddoe's group of 3,498 cannot be called a random sample of the overall population. Nevertheless, it is useful to compare the Beddoe group, especially those aged twenty-five to forty-nine, with the entire population. This age group included 2,801 men out of a total population of that age numbering 3.59 million. In the Beddoe group, 21.0 percent were born in Scotland, a significantly larger proportion than the 11.9 percent of all British males of that age living in Scotland in 1866. Since the Scots were, on average, taller and heavier than their counterparts from Wales and England, this distribution pushes the overall average upward. The results that follow consider average heights and weights adjusted for the proportions of men living in England and Wales compared to Scotland.[12]

Concerning age groups, the distribution is much more similar, as shown by comparing the Beddoe group with averaged proportions from the 1861 and 1871 censuses:

AGE	% BEDDOE GROUP	% OVERALL POPULATION
25–29	28.2	25.0
30–34	22.9	22.3
35–39	19.3	19.4
40–44	16.1	18.1
45–49	13.4	15.2

Although they made no use of the Beddoe manuscripts, Floud, Wachter, and Gregory consulted Beddoe's published study, noting

11 Beddoe, *Stature and Bulk,* 12–113. This total, 8,583, represents my count of the number of unique individuals included in Beddoe's central tables. In presenting those tables, Beddoe sometimes summed up information provided earlier, thereby duplicating it. I have tried to eliminate duplications, but Beddoe's language is not always clear. Statistics concerning lunatics, criminals, and others reported on pg. 113 are excluded from the figure of 8,583, as are men who fell outside Beddoe's age limits.

Heights are available for 3,497 subjects, weights for 3,484, and ages for 3,494. A sample of the excluded reports was analyzed to determine whether, as a group, the reports with rounded figures differ in their overall averages from the reports with more precise figures. Containing 434 individuals, the sample shows only trivial differences in age-standardized height, weight, and body mass index (BMI) from the Beddoe group, considering either the group as a whole or its Scots and English members separately.

12 This comparison and the next are based on data taken from Brian R. Mitchell, *British Historical Statistics* (Cambridge, 1988), 9, 12–13.

both that it discussed a nonrandom sample of the British population and that Beddoe's findings regarding average height "are remarkably close to our own estimates."[13]

The Beddoe group can also be compared to the overall population in socioeconomic status and occupation. Baxter estimated in 1868 that some 19.8 percent of the British population belonged to the middle and upper class, and 80.2 percent to the class of manual laborers. Using that broad division, the Beddoe group was weighted toward the working class, with 88.4 percent in that category. Since heights in the middle and upper class were greater, this distribution tends to reduce the average in the Beddoe group, compared to the whole adult male population.[14]

A more detailed comparison can be made for occupations, a category under which both census takers and Beddoe gathered information. Using Armstrong's division of occupations, one with nine categories, and considering only employed males in England and Wales, the comparison in Table 1 emerges. The Beddoe group contained similar proportions working in all categories. Table 1 also shows the average heights and weights in each occupational group for men age twenty-five to forty-nine. Noteworthy are the smaller size of men working in manufacturing than those in agriculture, the low heights and weights of domestic servants, and the larger size of men in public service and the professions in England and Wales. Members of the elite were significantly taller and heavier. Heights and body mass also varied by occupational category, both for all categories taken as a whole and for some individual categories when compared with the excluded occupation, agriculture.[15]

---

13 Floud, Wachter, and Gregory, *Height, Health and History*, 155. Clements and Pickett also regarded Beddoe's estimates of averages as close to actual circumstances, describing them as superior to the 1883 estimates of the Anthropometric Committee of the British Association for the Advancement of Science. E. M. B. Clements and Kathleen G. Pickett, "Stature and Weight of Men from England and Wales in 1941," *British Journal of Preventive and Social Medicine*, XI (1957), 55.

14 For R. Dudley Baxter's estimates, see Floud, Wachter, and Gregory, *Height, Health and History*, 79. The bias toward the working class may be more marked still, since I tended to err by assigning doubtful cases to the middle class. For example, farm bailiffs and farmers were assigned to the middle class.

15 W. Alan Armstrong modified Charles Booth's division of occupations, see "The Use of Information about Occupation," in E. Anthony Wrigley (ed.), *Nineteenth-Century Society: Essays in the Use of Quantitative Methods for the Study of Social Data* (Cambridge, 1972), 230, 253–281, 296–310. Occupations identified only as laborer could be assigned,

Table 1 Comparisons of Proportions by Occupation

	(ALL MALES)		(MALES 25–49 ONLY)		
	CENSUS PROPORTION	PROPORTION IN THE BEDDOE GROUP	HT. IN CM	WT. IN KG	BMI
Agriculture	22.6	31.7	170.45	67.47	23.2
Mining	6.6	10.6	171.19	67.62	23.1
Building	9.0	6.6	170.77	66.31	22.7
Manufacture	29.8	29.4	169.05	64.03	22.4
Transport	7.0	4.6	171.04	68.10	23.3
Dealing	8.9	6.2	172.12	70.77	23.9
Industrial Service	7.4	2.3	171.99	68.42	23.1
Public Service and Professional	6.0	4.7	173.46	68.59	22.8
Domestic Service	2.7	3.9	170.63	67.29	23.1

SOURCES   John Beddoe Collection, Special Collections, University Library, University of Bristol, Bristol; W. Alan Armstrong, "The Use of Information about Occupation," in E. Anthony Wrigley (ed.), *Nineteenth-Century Society: Essays in the Use of Quantitative Methods for the Study of Social Data* (Cambridge, 1972), 255–281.

Table 2 Height, Body Mass, and Occupational Selection

	BMI		HEIGHT
	NUMBER	COEFFICIENT	COEFFICIENT
Agriculture	872	omitted category	
Industrial Service	60	−.09194	1.53614
Domestic Service	118	−.10589	.18247
Public Service and Professional	122	−.42679	3.00918[a]
Transport	147	.05363	.58820
Dealing	162	.66227[a]	1.66816[a]
Building	176	−.49324[b]	.31702
Mining	360	−.11965	.74216
Manufacturing	708	−.83762[a]	−1.39977[a]
Other	76	.30923	3.52160[a]
Constant		23.17538[a]	170.44994[a]
Sum	2801		

[a]Significant at the .01 level.
[b]Significant at the .05 level.
SOURCES   See Table 1.

Regression results appear in Table 2. Manufacturing, public service and professional, dealing (Booth's term for retail trade), and the category "other," which includes such designations as "gentleman," show both substantial associations and associations that are statistically significant. An occupation in either public service or the category other adds more than 3 cm to height, compared to agricultural workers, whereas an occupation in manufacturing subtracts 1.4 cm. For body mass index (BMI), the largest associations occur for manufacturing and building, both negative, and dealing. These associations suggest the operation of a process of selection for height and weight or, in the case of body mass, perhaps a process of acquiring the weight characteristic of one's peers in an occupation. Birth, presumably, governed part of the selection, especially for men in the professions. But Table 2 suggests further that, in comparison to agriculture, men entered trades in manufacturing to some degree because of their anthropometric measurements.

The data about occupations also made it possible to calculate the average height and weight of the Beddoe group, and to calculate an adjusted average from the proportions of men counted in each occupational category in the censuses (interpolating from the censuses of 1861 and 1871). The Beddoe group produced overall values for men age twenty-five to forty-nine that are slightly smaller than the adjusted average values, 169.87 cm rather than 170.08, and 66.17 kg rather than 66.3. On these grounds, too, the Beddoe group tended slightly to understate height and weight.

The larger number of Scotsmen in the Beddoe group elevated anthropometric averages, whereas the smaller proportion of middle- and upper-class men and the distribution of occupations tended to lower them. Because it is more important to guard against an overstatement of height and weight, some of the comparisons made were adjusted for the disproportionate distribution by residence or place of birth, but no further attempt was made to correct for social class or occupation.

---

in the Booth divisions, either to industrial service, a category that includes accountants and bankers as well as laborers providing services to manufacturers, or to agriculture. Those living in rural communities have been assigned to agriculture, and those in towns to industrial services. Laborers were slighter than bankers and accountants. Table 1 omits 76 men assigned to the category "other" because the information about occupations was insufficient. They averaged 173.97 cm and 71.14 kg.

RESULTS   The records concerning these 3,498 men differ from the sources most commonly discussed in anthropometric history because they report on stature and bulk not toward the end of growth, around age twenty, but across a wider spectrum of age. Only a few men in the Beddoe group were less than twenty-three or more than fifty; Beddoe specified these limits in order to avoid being misled by men still growing or by those of advanced age who had lost height.[16] Figure 1 presents crude data for heights among men age twenty-five to forty-nine, whose average height was 170.61 cm (5 ft. 7.17 in.).

Assuming that all individuals were measured in 1866, Beddoe's subjects age twenty-five to forty-nine in 1866 were born between 1817 and 1841 and grew up in the period 1817–1841 to 1841–1866. According to Floud, Wachter, and Gregory, that period included major differences in nutritional status during growth years and, therefore, in final heights achieved by people who grew up during that time. In the way that they appear in Figure 1, however, Beddoe's findings give no evidence of such differences. They suggest, to the contrary, that across the period little or no variation occurred in nutritional status.[17]

Figure 2 provides crude data for weights. At age twenty-five to forty-nine the weights, like the heights, are nearly regular. Across the life cycle, however, weight increased, rising from an average of 64.8 kg (142.6 lbs.) at age twenty-five to 70.0 kg (154.3 lbs.) at age forty-nine. The men in this survey, like men in twentieth-century populations, tended to gain weight with age.

Figure 2 also shows the body mass, or Quetelet index. The body mass index is a standard measurement of weight by height in a simple formula devised by Quetelet, a Belgian statistician: $BMI = kg/m^2$, where BMI = body mass index, kg equals kilograms, and m^2 equals height in meters squared. Although other means of combining weight and height values have been developed, the Quetelet index is the one that is used most often and the one most appropriate for this study. It is valuable both as an

16   Some of Beddoe's subjects rounded their ages to numbers ending in 0 or 5, presumably to the 0 or 5 nearest their true age. No attempt has been made to allocate men at these ages because significant numbers of men rounded their age only when they were between ages 30 to 50, a time when growth was complete.
17   Floud, Wachter, and Gregory, *Height, Health and History*, 136–137. Some men may have been measured in 1865.

Fig. 1   Average Heights

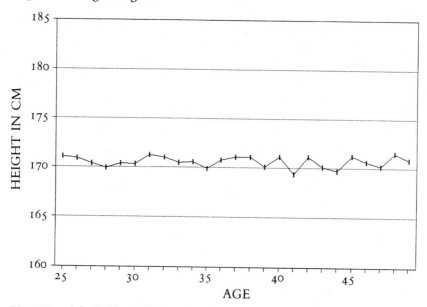

SOURCE   John Beddoe Collection, Special Collections, University Library, University of Bristol, Bristol.

Fig. 2   Average Weight and Body Mass

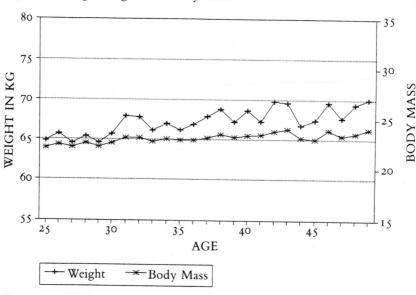

SOURCE   See Figure 1.

unbiased index of the relationship between height and weight, and as an index that has been shown to be statistically associated with survival prospects. As would be expected from the information given in the two previous figures, in which weight increased with age but height did not, Figure 2 shows that body mass increased with age.

The men in the Beddoe group were slight, significantly smaller than their counterparts in the modern population of Britain whose heights and weights were examined from a 1980 survey. Summarizing by age groups, Figure 3 shows the distribution of heights by age among British adult males in 1980, in the Beddoe group of 1866, and in an adjusted version of the Beddoe group that redistributes men from Scotland and England and

Fig. 3 Heights Compared

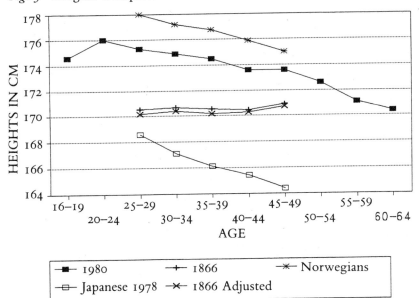

SOURCES   See Figure 1; Ian Knight and Jack Eldridge, *The Heights and Weights of Adults in Great Britain: Report on a Survey Carried Out on Behalf of the Department of Health and Social Security* (London, 1984), 9; Hans Th. Waaler, "Height, Weight, and Mortality: The Norwegian Experience," *Acta Medica Scandinavica*, Supp. 679 (1984), 12; Japan, Statistics Bureau, *Statistical Yearbook 1980*, 551 (averaging values for individual ages).

Wales in accord with proportions that prevailed in 1866. This figure provides three important points. First, the males of 1980 were taller than their counterparts of 1866. Adjusting men resident in England and Wales versus Scotland to make the Beddoe proportions agree with those of the population in 1866, however, has only a trivial effect on the age-specific averages. Second, in the 1980 sample, older men were shorter than their younger counterparts, a feature that shows the marked increase in heights in Britain during the twentieth century. Since the 1930s, each cohort of males has been taller than its parents. But, differences between cohorts are not prominent in the Beddoe group, suggesting that cohort effects were not strong in the period in which those men grew to maturity. Third, at higher ages, heights decline. Beddoe left off measuring height at ages above fifty, presumably because he knew about this feature of aging. The 1980 survey suggests that older males had not approached their potential heights as closely as younger counterparts and that they had also experienced height loss. In each age group, the 1980 population was substantially heavier than its 1866 counterparts. But, in both groups, men gained weight with age at about the same pace.[18]

Figure 4 compares Quetelet index values for the two populations. British males in 1980 not only exhibited higher propor-

[18] Ian Knight and Jack Eldridge, *The Heights and Weights of Adults in Great Britain: Report of a Survey Carried Out on Behalf of the Department of Health and Social Security Covering Adults Aged 16–64* (London, 1984).

W. F. F. Kemsley, "Body Weight at Different Ages and Heights," *Annals of Eugenics,* XVI (1952), 316–334, reported lower average heights and weights than those in the Beddoe group. The period of measurement, during World War II, may help account for the low weights, and it may also be that Kemsley overestimated the average weight of clothing, at 10 pounds, a value not much different from Beddoe's average deduction despite the interim introduction of interior heating in many buildings.

Using birth to allocate men into subgroups of English, Scots, and Welsh, only the English in the Beddoe group exhibited a strong change in height with age. Considering United States adults and Dutch conscripts, Roche found a stable ending age for growth across the period from the 1820s to the 1860s, which also suggests an absence of cohort effects. Alex F. Roche, "Secular Trends in Stature, Weight and Maturation," in *idem* (ed.), *Secular Trends in Human Growth, Maturation, and Development* (Chicago, 1979), 11–12. Regarding height decline at higher ages, W. E. Miall, M. T. Ashcroft, H. G. Lovell, and F. Moore, "A Longitudinal Study of the Decline of Adult Height with Age in Two Welsh Communities," *Human Biology,* XXXIX (1967), 445–454, detected only slight losses in height within the age range 25–55.

Fig. 4 Quetelet Values Compared

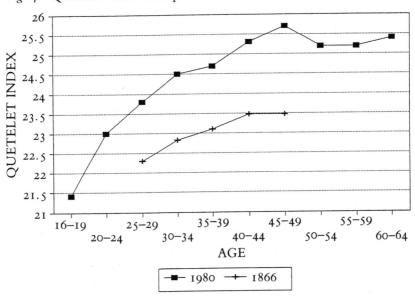

SOURCES   See Figure 1; Knight and Eldridge, *Heights and Weights of Adults in Great Britain,* 33.

tions of weight for height, but also gained body mass at a faster pace as they aged than did their 1866 counterparts. In 1980, older males were more likely to be overweight, which the British study defined as a Quetelet value exceeding 25. All age groups forty to forty-four and above were, on average, overweight in 1980. Yet, no age groups in the Beddoe group achieved that status. Significantly, no age group in either population achieved underweight status, defined as a Quetelet index value of 20 or less.[19]

The British survey of 1980 also makes a number of comparisons based on socioeconomic, residential, cultural, and health status, some of which can be repeated from data gathered by Beddoe. Considering only men age twenty-five to forty-nine, whose growth was complete and who were at ages when they would not appear to have experienced any loss of height, those

19   Knight and Eldridge, *Heights and Weights of Adults in Great Britain,* 33.

born in rural areas (population < 5000) achieved heights and weights greater than men born in towns. For example, their heights averaged 171.04 cm versus 169.54 cm. This difference was more marked for Scotsmen, among whom it was 1.62 cm, compared to 0.91 cm for Englishmen.

By finding the size of places of birth and residence, it is also possible to consider whether body mass varied with population size. Limiting the issue again to men age twenty-five to forty-nine, larger cities tended to produce shorter and slighter men and also to attract shorter and slighter men. The association between the size of birth cities, estimated from 1831 population data, and body mass is small; the same is true of the association with height. Between residence city size, estimated from 1871 census data, and body mass and height, however, the associations are larger. The more populous a residence city was, the more likely were the men in the Beddoe group living in it to be shorter and slighter.[20]

Since at least half of the men in the Beddoe group had moved away from their place of birth, it appears that the men who moved and those who did not alike sorted themselves by stature and weight into patterns of movement. Larger men seem to have moved to smaller cities in preference to larger cities, and slighter men to have moved in preference to larger cities. Taken in combination with the findings reported above about occupational categories, the implication is that shorter and slighter men migrated to urban jobs in manufacturing. In any case, migration

20 In this comparison, no effort has been made to adjust the threshold between rural and urban areas for growth in city size between 1831 and 1871. Population data for 1831 derive from John Gorton, *Population of Great Britain According to the Returns made to Parliament in 1831* (London, 1832); those for 1871 from Great Britain, House of Commons, Sessional Papers (1872) LXVI, pt. 1; (1872) LXVIII. Regressing age, 1831 city size, and 1871 city size on body mass for 1,533 men, and on height for 1,538 men, for whom the size of the place of residence in 1831 and 1871 is known, produces these coefficients:

	BMI	HEIGHT
age	.05015[a]	−.00232463
1831 population	−.000001625	−.000002399
1871 population	−.000006257[a]	−.000008784[a]
constant	21.26027[a]	170.23647[a]

[a]Significant at the .01 level.

Most of the missing information is for 1831 city size, and most of the missing values are probably villages. The results imply unrealistically low values for Londoners, suggesting that city size was not linearly related to BMI or height.

reduced body mass differentials between the town and the countryside. For men age twenty-five to forty-nine as a whole, the body mass differential dropped from 0.71 when birth locales are divided into rural and urban sites to 0.54 when residence locales are divided on the same grounds. Similar declines occurred in height and weight taken separately.

Comparing place of residence in 1980, the tallest Britons lived in southeastern England; Englishmen were slightly taller than Scotsmen and markedly taller than Welshmen. This difference in height was not true in the Beddoe group. On average, the Scots age twenty-five to forty-nine in the Beddoe group were taller than their English counterparts, by 3.71 cm, and taller than their Welsh counterparts, by 2.72 cm. Table 3 summarizes differences in average height, giving for 1866 both raw averages for the Beddoe group and averages adjusted to the division of population between rural and urban areas. Englishmen have gained height, which is especially noticeable in comparing younger adults in the 1980 sample with men of any age in the Beddoe group. It is less noticeable, however, when comparing older men in the 1980 sample with their counterparts in the Beddoe group, which implies that most of the interim height gain has occurred during the lifetimes of men measured in 1980.

Regarding Scotsmen, Beddoe himself provided three separate estimates of the average height of Scotsmen. The full number of

Table 3 Average Heights (Ages 25–49 in the Beddoe Group; All Adult Males in the 1980 Survey)

	1866	1980
Englishmen	169.86 cm	174.06 cm
Englishmen Adjusted (Rural/Urban Division)	169.78	
Scotsmen	173.57	173.0
Scotsmen Adjusted		
Rural/Urban	173.42	
Highland/Other	173.76	

SOURCES   Beddoe Collection; Knight and Eldridge, *Heights and Weights of Adults in Great Britain*, 12; C. M. Law, "Growth of Urban Population in England and Wales, 1801–1911," *Transactions of the Institute of British Geographers*, XLI (1967), 125–143; Great Britain, Parliament, *Sessional Papers*, 1871, LIX, 813.

individuals on whom his agents reported—1,446 men—averaged 173.75 cm; 537 military recruits averaged 170.94 cm (making them significantly shorter than civilians); and in a summary statement Beddoe estimated the average height for adults in Scotland at 5 ft. 7.5 in., or 171.45 cm, but did not explain how he arrived at this figure. It is identical to the average that Beddoe reported for townsmen, whom he regarded as shorter than their rural counterparts. Table 3 reports the average for the Beddoe group, which is slightly lower than the overall average of the 1,446 Scotsmen measured.

Both the Beddoe group and the overall 1,446 Scots include men who belonged to groups whose stature Beddoe recognized differed from the average. Some observers argued that Highlanders were taller than other Scotsmen, but Beddoe reached no firm conclusion on that issue; Beddoe knew that townsmen were shorter. Because the proportions of men from these different backgrounds in the Beddoe group differed from those in the entire population, it is useful to consider these two differences before deciding how to interpret Beddoe's findings. In the Beddoe group, Highlanders age twenty-five to forty-nine were slightly shorter than their counterparts born elsewhere in Scotland (173.03 cm versus 173.92 cm), and men born in rural areas taller (173.83 cm versus 172.21 cm). Table 3 gives actual and adjusted values. One recalculation, for Highlanders, pushes the overall average up slightly, whereas the other reduces it slightly. Both adjustments leave intact two conclusions. According to the evidence Beddoe gathered, which must be counted superior to his unexplained summary, Scotsmen were taller in 1866 than their English counterparts, and Scotsmen were taller in 1866 than their 1980 Scots counterparts.[21]

---

21 Beddoe, *Stature and Bulk*, 12–43, 152, 164 for the estimates; 159 for the evidence about townsmen. For a possible nutritional explanation for the loss of height, see Maisie Steven, *The Good Scots Diet: What Happened To It?* (Aberdeen, 1985), 19–26, 37. The author attributes the loss of height superiority, compared to English counterparts, to changes in diet.

In a private communication, Fogel reported that the average height of Union army recruits born in Scotland was 171.26 cm. Beddoe discounted the accuracy of military data for use in estimating overall population height, arguing that differences in economic incentives among regions distorted them. Beddoe, *Stature and Bulk*, 148.

The 1980 survey does not break height down by age and residence, so it is not possible to standardize the two populations for age. For Scotland, the threshold between rural and urban is a population of 10,000; for England and Wales, it is a population of 5,000.

Across the period from 1866 to 1980, crude death rates declined sharply in both regions. In England and Wales the rate fell from 23.4 deaths per 1,000 people in 1866 to 11.1 in 1975, and in Scotland from 22.2 to 12.1. Insofar as heights in the Beddoe group accurately reflected average heights in 1866, the implication is that adult males in England have gained height as well as longevity, but that their counterparts in Scotland have gained longevity but lost height.[22]

"UNDERHEIGHTEDNESS"   A principal question raised by anthropometric research, at least in the form pursued by Fogel, Komlos, Floud, and others, interprets evidence about stature as an indication of survival prospects. Historical populations with shorter heights, it is suggested, had diminished survival prospects. Whereas modern nutritionists usually identify underweight or overweight as health problems, anthropometric historians have coined a concept that might be termed "underheight." Heights substantially below the level attained by modern counterpart populations having a similar genetic composition are interpreted as evidence of poor nutrition during growth, a deficit that influenced survival throughout life. This hypothesis cannot be tested directly because of the difficulty of comparing historical and modern populations on terms that allow nutrition during growth to be isolated as a determinant of survival in adulthood. In modern populations, it is known that people with low heights or unusually low or high weights have lower survival prospects than their counterparts who are sized toward the mean. Although no historical studies have yet been completed in which adult height has been linked to survivorship in a large population, it is plausible to suppose that people in the past who were short or whose weights deviated from the mean weight also had lower survival prospects. But here is the problem. Are survival prospects reduced by deviation from the modern standards of height and weight, operating with a timeless effect? Or are they reduced by deviation from the averages that obtain at any given time?

Compared to modern height distributions, most historical populations have more people who seem short. In effect, the anthropometric historians have implied that the bias toward shortness that shows up in this comparison is revealing about survival

22 Mitchell, *European Historical Statistics, 1750–1975* (New York, 1981), 123, 134.

prospects. What it reveals is that a larger proportion of the historical population suffered the liability of underheightedness. Mortality was high because so many people were short, itself a consequence of poor nutrition in childhood. But, in modern experience, shorter populations have often achieved survival prospects equivalent to or greater than those of taller populations (see Fig. 3). For example, the Japanese achieved life expectancies equivalent to those in Western nations before gaining the stature of their Western counterparts. Similarly, Mediterranean populations have achieved life expectancies equivalent to their counterparts in Britain without achieving heights that are equivalent. There was no cross-national optimum height in the period 1960–1980, when Swedes and Japanese, each toward opposing ends of the spectrum of adult heights, led the world in life expectancy. On those grounds, it seems unlikely that any optimum height obtains across time even within the same population.

Here, too, it is not possible to link a historical population that was measured for height with survival experience after the measurement. But it is possible to add weight to the consideration, so that body mass index values can be calculated rather than estimated. Because Quetelet index values relate height to weight, they provide a proportional measure that makes it possible to avoid the absolute comparison between historical and modern heights.

HEIGHT, WEIGHT, AND HEALTH   Waaler's investigation of Norwegian experience probes the association between body mass and survival for a population distributed across the age spectrum. His study forms the basis for the comparison that follows. But this comparison, too, operates under an assumption that the body-mass relationships found to obtain in Norway during 1963–1975 obtain for other populations and other periods, something about which Waaler himself expressed misgivings. Among 1.7 million Norwegians age fifteen and above measured for height and weight as part of compulsory national screening for tuberculosis, 176,574 died in the period 1963–1979. Those deaths, distributed by sex, age, Quetelet index, and height by itself, provide the principal results of Waaler's study. Waaler found that, for most age groups, survival prospects increased with height. For example, males age thirty to thirty-four and 160–164 cm in height (about 5 ft. 4 in.)

were nearly twice as likely to die in the study period as those 180–184 cm tall (about 6 ft.). This finding has proved of most interest to anthropometric historians. Waaler also examined survivorship by body mass (that is, height-for-weight). His findings for males are reproduced in Figure 5, which shows that low death rates (given in the vertical column in a log scale) are associated with Quetelet index values toward the mean. At the lower ages in this comparison, twenty to forty-nine, the difference in survival prospects is so great as to produce a series of bathtub-shaped curves, in each case with a broad base. In that base area, differences in survival prospects are evident, but they are comparatively small. The differences are large only at the extremes, where individuals had either markedly low or high weight-for-height. For example, a male age 45–49 with a Quetelet index value of 33 was more than twice as likely to die as a male of the same age with a value of 25.[23]

In order to compare these findings with the Quetelet index values of men in the Beddoe group, consider Figure 6. It shows the range of Quetelet index values that Waaler found to be associated with lower mortality, at the lower bound always a value of 19, and at the higher bound a value rising with age from 27 to 30. Two curves appear within that range. One shows the distribution of average values among males in the Norwegian study population. The other depicts average values calculated for the Beddoe group. On average, the men in Waaler's study fall closer to the middle of the range of desirable Quetelet index values, but the Beddoe group also falls toward the middle of that wide range. Compared to the men in Waaler's study, the Britons that Beddoe and his collaborators measured in 1866 were nourished toward lower average heights and body mass. But, the body mass that they achieved as adults appears to be associated with good survival prospects.

Costa's study of a small group of 377 veterans of the Union Army in the American Civil War promotes the same conclusion. The lowest mortality risk in her study group was associated with a Quetelet index value of 22 which, unlike the Waaler results, was decisively more favorable for survival than slightly higher or

---

23 Waaler, "Height, Weight, and Mortality," 3–4. These proportions are inferred from the figure on p. 13. Waaler does not provide actual values.

Fig. 5 Survivorship by Body Mass

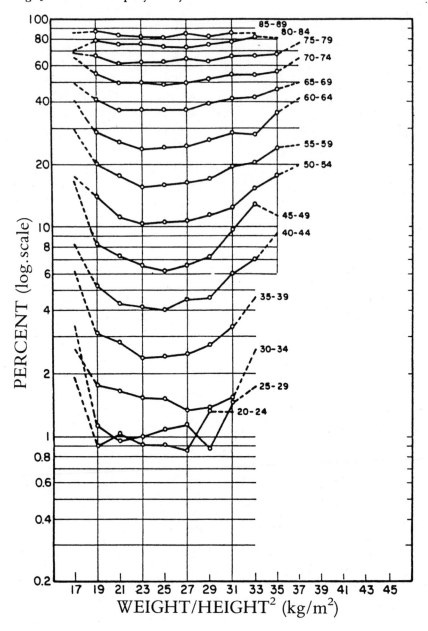

SOURCE   Waaler, "Height, Weight, and Mortality," 20.

Fig. 6 Quetelet Values Compared

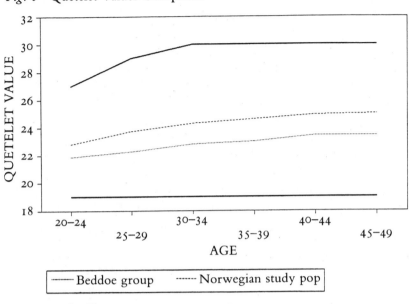

SOURCE   See Figure 3.

lower values. Like the men in the Beddoe group, the Union Army veterans died after 1865. If the comparison across space but not time is valid, Costa's finding suggests that the men in the Beddoe group averaged close to an ideal body mass, in terms of survivorship.[24] The Quetelet values in Table 1 suggest further that heights varied more markedly across occupations than did body mass. Men who, on grounds of underheightedness, have faced abridged survival prospects appear, when body mass is considered, to have had nearly optimal survival prospects.

Waaler's study of modern experience is noteworthy, among other features, for its suggestion that humans possess "a large tolerance for weight variations" within which mortality risks change little. Other sources of advice, given by panels of nutrition scientists, suggest that optimal weights should be lower. These standards have influenced the interpretation of body mass in the

24 Dora L. Costa, "Determinants of Older Age Mortality: Some Preliminary Evidence from the Union Army Records," unpub. paper (Chicago, 1991).

1980 British study. For that study, four groups were singled out: (1) those deemed underweight, with a Quetelet index of less than 20; (2) those deemed to have desirable values, specified at 20–24.99; (3) those deemed overweight, with values of 25–29.99; and (4) those deemed obese, with values of 30 or greater. These standards imply that optimal weights should be considerably lower than those suggested by Waaler's study. Table 4 compares the 1866 group and the 1980 British sample by the proportions of men within each of these boundaries. In both populations, people deemed overweight and obese make up larger proportions than those deemed underweight, although the excess is far greater in the 1980 sample than in the 1866 group. In both cases, excessive weight appears to constitute a greater health problem than low weight. Equally striking is the concentration of members of the 1866 group in the range considered the healthiest. Only 30.4 percent of that group fell outside the range considered optimal, whereas nearly half the 1980 sample falls outside that range.[25]

Finally, Figure 7 compares the heights and weights of British males age sixteen to sixty-four in the 1980 survey and those of the Beddoe group to the heights and weights recommended by panels of British and American nutritionists. In that comparison, the Beddoe group appears to have been slightly overweight, whereas the 1980 survey population was decidedly overweight.

Table 4 Distribution of Quetelet Index Values in Two Groups

QUETELET INDEX VALUES	UP TO 20	20–24.99	25–29.99	30+
1866 Group	13.4%	69.6%	15.3%	1.7%
1980 Sample	7.2	50.8	35.8	6.3

SOURCES   See Table 3.

25 Waaler, "Height, Weight, and Mortality," 47. Passmore and Eastwood, *Human Nutrition,* 521, reproduce the recommendations of Anglo-American panels, which are discussed further below. They are often described as superior to standards set on the basis of the experience of insureds because the latter also distinguish by body frame, which is arbitrary.
    Extreme values occur rarely; most men had values in the low 20s. These comparisons and Costa's evidence assume that desirable Quetelet index values remain more or less constant over time.

Fig. 7 Recommended and Actual Weights

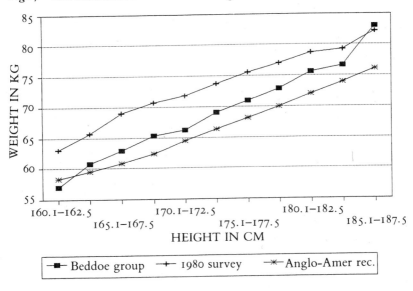

SOURCE   See Figure 3.

Although their survivorship remains unobserved, the men in the Beddoe group likely died earlier in life than their counterparts in late twentieth-century Britain. But, did they die earlier because they were underheighted? If an answer to this question is reached by comparing their adult heights to the heights of their modern counterparts, then there are grounds for supposing that the *English* males in the Beddoe group were nutritionally deprived in ways that may have played a significant role in their survival. They were so much shorter that it is necessary to conclude that they reached adulthood at a height well below their potential, a deficiency that must be due to inadequate nutrition. Even so, it would remain uncertain whether the inadequacy consisted of a deficient supply of calories or a poorly balanced diet, one notably short in elements associated with growth. When the comparison is extended to *Scots* in the Beddoe group, however, the opposite conclusion is warranted. The Scots seem to have been better nourished in 1866 than their counterparts in 1980 and, if the comparison made on the basis of height is to be sustained, then their life expectancy in 1866 should exceed that in 1980, which is far from being true.

When the analysis takes up body mass index rather than height, the evidence drawn from Beddoe's research suggests that the men in his study were smaller in proportion to their late twentieth-century counterparts, but not at greater risk. Judging by twentieth-century standards, those who prefer Waaler's estimates of the association between body mass and survivorship will find that the Beddoe group is slightly less favored than modern populations, which are heavier and have higher Quetelet index values. Those who prefer the more conservative advice of the Anglo-American nutritionists will find that Beddoe's group is favored. Its members were closer to the slender ideal recommended by present-day nutritionists. In either case, there are no grounds for supposing that nutritional deficiency in adulthood played a significant role in the higher mortality of adult males in Britain in the 1860s. Judged by a small body of evidence from that period, most men in the Beddoe group had nearly ideal body mass.

When stature alone is considered in comparison with mortality, the comparison has often been taken to suggest that mortality decline may have been associated with whatever factors have promoted gains in stature. But, weight matters. The addition of information about weight, which allows calculation of body mass, calls into question the use of height as a gauge of quality of life, nutritional status, and mortality risk. The favorable body mass of men in the Beddoe group challenges the conclusions of anthropometric historians, who have based their findings and interpretations primarily on information about height.

Massimo Livi-Bacci

Fertility, Nutrition, and Pellagra: Italy during the Vital Revolution

During the last decades of the nineteenth century, fertility began its secular decline in several regions of the north and center of Italy, at a faster rate in the urban and semi-urban areas and more slowly elsewhere. Fertility control spread to other regions in the area and, with the return to normalcy after World War I, the process became firmly rooted. The story has been written elsewhere and does not need to be told here.

There was, however, an interesting exception to this classical development: Veneto, a large region with some populous adjoining areas, did not follow the course of the other northern regions. At the beginning of this century it saw a significant increase in marital fertility despite the contemporary diffusion of contraception in the urban centers and, quite probably, in some non-urban social strata. In this same area, in the second half of the nineteenth century, the gradual deterioration of the peasants' diet had brought to its height the incidence of pellagra, a chronic disease with seasonal relapses caused by a dietary deficiency of niacin, called also PP vitamin (Pellagra-Preventive) of the B group. By the beginning of this century, the general improvement in the economic condition of the rural population and in its nutritional standard rapidly reduced the incidence of the disease while, at the same time, fertility rose.[1]

Before proceeding further, something more must be said about the etiology of pellagra, with its symptoms of weakness, apathy, loss of appetite, and neurasthenia. In later stages of the disease appear the classic three D's: dermatitis, diarrhea, and dementia, frequently followed by a fourth one: death. Dermatitis

Massimo Livi-Bacci is Professor of Demography at the University of Florence. He is the author of *A History of Italian Fertility during the Last Two Centuries* (Princeton, 1977).

1 For an analysis of the history of fertility in Italy, see Livi-Bacci, *A History of Italian Fertility during the Last Two Centuries* (Princeton, 1977).

begins with an erythema as in a sunburn; lesions then appear on various parts of the body—the hands, wrists, elbows, under the breasts, and on the knees and feet—and particularly in parts of the body exposed to the sun. The digestive system is affected with anorexia, dyspepsia, vomiting, and, in the acute stage, watery diarrhea. Psychic symptoms are present at all stages of the sickness, and they become acute in the final stages: insomnia, dizziness, and irritability at first; neurasthenia, confusion, and hallucinations in the final stage. Death inevitably follows unless intensive treatment is administered.[2]

As said above, a niacin deficient diet is a root cause of pellagra. Niacin is a common B group vitamin present in some foods either in low quantities or in quantities that cannot be absorbed. In general, a diet based on maize—*polenta* and its varieties in Italy—is poor in niacin. With little or no supplementation of milk, meat, and vegetables, it was at the base of the disease. The diffusion of pellagra in Europe followed the diffusion of the cultivation of maize and the popularization of its consumption.

The hypothesis that changes in fertility around the turn of the century were associated with the rise and fall of pellagra, itself a consequence of the changing nutritional and dietary patterns of the population, is advanced in this article, raising again the much-debated nutrition fertility issue. That malnutrition can impair the functions of the human reproductive process, particularly during famine and starvation, is an accepted fact; opinions diverge much more on the evaluation of the dimensions of the fertility depressing effects of chronic malnutrition.

Bongaarts, in a review of the evidence drawn from contemporary populations, concludes that "moderate chronic malnutrition has only a minor effect on fecundity, and the resulting decrease in fertility is very small." Among the components of fecundity, menarche and the duration of postpartum amenorrhea appear to be most affected, whereas the evidence concerning other components, such as age at menopause, permanent sterility, regularity of ovulation, and intrauterine death, appear insufficient or contradictory. Menken, Trussell, and Watkins affirm that "the

2 W. R. Aykroyd, *L'elimination des maladies de carence* (Geneva, 1970); D. A. Roe, *A Plague of Corn: The Social History of Pellagra* (Ithaca, 1973); Alberto Fonnesu, "Vitamine e disturbi da deficienza vitaminica," in Giuseppe Favilli (ed.), *Trattato di Patologia Generale* (Milan, 1968), II, 1548–1563.

evidence for a direct, strictly biological link is not convincing. . . . Reproductive function would appear to be rather impervious to outside environmental insult."[3]

However, two points deserve to be stressed. First, contemporary studies relate to fecundity and fertility levels of poorly nourished and well-nourished women, the discriminant being the difference in the amount of caloric intake and not in the quality and composition of the diet. A study of the fecundity impact of diets leading to chronic pathological consequences—such as pellagra—might yield different results. Second, if the biological link is weak, the social one may be strong; indeed the effect of varying nutritional patterns on stress, libido, sexual intercourse frequency, and voluntary abstinence may be considerable.[4]

The historical documentation available does not permit a detailed analysis of the fertility mechanisms of the population under scrutiny, much less the linkage of individuals' fertility performances with individual nutritional levels. The case is built, therefore, upon circumstantial evidence. First, I describe the peculiarity of fertility changes in Veneto and adjoining areas and discuss its features and its demographic implications. Second, the history of pellagra and of its determinant—overconsumption of maize—is recounted. Third, the geographical and statistical association of pellagra with fertility changes is examined.

THE RISE OF MARITAL FERTILITY BEFORE WORLD WAR I   The differential acceleration of natural growth during the vital revolution was, in the nineteenth century, the main factor of population redistribution in Western Europe; between 1820 and 1900 the combined population of England and Germany increased from 25.4 to 36.9 percent; that of France fell from 26.2 to 19.1 percent; and that of Italy remained constant. Indeed, during the two centuries preceding 1970, natural growth in Italy had been remarkably constant, oscillating between .6 and .8 percent per year, with a slight acceleration to slightly over 1 percent around the turn of the century. However, moderate acceleration of natural growth

3 John Bongaarts, "Does Malnutrition Affect Fecundity? A Summary of Evidence," *Science*, CCVIII (1980), 568. Jane Menken, James Trussell, and Susan Watkins, "The Nutrition Fertility Link: An Evaluation of the Evidence," *Journal of Interdisciplinary History*, XI (1981), 440.
4 *Ibid.*, 440–441.

was not universal; in Veneto a decline in natural growth was conspicuous and the difference between the birth rate and the death rate fluctuated between 1.5 and 2 percent from the end of the 1880s to the end of the 1920s, as against .8 or .9 percent for the rest of the country (Figure 1). The area of rapid growth also comprised parts of adjoining Lombardia and Emilia, with a total population of close to 5 million, about the size of the average national population at the same date of the four Scandinavian countries, Belgium, the Netherlands, and Switzerland.[5]

Table 1 reports some relevant demographic indicators for the Veneto region from 1871 to 1931. The indicators reveal a general stability in the birth rate and a continuous decline in general and

Fig. 1 Birth and Death Rates in Veneto and in the Remainder of Italy, 1871 to 1931

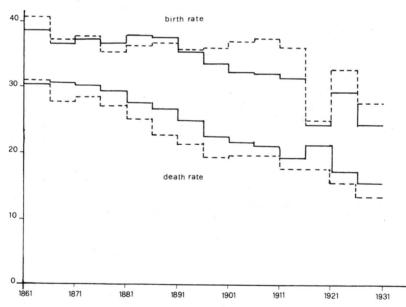

5 On the acceleration of natural growth during the demographic transition, see Jean Claude Chesnais, "L'effet multiplicatif de la transition démographique," *Population*, VI (1979), 1138–1144; E. Anthony Wrigley, "The Growth of Population in Nineteenth-Century England: A Conundrum Resolved," *Past & Present*, 98 (1983), 122.

Table 1 Demographic Indicators for Veneto, 1871–1931

YEAR	POPULATION	BIRTH RATE	DEATH RATE	RATE OF NATURAL INCREASE	INFANT MORTALITY
1871	2643	37.6	28.3	9.3	237.0
1881	2814	34.4	26.0	8.4	200.7
1891	2970	35.1	22.4	12.7	180.8
1901	3134	36.9	20.0	16.9	151.6
1911	3527	37.0	18.3	18.7	133.8
1921	3957	33.3	15.9	17.4	116.0
1931	4123	26.2	12.5	13.7	87.5

NOTE: Rates are computed on the basis of three-year averages of events centered on the census date.

infant mortality. The trend of the birth rate, showing a slight increase at the beginning of the century, is worth investigating more closely. Unfortunately, birth statistics by age of mother and birth order are not available before 1929 and therefore the analysis of fertility must rely on aggregate indicators. However, the standardized indices of general, marital, and non-marital fertility are, at this stage, adequate to investigate the trends of fertility; these measures are supplemented by a few indicators of nuptiality (Table 2).

I_f, I_g, I_h, and I_m are the standardized indices used throughout the Princeton European Fertility Project and do not need extensive description here. I'_g is the corrected index of marital fertility used throughout the Italian study. It is defined as I_g multiplied by the ratio of married females to married males, in order to eliminate the effects of an unbalanced sex ratio in the reproductive ages due to male emigration. Both I_g and I'_g show evidence of an increase in marital fertility before World War I: the rise of I'_g from the minimum (1881) to the maximum (1911) is 18.4 percent; the increase of the mean level of I'_g between 1871 and 1881 and between 1901 and 1911 is less but still very significant at 14.4 percent. Even after the end of the war, Veneto's marital fertility was higher than in the latter part of the nineteenth century, and this in spite of birth control being well established in the large urban centers. The contrast with the change of I'_g in the other Italian regions is noteworthy: in Lombardia and Emilia, which

Table 2 Indicators of Fertility and Nuptiality, Veneto, 1871–1931

YEAR	INDEX OF GENERAL FERTILITY	INDEX OF MARITAL FERTILITY		INDEX OF THE PROPORTION MARRIED (I_m)	PERCENT FEMALES SINGLE, AGE 50–54	MEAN AGE AT FIRST MARRIAGE (FEMALES)	INDEX OF ILLEGITIMATE FERTILITY I_h
		I_g	I'_g				
1871	.412	.682	.688	.586	9.8	24.7	.028
1881	.379	.651	.683	.546	10.0	24.4	.051
1891	.400	.698	.712	.540	..	..	.050
1901	.419	.743	.760	.534	10.2	23.8	.049
1911	.400	.738	.809	.512	10.5	23.6	.046
1921	.348	.704	.712	.457	11.3	24.3	.049
1931	.265	.527	.565	.470	11.8	24.2	.033

NOTE: Indexes of fertility and nuptiality have been computed on the basis of three-year averages of events centered on the census date. For 1921 the average of 1921–26 has been considered and the census population has been reported at the end of 1923.

shared some of the nutritional patterns of Veneto, there was a slight increase of 2 to 3 percent between 1871 and 1881 and between 1901 and 1911; in the other regions of the center and of the north there was a fall of 11 percent; in the south there was no change at all. It is only at the end of the 1920s that natural fertility patterns were rapidly abandoned by the population of Veneto, some half a century after Liguria and Toscana and considerably later than in other areas of northern Italy.[6]

The other indicators of fertility, I_f and I_h, show a remarkable stability, whereas the measures of nuptiality indicate that no major revolution took place during the period under consideration. Nuptiality is not independent of marital fertility, particularly when its level is high and contraception is absent. However, there are no changes in nuptiality that can account, even partially, for the changes in marital fertility; the mean age at first marriage for women fluctuated around twenty-four years and the proportion remaining single between the ages of fifty and fifty-four among women experienced only a slight increase. The 13 percent decline of I_m between 1871 and 1911 was largely due to the numerical imbalance between males and females caused by selective migration of men; a decline of a similar order of magnitude (10 percent) can be observed in the other regions of the north.

The rise in marital fertility is real and not a statistical artifact. Birth registration was virtually complete. Census coverage and quality improved over time but certainly cannot be held responsible for false indications of an increase in fertility rates. Emigration certainly had a depressive effect on fertility, an effect that is in part eliminated by the calculation of I_g'; on no account should it be invoked to explain the rise in fertility. Indeed both seasonal and, particularly, permanent emigration increased at the end of the nineteenth and at the beginning of the twentieth century, causing an alteration in the demographic and social structure before World War I with a negative impact on fertility. Yet I_g and I_g' reached their maximum during those years. Other standard demographic factors cannot be invoked to explain the rise in

6 Livi-Bacci, *Italian Fertility*, 56, 81–83. The general marital fertility rate in Veneto was 284.5 per 1,000 in 1901 for the small *comuni* with less than 30,000 inhabitants; 222.5 per 1,000 for the *comuni* with 30,000 to 100,000 inhabitants; 186.5 per 1,000 for Venezia, the only *comune* with more than 100,000 inhabitants. *Ibid.*, 122. (The *comune* is the smallest administrative unit.)

fertility. Infant mortality was rapidly falling and there was no increasing replacement or insurance effect to explain the increased marital fertility. Both between 1880 and 1882 and between 1910 and 1912 infant mortality in Veneto was lower than in the rest of Italy and declined between the two dates at a slightly faster rate.[7]

Finally, a sharp decrease in breast-feeding incidence, intensity, and duration is sometimes invoked as a possible source of the fluctuation and increasing natural fertility during the demographic transition. In Italy, breastfeeding was still universal at the end of the nineteenth century and an official inquiry at the end of the 1920s showed that breastfeeding was still widespread and the Veneto was no exception.[8]

A final point concerns the geographical extent of the rise in fertility at the beginning of this century, here examined only for the Veneto region. I have indicated that the acceleration of natural growth took place in other areas contiguous to Lombardia and Emilia. Figure 2 shows the percent variation of provincial I_g from 1881 to 1911. If we exclude two isolated cases in the south, the provinces with an increase exceeding 10 percent are all in the northeastern portion of the country: two of the nine provinces of Lombardia; six of the eight provinces of Veneto; and five of the eight in Emilia. The rise in fertility in Emilia needs some qualification, since there is evidence that illegitimacy in the 1870s and 1880s was unduly inflated by the classification as illegitimate of the children of many couples married only by religious rite, a classification that depressed recorded marital fertility. The eight provinces which, in Lombardia and Veneto, had an increase of 10 percent or more were subdivided into sixty-eight smaller administrative units (the *circondario*), and only three of these experienced a decline between 1881 and 1911, one case being the circondario comprising the city of Venice.[9]

7 Intercensal net migration was 8,000 a year between 1871 and 1881 and 20 to 25,000 per year between 1881 and 1911. Official statistics of emigrants' departures show some 20,000 departures per year between 1876 and 1880; 40,000 between 1881 and 1885; 80,000 between 1886 and 1890; and about 100,000 per year between 1891 and 1914. See, for detailed data, Commissariato Generale dell'Emigrazione, *Annuario Statistico dell'Emigrazione Italiana dal 1876 al 1925* (Rome, 1926). Infant mortality rates for Italy were 206.2 from 1880 to 1882 and 141.4 from 1910 to 1912.

8 Livi-Bacci, *Italian Fertility*, 69–73. Detailed results of the official enquiry can be found in Istituto Italiano di Statistica (ISTAT), *Movimento della popolazione secondo gli atti dello stato civile nell'anno 1928* (Rome, 1932), 157, 178.

9 Provincial variations in fertility, measured here with I_g, underestimate the real rise,

Fig. 2 Provinces of Northern Italy with an Increase of Ig between 1881 and 1911 exceeding 10 Percent

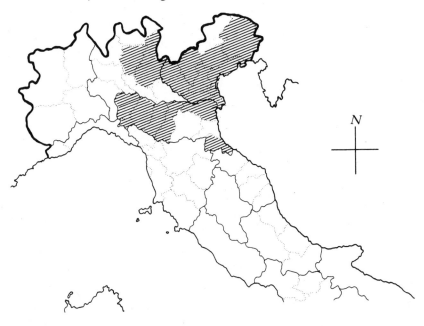

FLUCTUATIONS IN NATURAL FERTILITY   A rise in marital fertility, in general preceding a sustained decline, has occurred in many less developed countries: in Korea, in Taiwan, among some Asian populations in the Soviet Union, and in West Africa. "Such increases," observed Coale, "result from shortened or less intensive breastfeeding, from reduction in the frequency of separation of spouses because of a decline in seasonal migration, from abandonment or curtailment of postpartum abstinence and from effective treatment of pathological sterility." In the more developed populations this phenomenon has attracted less attention. Quoting Coale again: "a little noted feature of the transition to a declining birth rate is that fertility of married women often rose before a major reduction began. Such a rise was common in the départe-

---

since the excess of married females over married males because of emigration has increased over time, reaching a maximum before the war. See Livi-Bacci, *Italian Fertility*, 141–142. On illegitimacy and classification of births, see *ibid.*, 69–73.

ments of France . . . it was also apparent in Denmark, England and Wales, Germany and some regions of Italy."[10]

There are many reasons why the rise in fertility has passed unnoticed. Since this rise occurred mainly during the nineteenth century, observers and scholars have been interested, above all, in detecting a pattern in the fall of marital fertility as an indicator of spreading birth control and of demographic modernization. The rise in fertility was often attributed to the poor quality of the data; to an improved completeness of registration; and to random fluctuations in the factors of natural fertility. Seldom has such a rise been recognized as a real change in one or more of the components of natural fertility.

Of great interest is a recent article by Knodel and Wilson. They examined the reproductive histories of couples in fourteen German villages married between 1750 and 1899. The absence of change in overall indicators of natural fertility (such as I_g) is deceptive because the decline in marital fertility rates at older ages is compensated for by an increase at the younger ages and therefore "the earlier onset of voluntary fertility control was masked in the measures of observed fertility by a substantial and concurrent rise in the underlying level of fertility." The underlying level of marital fertility is measured by the parameter M of the Coale and Trussel equation. When the separate components of fecundity are examined, the authors find firm evidence of a rise in fecundability—the probability of conceiving; less conclusive evidence of a decline in the non-susceptible period following birth; and little or no change in primary sterility. As to the causes of the rise in fecundity, the authors advance a few tentative hypotheses: a decline in intrauterine mortality; improved nutrition or changes in infant feeding practices; or a combination of these factors.[11]

POPULARIZATION OF MAIZE AND THE APPEARANCE OF PELLAGRA
The case of northeastern Italy, unfortunately, cannot be investi-

10 Ansley J. Coale, "Recent Trends in Fertility in Less Developed Countries," *Science*, CCXXI (1983), 829. For an extensive survey of fertility rise during the transition, see Moni Nag, "How Modernization Can Also Increase Fertility," *Current Anthropology*, XXI (1980), 571–580.
11 John Knodel and Christopher Wilson, "The Secular Increase of Fecundity in German Village Populations: An Analysis of Reproductive Histories of Couples Married, 1750–1899," *Population Studies*, XXXV (1981), 53–84.

gated with the same richness of detail available for the fourteen German villages; it is possible, however, to gather some interesting circumstantial evidence on the possible underlying causes for the rise in marital fertility at the beginning of this century. My intention is to prove that there is a connection between fertility and nutrition, and that the history of pellagra is the symptom, if not the proof, of that connection.

The history of pellagra is closely related to the history of maize in Spain, France, Italy, and in several areas of Eastern Europe. Maize was already known in Veneto in the sixteenth century, and its diffusion increased in the seventeenth, spreading to Lombardia. The popularization of corn in Romagna (part of the Emilia region) took place in the latter half of the eighteenth century, when it was still relatively rare in Toscana. From the end of the eighteenth century the cultivation and consumption of corn rapidly increased in the north and in the center of the country. The worsened living conditions of the rural populations at the end of the eighteenth century, the consequences of the Napoleonic Wars, and the profound subsistence crisis of 1816/17 were all powerful incentives to the cultivation of maize. Its high productivity and nutritional value and its relatively low price made it particularly attractive to the impoverished peasants. Maize became increasingly popular in the form of bread and, particularly, polenta, becoming practically the exclusive food of the very poor. In the years of poverty, when the price of wheat rose, maize became its universal substitute; diets already poor in nutritional value were further impoverished and imbalanced, and pellagra increased. Many writers have emphasized the fact that the modernization of agriculture in the lowlands of northern Italy was responsible for the proletarization of a large part of the rural population and for a downgrading of their nutritional patterns. Maize was grown on the farm mainly for direct consumption, whereas the other products were sold on the market.[12]

12   On the history of the cultivation of maize in Italy and of its role in nutrition, see L. Messedaglia, *Il mais e la vita rurale in Italia* (Piacenza, 1927). See also, *idem, Per la storia dell'agricoltura e dell'alimentazione* (Piacenza, 1932). One of the many examples of fluctuations of pellagra is its increase in Veneto in 1880 after the scarce harvest of 1879. See Emilio Morpurgo, "Relazione sulla XI Circoscrizione," in *Atti della Giunta per l'inchiesta agraria* (Rome, 1882), IV. On the living conditions of the rural population, see Giorgio Porisini, "Agricoltura, alimentazione e condizioni sanitarie. Prime ricerche sulla pellagra in Italia dal 1880 al 1940," unpub. ms. (Bologna, n.d.).

The increasing presence of corn in the daily diet was accompanied, in the area of investigation, by general deterioration in real income and in nutritional patterns in the 1860s and 1870s; the monumental parliamentary *Inchiesta Agraria* carried out in the early 1880s leaves no doubt about this decline. The agrarian crisis of the 1880s, triggered by the devastating competition from North American products, added new difficulties to a situation of grave poverty and widespread destitution. Only at the end of the century was there a general improvement in the living conditions of the rural population, with a sustained trend until World War I. Official surveys and private investigations confirm the corresponding improvement in diet. Official estimates of the per capita daily caloric intake for the entire population show a decrease from 2,647 between 1871 and 1880 to 2,197 from 1881 to 1890 and 2,119 from 1891 to 1900 and a rise to 2,617 from 1901 to 1910; unfortunately the statistics on which these estimates are based leave much to be desired.[13]

Since maize was mainly consumed where it was grown, and only a small part of the total production was traded even domestically, there was a correspondence between the geography of production and the geography of consumption. In the latter part of last century over half of the total production came from Lombardia, Veneto, and Emilia, and about 80 percent from the seven regions where pellagra was present. With the beginning of the new century an increase in the use of maize for cattle feed and in the growth of internal and international trade lessened the correspondence between area of production and area of consumption.[14]

Pellagra follows the track of maize; it appears in Spain, probably at the end of the seventeenth century, where it was systematically described by Gaspar Casal, an Asturian physician. The

13 The *Giunta per l'Inchiesta Agraria* was a parliamentary commission created to inquire into the conditions of the rural population; it was chaired by Stefano Jacini, an economist and a senator. See *Atti della Giunta per l'Inchiesta Agraria* (Rome, 1881–1884), 15 v. The material on the living conditions of the rural population in the pellagra area is very rich. See particularly *ibid.* (1882), VI, pts. 1 and 2, concerning Lombardia and the general report by Jacini himself; see also *ibid.*, IV, on Veneto. On the agrarian crisis of the 1880s, see Gino Luzzatto, *L'economia italiana dal 1861 al 1914* (Milan, 1963), 218 ff; Mario Romani, *Un secolo di vita agricola in Lombardia* (Milan, 1963), 50. On the improvement of the living conditions at the turn of the century, see Riccardo Bachi, *L'alimentazione e la politica annonaria in Italia* (Bari, 1926), 18 ff: Romani, *Un secolo.* Statistics on caloric intakes can be found in ISTAT, *Sommario di statistiche storiche dell'Italia, 1861–1975* (Rome, 1976), 161.
14 Porisini, "Agricoltura," 17.

spread of the disease in Lombardia and Veneto, its characteristics, and its presumed causative factors have been widely observed, systematically described, and continuously discussed since the end of the eighteenth century. Works on pellagra have been published since 1769; the names of Frapolli and Strambio, authors of famous books on pellagra, came to be known throughout Europe. Contemporary writers observed its rapid diffusion, accelerated after the subsistence crisis of 1816/17. During the nineteenth century pellagra crossed the Po River and became endemic in many provinces of Emilia and, to a lesser extent, in some areas of Marche, Umbria, and Tuscany. The southern part of the country, where maize was virtually absent from the diet, remained untouched by the disease. The diffusion and prevalence of pellagra reached a maximum in the 1870s and 1880s; remained at high levels until the beginning of this century; rapidly declined in the ten to fifteen years preceding World War I; and disappeared in the 1920s. Yet, in the second half of the nineteenth century pellagra was a national social problem, and politicians, administrators, and medical people were mobilized by growing public concern to find effective preventive and curative measures.[15]

The association of pellagra with the consumption of maize was clearly perceived from the time of its initial appearance. Before the studies by Funk, who hypothesized that vitamin deficiency was at the base of pellagra, several theories on the causal relationship between a maize-based diet and the disease were advanced. One popular theory stated that pellagra was an intoxication caused by decayed maize; it was first advanced by Balardini in 1844 and vigorously sustained by Lombroso, who influenced

15 Ministero di Agricoltura, Industria e Commercio (MAIC), "La pellagra in Italia," *Annali di Agricoltura*, XVIII (1879), Appendix. The area of diffusion in Spain comprised Galicia, Asturias, Navarra, Aragon, Castilla la Nueva, and Castilla la Vieja. Pellagra in Spain never reached the intensity it did in Italy; in 1900, the number of deaths in Spain from pellagra amounted to little more than 10% of the number registered in Italy. In France, pellagra appeared in the first half of the nineteenth century in the Landes and part of Gironde, Hautes and Basses Pyrénées, Haute Garonne, and Aude. For the social history of pellagra in Italy see Porisini, "Agricoltura"; Roberto Finzi, "Un esempio di malattia da carenza: la pellagra," unpub. ms. (1981). Gaspar Casal, *Mal de la rosa. Su historia, causa, easos, curación* (Barcelona, 1936). This work, originally written in Latin in 1735, was published posthumously in 1762, three years after the death of the author. Francesco Frapolli, *Animadversiones in morbum vulgo pellagra* (Milan, 1771). Gaetano Strambio, *De pellagra Cajtani Strambio M.D. observationes in Regio pellagrosorum Nosocomio factae a Calendis Junii 1784 usque ad finem anni 1785* (n.d. and n.p.).

the course of public action in the last decades of the nineteenth century. A second theory hypothesized the existence of an endogenous intoxication caused by dysfunctions in the process of assimilation of a cornmeal-based diet. A third theory claimed that the etiology of pellagra was associated with the insufficient nutritional content of a maize-based diet. Whatever the theory in vogue, direct experience and daily observations were in absolute agreement with the scientific opinion that an exclusive or semi-exclusive maize diet was the cause of pellagra. And since the maize diet was typical of the poor, rural classes, the combination of polenta and misery was rightly held responsible for the diffusion of the disease.[16]

Current experience has shown that an improvement in diet, particularly in the early stage, causes a retreat of the disease; that in years of economic depression, soaring prices, and bad harvests, the substitution of less expensive corn for the consumption of wheat brings about a recrudescence of pellagra; and that whenever corn is introduced in a new area, the deadly disease slowly makes its appearance.

DIFFUSION AND PREVALENCE OF PELLAGRA IN ITALY   For the last quarter of the nineteenth century, the diffusion and prevalence of pellagra can be traced with the aid of two complementary sources, neither of which is immune from serious distortions. The first source is a series of surveys—the first two taken in 1879 and 1881—ordered by the ministry of agriculture and carried out on behalf of the *prefetture* (the provincial state authorities) by medical and other public personnel in the various *comuni*. In 1881 the person responsible for the survey in each *comune* had to file a form containing the data on the number, sex, age, and profession of the pellagrins. Provincial health boards had to examine and approve the reports before transmitting the results to the Ministry in Rome. Although the symptoms of the pellagrins were often visible and the identity of those afflicted was often well known

16 C. Funk, "The Etiology of the Deficiency Diseases . . .," *Journal of State Medicine*, XX (1912), 341–368; G. Balardini, *Della Pellagra, del grano turco quale causa precipua* (Milan, 1845); Cesare Lombroso, *La pellagra e il mais in Italia. Lettura d'igiene popolare* (Turin, 1879). For the theories on the etiology of pellagra, see Vincenzo de Giaxa, "La pellagra," in Oddo Casagrandi (ed.), *Trattato Italiano d'Igiene* (Turin, 1927), VI, pt. 6. Porisini, "Agricoltura," 23–31; Finzi, "Un esempio."

in small rural communities, several health boards considered the results to be largely an underestimation of reality. The reasons were various: in some areas there were no medical personnel; pellagra was difficult to detect in the early stages; and there was a widespread reticence to make manifest a disease which was known to undermine the working efficiency of the individual. In short, the surveys underestimated the number of pellagrins on the one hand while, on the other, the criteria followed in estimating their number varied considerably from area to area. In some extreme cases, *comuni* notoriously afflicted by pellagra were declared immune.[17]

The second source consists of the cause of death statistics which were initiated in Italy in 1881 in a number of large *comuni*, comprising one third of the total population, and were extended to the entire country in 1887. Cause of death statistics, particularly in the first years, were subject to criticism and they illustrate only the tip of the iceberg as far as the disease is concerned.[18]

The first surveys—with their biases and distortions—were taken at the zenith of the epidemic. Indeed, some early surveys taken in Lombardia claimed 20,282 pellagrins in 1839 and 38,777 in 1856, numbers that grew to 40,838 in 1879. In 1870, Balardini gave a total count of 14,502 pellagrins in the province of Brescia (which had the highest prevalence in Lombardia), compared with 10,924 in 1856, and 6,939 in 1839. This quantitative evidence, together with abundant documentary evidence of other kinds, indicates that the gravity of the disease in Lombardia reached a maximum in the 1870s. In Veneto the maximum probably occurred in the 1880s: earlier surveys in the mid-1850s claimed some 15,000 to 16,000 pellagrins, little more than one fourth the number in 1881. Between 1881 and 1899, the prevalence of pellagra declined rapidly in Lombardia and Emilia and less rapidly in Veneto; the rise in other regions, where the prevalence always remained relatively low, reflected a further geographical spread

17 The results of the first survey are published in MAIC, "La pellagra." The results of the second and more careful survey of 1881 can be found in MAIC, "La pellagra in Italia. Provvedimenti e statistica. Pt. II: Statistica dei pellagrosi esistenti in Italia nel biennio 1880–81," *Annali di Agricoltura*, XLIV (1885). On the underestimation of pellagrins, see the explicit comments made by the Health Boards of Pavia, Como, Cremona, Rovigo, and Modena in *ibid.*

18 Direzione Generale di Statistica (DIRSTAT), *Statistica delle cause di morte*, yearly volumes since 1881.

of the disease (Table 3). In 1910 the prevalence of pellagrins was reduced to little more than one fourth the level of 1881. Later surveys, in the 1920s, show that pellagra had practically disappeared; only 1,466 cases, mainly chronic elderly cases, were enumerated in 1926.[19]

Death statistics confirm the trend which, because of the late start of the statistics, can be followed only after 1887, when the zenith of the epidemic was over (Table 4). Between 1887 to 1891 and 1912 to 1916, the mortality rate from pellagra declined from 152 per 100,000 population to 23 in Lombardia; from 228 to 60 in Veneto; from 118 to 12 in Emilia; and from 40 to 8 in the other four regions stricken by the disease. During the same period there was a rapid aging of the distribution of deaths from pellagra, as is to be expected from a chronic disease with declining incidence. The partial statistics from 1881 to 1886 show that mortality from

Table 3   Pellagrins according to Various Official Surveys, 1879, 1881, 1899, and 1910

AREA	1879	1881	1899	1910
		Number		
Lombardia	40,838	36,630	19,547	8,231
Veneto	29,836	55,881	39,892	20,303
Emilia	18,728	7,891	4,617	1,808
4 Regions[a]	8,229	3,467	8,267	3,319
Other Regions	–	32	146	208
ITALY	97,855	104,067	72,603	33,869
	Pellagrins per 100,000 population			
Lombardia	1,109	995	465	172
Veneto	1,060	1,986	1,869	576
Emilia	858	361	189	67
4 Regions[a]	121	51	109	42
Other Regions	–	–	1	1
ITALY	344	366	224	98

a   The 4 regions are Piemonte, Toscana, Marche, and Umbria.

SOURCES: Survey of 1879: MAIC "La pellagra" (1879), n. 18. Survey of 1881: MAIC "La pellagra" (1885). Survey of 1899: "Inchiesta sulla pellagra nel Regno e sui provvedimenti diversi per la cura della stessa," *Bollettino di Notizie Agrarie*, XXII (1900), n. 31. Survey of 1910: G. Porisini, "Agricoltura, alimentazione e condizioni sanitarie: Appendice Statistica," unpub. ms. (Bologna, n.d.).

19   Data for 1839 are quoted by Jacini, "La proprietà fondiaria e le popolazioni agricole in Lombardia," *Biblioteca dell'Economista*, II (1861), 361. For the survey of 1856 and for Brescia and Veneto, MAIC, "La pellagra" (1879). For 1926, Ministero dell'Interno, *Relazione al Consiglio Superiore di Sanità, 1 Luglio 1926–30 Giugno 1927* (Rome, 1928), I.

Table 4 Deaths and Death Rates by Pellagra, by Region, 1887–91 to 1927–31

PERIOD	DEATHS BY PELLAGRA					DEATH RATE BY PELLAGRA PER 100,000 POPULATION				
	LOMBARDIA	VENETO	EMILIA	4 REGIONS[a]	TOTAL 7 REGIONS[b]	LOMBARDIA	VENETO	EMILIA	4 REGIONS[a]	TOTAL 7 REGIONS[b]
1887–91	5,938	6,679	2,686	2,862	18,263	152	228	118	40	113
1892–96	5,705	5,528	2,690	2,834	16,917	141	184	115	39	101
1897–01	4,645	5,547	3,413	3,664	17,472	111	179	142	49	102
1902–06	3,175	4,355	1,605	2,445	11,767	72	135	64	32	66
1907–11	1,850	2,989	733	1,214	6,923	40	87	28	16	37
1912–16	1,131	2,180	322	652	4,349	23	60	12	8	23
1917–21	820	1,047	167	330	2,408	16	27	6	4	12
1922–26	224	280	60	123	710	4	7	2	2	3
1927–31	98	204	40	46	403	2	5	1	1	2

a The 4 regions are Piemonte, Toscana, Marche, and Umbria.

b The total number of deaths for the 7 regions is the total for Italy and contains about 1 percent of the deaths of Liguria, Lazio, and Abruzzi.

SOURCE: DIRSTAT, *Statistica delle cause delle morti* (1887–1931).

pellagra must have been higher in the early 1880s; other indicators prove that it must have been on the rise during the 1870s.

Summing up the evidence, we can state that the incidence of pellagra and its geographical diffusion increased and reached a high point in the 1870s and 1880s. The disease then started a vigorous decline at the turn of the century; fell to low levels before World War I; and disappeared as a major social disease in the 1920s. The decline must have been earlier and faster among the younger age groups in the population.

CHANGES IN MARITAL FERTILITY AND PELLAGRA   In the early 1880s, fertility was still at natural levels in most of Italy, with a few isolated areas in the north and in the center experiencing declining fertility. The province of Bergamo (Lombardia), with its 400,000 inhabitants, was subdivided into three *circondari* (districts): Clusone, in 1881, had the highest I_g (.814) and the lowest incidence of pellagra (9 per 1,000); Treviglio had the lowest I_g (.703) and the highest level of pellagra (29 per 1,000); Bergamo, the third *circondario*, had intermediate levels of fertility (.748) and of disease prevalence (21 per 1,000). Thirty years later the incidence of pellagra had dropped to very low levels, but fertility, when compared with the levels of 1881, showed a maximum increase in Treviglio (20 percent), where pellagra had the highest incidence; a minimum increase (3 percent) in Clusone, where pellagra had the lowest incidence in 1881; and an intermediate increase (12 percent) in Bergamo, which had intermediate levels of pellagra.

The example of the province of Bergamo illustrates the type of relationship that existed between marital fertility and pellagra during the three or four decades around the turn of the century.

Figure 3 charts the diffusion of pellagra according to the official 1881 survey. If Figure 3 is compared with Figure 2, which reports the areas with an increase in marital fertility between 1881 and 1911, one notes a striking coincidence between the pellagra-stricken areas and the areas that show an increase of marital fertility. Pellagra or, better, officially recorded pellagra, had the highest prevalence in the provinces of Belluno, Padua, and Treviso in Veneto (more than 30 per 1,000 of the total population), and high incidence (between 10 and 30 per 1,000) in the other provinces of Veneto (Verona excluded) and in four provinces of

Fig. 3 Prevalence of Pellagra in Northern Italy, 1881

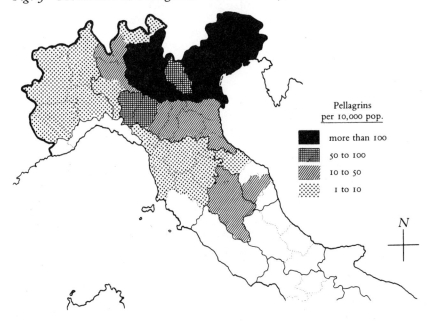

Lombardia (Brescia, Bergamo, Cremona, and Mantova). Minor but significant levels prevailed in the other provinces of Lombardia, in Emilia, and in two provinces of Marche and Umbria.

The relationships between pellagra and fertility can be specified at the level of the smaller administrative units, the *circondari*. Because of reservations about the quality of pellagra surveys, the results have to be taken with due caution. The analysis has also been limited to the *circondari* of Lombardia and Veneto, excluding the third region seriously afflicted by the disease—Emilia—since here the variations over time of I_g were biased by the distortion in the classification of births by legitimacy.

Table 5 reports the average incidence of pellagra for the *circondari* falling in various classes of I_g (1881). There is a clear (although imperfect) inverse association: the *circondari* with low I_g (below .650) had an incidence of pellagrins three times as high as those with high fertility (I_g above .750).

Table 6, however, is more interesting; it relates variations of I_g between 1881 and 1911 to the average incidence of pellagra in

Table 5   Index of Marital Fertility and Prevalence of Pellagra, 1881, in
111 Districts of Lombardia and Veneto

LEVEL OF I_g	DISTRICTS	AVERAGE LEVEL OF I_g (1880–82)	PERSONS WITH PELLAGRA PER 100,000 (1881)
−.600	30	.571	191
.600–.649	33	.628	179
.650–.699	17	.677	155
.700–.749	20	.723	175
.750–.799	9	.778	86
.800 and over	2	.854	58
Mean	–	.653	168

Table 6   Variation of the Index of Marital Fertility, 1881 to 1911, and
Prevalence of Pellagra in 1881, in 103 Districts of Lombardia
and Veneto

PERCENT VARIATION OF I_g, 1880–82 TO 1910–12	N. OF DISTRICTS (103)	AVERAGE VAR. OF I_g 1880–82 TO 1910–12	LEVEL OF I_g 1910–12	PERSONS WITH PELLAGRA PER 100,000 (1881)
−10 and over	9	−20.8	.544	23
−10 to 0	15	− 5.5	.643	112
0 to +10	27	+ 5.6	.698	116
+10 to +20	29	+15.9	.721	166
+20 to +30	12	+24.1	.790	323
+30 and over	11	+38.0	.836	377
Mean	–	+10.2	.710	174

1881. The relationship is a direct one: the highest increase of I_g
took place in the *circondari* where pellagra had the maximum
incidence in 1881; the few *circondari* of the two regions which
experienced a decline in marital fertility had a low incidence of
the disease. Table 6 also shows the level of I_g for 1910 to 1912
according to classes of variation of I_g for 1880 to 1882 and for
1910 to 1912 and the mean incidence of pellagra in 1881. In a
regime of natural fertility, if pellagra were the only source of
fertility differences, one would expect that the elimination of
pellagra (as almost happened before World War I) would remove
all source of variation in fertility. But this was not the case; in
Table 6, I_g for 1910 to 1912 is positively associated with the level

of pellagra in 1881 (which was *negatively* associated with I_g for 1880 to 1882, as shown in Table 5).

This fact, however, is not surprising, since pellagra is not the only source of fertility variation during the period examined. Oversimplifying a very complex reality, we could say two classes of factors affect fertility over the period under investigation: first, factors affecting natural fertility (mainly pellagra); and second, factors determining the diffusion of fertility control. Although the evolution of the first factor determines the decrease in the variation of natural fertility levels, the second factor introduces a new source of variation (indeed, during the period, the diffusion of fertility control is evident in several areas). But both factors are also inversely associated—development was more rapid in the areas with better living conditions in 1881 and lower pellagra— and this fact explains why the negative association of pellagra (1881) with I_g (1880–82) becomes positive when pellagra (1881) is associated with I_g (1910–12).[20]

When the other indicator of the incidence of pellagra (the pellagra-specific mortality rate) is used, similar results are obtained. However, since death statistics by cause are only available from 1887 at the provincial level, all provinces with a significant death rate from pellagra have been considered. There are twenty-nine in all, including some provinces of Marche and Umbria and Emilia. Table 7, in full conformity with the results of Tables 5 and 6, shows the existence of a negative association between death rates by pellagra from 1887 to 1889 and marital fertility from 1880 to 1882 and a strong positive association between pellagra levels from 1887 to 1889 and marital fertility from 1910 to 1912.

The results are interesting but probably inconclusive; data on pellagra are far from flawless, although the agreement between two independent sources (surveys of pellagrins and death statistics) is reassuring.

---

20 The poor quality and doubtful completeness of the data on pellagra prevalence does not call for refined measures of the association between pellagra and fertility. The correlation coefficients for the *circondari* of Lombardia and Veneto between I (1881) and the prevalence of pellagra (1880–82) is weakly negative (r = −.141) and higher for Lombardia (35 *circondari*, r = −.290) than for Veneto (76 *circondari*, r = −.122). The correlation coefficient between the variation of I_g between 1880 to 1882 and 1910 to 1912 and the pellagra prevalence of 1881 is +.541 for the pooled *circondari* of the two regions and higher for Lombardia (+.711) than for Veneto (+.470).

Table 7 Index of Marital Fertility, 1881 and 1911, and Death Rate by Pellagra, 1887–89, in 29 Provinces

LEVEL OF I_g	NUMBER OF PROVINCES (29)[a]	AVERAGE LEVEL OF I_g	DEATHS OF PELLAGRA PER 100,000 INHABS.
		1880–82	(1887–89)
−600	7	.597	26.6
600–649	11	.619	33.7
650–699	6	.670	32.8
700–749	3	.727	20.0
750 and over	2	.759	19.0
		.641	29.4
		1910–12	
−600	5	.552	17.0
600–649	6	.629	20.7
650–699	7	.674	26.6
700–749	8	.728	36.6
750 and over	3	.806	54.7
		.672	29.4

a   The 29 Provinces belong to Lombardia (8), Veneto (8), Emilia (8), Marche (4), and Umbria (1).

Three aspects of the relationship between fertility and pellagra should be emphasized. The first concerns the striking coincidence between the pellagra-stricken areas and the area where marital fertility rose during the three or four decades preceding World War I. The second is the negative association between the level of marital fertility from 1880 to 1882 and the contemporary incidence of pellagra. The third is the obvious positive association between the rise in marital fertility and the level of pellagra during the 1880s. The areas where pellagra was highest in the 1880s and from which it disappeared before the war were also the areas with the largest increase in marital fertility.

IN SEARCH OF A CAUSAL LINK   Are the diffusion of pellagra in the 1870s and 1880s and its rapid decline at the beginning of this century sufficient elements to explain the rise in marital fertility in northeastern Italy? In theory, it is clear that endemic and chronic disease with the etiology of pellagra must have had a depressive effect on natural fertility. Weakness, apathy, and neurasthenia in the initial stage of the disease might easily have caused a loss of libido and affected the frequency of sexual intercourse. The digestive afflictions at a more advanced stage of the disease might have affected fecundability in various ways, particularly through pregnancy wastage. Although the effects of pellagra have not been specifically studied, the existence of a depressive effect on fertility is a logical deduction, given the medical implications of the disease.

Information that is not irrelevant can be derived from pellagra's death statistics. In the reproductive ages, female excess mortality is very high: the female to male ratio in the twenty to forty age group is two to three female deaths for every male death, compared to a general ratio below one for all ages combined. The high vulnerability of women at these ages is doubtless the result of the exacting biological requirements for reproduction. Data on morbidity are rare and less solid, but a high incidence of the disease among young women is often reported.

Some doubts as to the strength of the association between pellagra and fertility may arise after a consideration of the relatively low prevalence of the disease even in the areas of maximum diffusion (5 to 10 percent in some *circondari*). Even allowing for a conspicuous underestimation of pellagra—and for the possibility that the official number of pellagrins was underestimated by a factor of 2 or 3 as was widely believed—it is prudent to assume that the rise in fertility cannot wholly be attributed to the decline in the disease.[21]

One possible hypothesis is that pellagra was a symptom of a general state of malnutrition that, in the majority of cases, did not induce or cause pathological dysfunctions. There is a consensus that the second half of the nineteenth century saw falling standards of living for large sections of the rural masses, particularly in the area of our concern, and that only at the end of the century did a sustained improvement take place. Vast sectors of the population that had survived on poor diets easily crossed the borderline leading to pathological consequences in years of bad harvests and economic straits.

But, before accepting the malnutrition scenario, we must overcome one logical obstacle: in the pellagra area, malnutrition was not linked to higher than average mortality. Figure 1 shows that general mortality was lower in Veneto than in the rest of the

21   Morpurgo, "Relazione," 172–176.

country, and the same can be said of infant mortality. Can a lower than average mortality be reconciled with a higher than average level of malnutrition? Table 8 shows that a reconciliation between the two facts may be possible; indeed, in spite of a lower general mortality, the pellagra area had a higher incidence of recruits rejected at the military draft for debility, congenital weakness, and malformation—typical causes of ineligibility for service linked to poor living and nutritional conditions. Poor nutrition was also linked to a higher-than-average mortality rate from rickets.

Malnutrition is a complex phenomenon and unless more circumstances are specified, such as its relationship to particular diseases, it cannot offer more than generic explanations of aggregate trends and differences. It is enough, at this stage, to say that malnutrition was not inconsistent with a moderate death rate.[22]

The elimination of pellagra and the improvement in nutritional standards removed a series of depressing effects on fertility. They are most likely the cause of the increase in marital fertility in northeastern Italy before World War I. This hypothesis is sustained by the analysis of aggregate series; as to the mechanisms through which nutrition affected fertility—biological or social, or a mix of the two—nothing can be said on the basis of the aggregate available data.

Table 8 Proportion Rejected at Military Draft (Cohorts 1843–56) and Indicators of Mortality (1887–89) by Region

AREA	PERCENT REJECTED FOR DEBILITY AND WEAK CONSTITUTION[a]	DEATH RATE (PER 1,000)	INFANT MORTALITY RATE (PER 1,000)	DEATH RATE FOR RICKETS (PER 100,000)
Lombardia	8.67	25.4	196.6	1.1
Veneto	7.84	23.0	184.9	1.5
Emilia	4.80	26.4	222.2	2.2
Other Regions	4.76	27.6	189.5	0.7
Italy	5.53	26.8	192.4	1.0

a SOURCE: Giuseppe Sormani, "Geografia nosologica d'Italia," *Annali di Statistica*, VI (1881).

22 Contributions and discussions at a 1982 conference on hunger and history give a good account of the complexity of the interaction between nutrition and mortality. See the special issue, "Hunger and History: The Impact of Changing Food Production and Consumption Patterns on Society," *Journal of Interdisciplinary History*, XIV (1983), 199–534.

Susan B. Hanley

Urban Sanitation in Preindustrial Japan

The sudden increase in Japan's urban population in the century and a half from the 1580s to the mid-1700s may well have had no parallel in world history prior to industrialization. Edo, renamed Tokyo in 1868, was a cluster of fishing villages around a castle in 1590, but, during the eighteenth century, it is readily acknowledged to have been one of the largest, if not the largest, city in the world. Even by 1700, Edo was certainly larger than any European city, including London at 575,000, and rivaled or exceeded in population the largest of the Chinese cities at the time, Peking. But urban growth was not limited to Edo; cities sprang up throughout the country from the late sixteenth century on and both Kyoto and Osaka had populations in the hundreds of thousands. By the late eighteenth century, Japan had about 3 percent of the world's population, but it is estimated to have had more than 8 percent of the people in the world who lived in cities of more than 10,000. By this standard, about 10 percent of the total population of Japan was urban in 1800.[1]

To support a metropolitan population, food and other daily necessities must be adequately supplied, and demands for housing, water, transportation, a monetary system, and numerous other requirements must be met. Even if all other requirements are

Susan B. Hanley is Professor of Japanese Studies and History at the University of Washington, Seattle, and is editor of the *Journal of Japanese Studies*. She is coauthor of *Economic and Demographic Change in Preindustrial Japan, 1600–1868* (Princeton, 1977).

The author wishes to thank William B. Hauser, Joel A. Tarr, and Kozo Yamamura for helpful suggestions and Robert J. Smith for the invitation to the Social Science Research Council workshop on the Japanese city for which this research was begun.

1 Ōishi Shinzaburō, "Kyodai toshi Edo no jinkō wa dore kurai ka," *Rekishi to jimbutsu*, CX (1980), 76–81; E. Anthony Wrigley, "A Simple Model of London's Importance in Changing English Society and Economy 1650–1750," in Philip Abrams and Wrigley (eds.), *Towns in Societies* (Cambridge, 1978), 215; G. William Skinner (ed.), *The City in Late Imperial China* (Stanford, 1977), 29. Gilbert Rozman, *Urban Networks in Ch'ing China and Tokugawa Japan* (Princeton, 1973), 6, estimates Japan to have been 10% urban while Sekiyama Naotarō, *Kinsei Nihon no jinkō kōzō* (Tokyo, 1957), 239, considers 12% of the population to have been urban.

satisfied, however, if sanitation is inadequate, one would not expect the population of a city to reach a million, much less be maintained at this figure over centuries. Yet Edo, which lacked modern water supply and sewage systems, and which relied primarily on manpower or boats to carry away garbage, refuse, and other human wastes, is estimated to have had a population in the range of a million from about 1700 on. How did Japan manage to maintain such an enormous urban concentration of people for two centuries prior to industrialization?

Numerous studies have discussed urban sanitation and water systems in the West, as well as the negative rate of natural increase in the population of urban areas in premodern times. However, scholars in Japan have begun to research these subjects only in the last decade, and no one has attempted to evaluate as a whole the various aspects of sanitation in premodern Japanese cities and their significance in Japanese history. Here my focus will be on the problem of sanitation in the major metropolises of Japan from approximately 1590 to 1890 and will include an assessment of the sanitation standards in light of Western standards for the same centuries. This is not intended to be an exhaustive study that will provide full evidence, but one that provides a new perspective on Japan and, through comparison, on the West as well.

The lack of interest in these topics in Japan results primarily from the political-institutional focus that historians traditionally have had. Perhaps equally important is the fact that Japanese have not had to contend with the urban problems that Westerners faced in early modern times. Thus, the wealth of personal observations, proposals for improvement, and other materials so widely available in the West from at least the early nineteenth century are, by and large, lacking for Japan. But from Japanese laws, regulations, and political concerns, a good deal of information can be extracted about Edo's water supply and waste disposal systems and on Osaka's system for disposing of night soil.

This article examines how the premodern Japanese provided a water supply system for urban residents and developed systems to rid the cities of waste, ranging from garbage and rubbish to water and human excreta, or night soil. It also looks at Japanese customs that had an effect on levels of sanitation and disposal of night soil and compares urban conditions in Japan with those in the West. The article is divided into four main parts: 1) a brief summary of the growth and changes in the city population in the Tokugawa period (1600–1868); 2) a description of Edo's water supply system and brief comparison with how other Japanese cities were supplied; 3) an analysis of how the cities handled the crucial problems of waste disposal; and 4) a comparison of sanitation and hygiene in Japan from the seventeenth through the nineteenth centuries with sanitation levels in Western cities. The implications of the findings and their possible relationship to the course of industrialization in Japan are discussed in the conclusion.

THE URBAN POPULATION IN THE TOKUGAWA PERIOD   The growth of Edo in the seventeenth century was the most remarkable event in Japan's urban history. In the sixteenth century, the site was occupied only by a number of small fishing villages and a castle, but it was strategically located on one of the largest bays in Japan and at the edge of its largest plain. Here, in 1590, the founder of the Tokugawa Shogunate began to build his new administrative capital. Edo grew so rapidly in the seventeenth century that the first survey of its population taken in 1678 listed a total commoner population of 570,361. In the period from 1734 to 1867, Edo's commoner population was always above 500,000, with a low of 501,166 in 1743 and a peak of 559,497 in 1844. However, there also existed a large unregistered population in Edo, estimated at 80,000 in the second half of the nineteenth century. Thus, a figure of 600,000 for the commoner population of Edo for much of the Tokugawa period is a reasonable estimate.[2]

Added to the commoner population must be that of the samurai class and their servants. Since the number of people connected with the warrior class was not included in the surveys of urban population, we have to "guesstimate" the number of people who occupied two thirds of the space of the city. The direct retainers of the Shogun numbered approximately 22,500 in the beginning of the eighteenth century and 26,000 at the start of the nineteenth. At a minimum, these retainers plus their households would have added 100,000 to Edo's population. But most of the space in Edo allocated to the samurai was taken up by the official residences of the 260-odd daimyo who each maintained a

---

2   See Takeuchi Makoto, "Edo no chiiki kōzō to jūmin ishiki," in Toyoda Takeshi et al. (eds.), *Nihon no hōken toshi* (Tokyo, 1983), II, 300; Ōishi, "Kyodai toshi Edo," 77–80.

residence and one or two additional establishments in the city. The daimyo had to spend half of their time in Edo to "pay attendance upon the Shogun," but in reality this requirement enabled the Shogun to keep an eye on them—a polite hostage system. Although some of the smallest daimyo probably had only a hundred or so people in residence in Edo, some of the largest had thousands. The largest daimyo, the Maeda of Kaga, maintained a regular staff of about 1,000 retainers, who with their families constituted at least 4,000 permanent residents. When the daimyo himself was in residence, it is estimated that as many as 8,000 people were in attendance. Thus even a conservative estimate of the daimyo population would require adding a few hundred thousand to the population of Edo, and this number does not include servants.[3]

To estimate Edo's population, from a base of 600,000 commoners, we would have to add a very conservative estimate of 100,000 for the Shogun's direct retainers, a minimum of 200,000 in the samurai class from the daimyo establishments, plus an unknown number of servants. Clearly a total of 1 million for Edo's population is not wild speculation. Edo was certainly much larger than London in 1700 and rivaled it in population in 1800.

Not only was Edo larger than any European city, but both Osaka and Kyoto were larger than the European capitals of Vienna, Moscow, and Berlin even at the beginning of the nineteenth century and were surpassed in size only by London and Paris. After the Battle of 1614/15, Osaka was built to become the commercial entrepôt of Japan. At its peak in 1763, it had a commoner population of 418,537. Even after Edo gradually took over many of the marketing and financial functions of Osaka, the city remained the second largest in the country with a population of 314,370 in 1858. Kyoto, the seat of the emperor, had a population recorded at 410,000 by 1534, and then, as other urban areas grew,

---

3 The samurai were originally warriors, but by the Tokugawa period this was the general term for the warrior estate or class. During the Tokugawa period, the daimyo were regional military lords who held domains assessed at 10,000 or more *koku* (a unit of rice, approximately 5 bushels). The direct retainers of the Shogun were his vassals: a minority of daimyo (*fudai*), the bannermen (*hatamoto*), and the housemen (*gokenin*). For information on the samurai, see Kozo Yamamura, *A Study of Samurai Income and Entrepreneurship* (Cambridge, Mass., 1974), 10; Naitō Akira, "Edo no toshi kōzō," *Edo jidai zushi* (Tokyo, 1975), IV, 169; Toshio G. Tsukahira, *Feudal Control in Tokugawa Japan: The Sankin Kōtai System* (Cambridge, Mass., 1966), 95.

its population fell into the mid-300,000 range from the late 1660s on.[4]

Japan's urban growth in the seventeenth century was not limited to the three largest metropolises; equally important in the long run was the proliferation of the castle towns in the same period. From the last quarter of the sixteenth century and into the seventeenth, numerous cities sprang up in the Japanese countryside. These originated as the headquarters of major daimyo and were known as castle towns, because at the center of each was the castle, which served as the domain's administrative center. Quartered here were the daimyo's forces, and to supply them there was a need for merchants and artisans. A domain's castle town usually maintained about 10 percent of the domain's total population. The commoner population of the major castle towns ranged from 10,000 up to more than 60,000 (Kanazawa) and, although their commercial activities began to be taken over by smaller towns in outlying areas in the late Tokugawa period, most of these towns remained vital centers. Half of the sixty most populous cities in Japan today originated as castle towns during the late sixteenth century.[5]

Japan also had a score of ports by the sixteenth century that ranged in size from 10,000 to 50,000, and an even larger number of cities or towns with populations in excess of 5,000. With the establishment of formal shipping routes in the Tokugawa period, the number and size of port towns increased. By the late eighteenth and nineteenth centuries, villages in the countryside had become towns, and towns had grown into cities. After the formation of the castle towns, Japan was no longer dominated by its capital, and two centuries later, with the growth of outlying centers, the castle towns were no longer the only urban areas in many domains. The Tokugawa period witnessed not only the rise of one of the largest cities in the world, but also the urbanization of Japan.[6]

4 Sekiyama, *Kinsei Nihon*, 220, 232; Osaka-shi Sanjikai, *Osaka shishi* (Tokyo, 1927), I, 482–483, 602, 880–882; (1928), II, 107, 180–181, 546, 758–759.
5 See John W. Hall, "The Castle Town and Japan's Modern Urbanization," in *idem* and Marius B. Jansen (eds.), *Studies in the Institutional History of Early Modern Japan* (Princeton, 1968), 169–188; Thomas C. Smith, "Pre-modern Economic Growth: Japan and the West," *Past & Present*, 60 (1973), 127–160; Jansen and Rozman (eds.), *Japan in Transition* (Princeton, 1986), 273–374.
6 For discussions of pre-Tokugawa urban development, see Toyoda, *Chūsei Nihon shō-*

EDO'S WATER SUPPLY SYSTEM   When Tokugawa Ieyasu selected Edo for his capital, he recognized from the outset the problem of obtaining an adequate water supply and ordered a former retainer, Ōkubo Tōgorō Tadayuki, to construct a water supply system. In 1590, Ōkubo first went to Edo to assess the situation and make plans. The system he began was so large in scale and so successful that it has been compared to that of the Romans.[7]

Although Edo was strategically situated, much of it was on low, marshy ground near the sea. The potable water was originally obtained from ponds and underground springs, but wells had to be deep because of the depth of the aquifer. The first system constructed, the Kanda system, drew its water from the Inokashira spring east of the city. Water was carried to the city limits mainly in exposed aqueducts, and then in underground aqueducts or wooden pipes within the city. The Kanda system was over forty-one miles in length and had 3,663 subsidiary ducts which drew water from the main source and distributed it to various parts of the city. Whenever possible, natural waterflow was used, but the Japanese did increase pressure at selected points to lift water from one level to another. However, the Kanda system was designed for delivering water to the lower-lying sections of the city, so that natural waterflow was usually sufficient. A problem with this system was that the water from the Inokashira spring was limited in quantity and, if too much was pumped out, the quality suffered—the water turned muddy. By the mid-seventeenth century, this system was inadequate for the growing city's needs, and a new system was begun in 1652.[8]

The second system took its water from the Tama River. Well over fifty miles in total length, it was larger than the Kanda system and carried a far greater volume of water. The Tama River system brought water up to the Yotsuya gate of Edo castle, a distance of nearly twenty-seven miles, supplying first of all the Shogun and then the nearby areas, Kōjimachi, Yotsuya, Kyōbashi, and Aka-

gyō-shi no kenkyū (Tokyo, 1952), 364–386; Sasaki Ginya, Shōgakkan Nihon rekishi (Tokyo, 1975), XIII, 260–271; Yagi Akio, "Chūsei no shōkōgyōsha to toshi," in Nakamura Kichiji (ed.), Taikei Nihon-shi sōsho (Tokyo, 1965), VIII, 328–345.

7 Higuchi Kiyoyuki, Edo (Tokyo, 1968), IV, 233.

8 Descriptions of Edo's water supply system are to be found in Horikoshi Masao, Ido to suidō no hanashi (Tokyo, 1981); Sabata Toyoyuki, Suidō no bunka: Seiō to Nihon (Tokyo, 1983); Itō Kōichi, "Edo no suidō seido," in Nishiyama Matsunosuke (ed.), Edo chōnin no kenkyū (Tokyo, 1978), V, 283–308; Higuchi, Edo, IV, 231–247.

saka. When first constructed, there was sufficient water to serve the city and also to irrigate rice paddies in Musashino, a farming area west of Edo. However, as the city expanded, the use of the Tama River system's water for irrigation had to be curtailed.

The Tama River system proved to be inadequate, not so much because of the insufficiency of water, but because of the difficulties of raising the water to higher ground as the city expanded outward. A major stimulus for continued construction of water systems was also the problem of frequent and devastating fires in Edo, which was largely constructed of wood. In the great Meireki fire of 1657, approximately two thirds of the city was destroyed; deaths were estimated in the tens of thousands. Subsequently, a policy was implemented to decrease the density of the population at the center, and many samurai mansions and temples were relocated on the outskirts of the city, leaving open spaces within the city to serve as fire breaks. Four new water systems were added—the Honjo, Aoyama, Mita, and Sengawa—all of which relied on the Tama River for their water supply and were really subsidiary to the main system. These newer systems seem not to have been entirely satisfactory for, by the mid-nineteenth century, Edo relied primarily on the original Kanda and Tama River systems. Since the Kanda system now received some of its water supply from the Tama River, Edo's water supply came mainly from that one river.

During the century that it took to build Edo's water systems, the engineering techniques became increasingly sophisticated. In the early part of the seventeenth century, ditches were the most common conduit outside city limits. For its underground aqueducts, the Kanda system used square pipes of red pine, but other early systems had pipes made of other kinds of wood, stone, earth, and bamboo. By the time the Tama River system was constructed, the engineers designing it were using triangulation, which made accurate surveying possible and helped solve the problems created by differing heights of land. Siphons were used to draw water up into Edo castle from the ducts of the Tama River system. The newer the system, the more pipes it had rather than open channels, and thus much more of the later systems were underground.[9]

9 Higuchi, *Edo*, IV, 244.

The government was not only responsible for the building of the water systems supplying Edo, but it also tightly regulated their use. No individual was permitted to draw water directly from the main system unless he were a samurai of high status, usually a daimyo or a high-ranking retainer of the Shogun. The public was supplied with water from wells built into the aqueduct system; people were required to go to the nearest well and draw water there rather than tap the nearest duct themselves. This control ensured an adequate flow of water and proper maintenance of the system.

Clearly Edo was a special case. Its water supply system was designed at the same time the city was, and the system was expanded as the city grew. Edo's system was vastly superior to the water supply systems in all other Japanese cities, most of which relied on rivers and wells for their water supply. However, with the building of the castle towns from the late sixteenth century on, water supply systems were constructed in various regions, no longer primarily for irrigation but to supply drinking water to urban populations. The first major system built primarily to supply drinking water was the Kanda, followed by systems constructed for cities not only in central Japan but also in such far-flung places as the southern tip of Kyushu. Many were built in the early seventeenth century, followed by continued construction of new systems throughout the Tokugawa period. In addition to systems designed specifically for supplying cities with potable water, numerous irrigation projects supplied drinking water as well.[10]

WASTE DISPOSAL IN OSAKA AND EDO   The methods developed for disposing of various kinds of wastes in both Edo and Osaka can be documented through regulations, contracts, and records of challenges or conflicts. The number and variety of the sources indicate that from the mid-seventeenth century on, waste disposal was a major concern for urban administrations. Osaka provides the best example of how different sewage disposal was in Japan, in contrast to Western nations, whereas Edo illustrates how complex waste disposal in a premodern Japanese metropolis was and how the problems were managed.

10   Horikoshi, *Ido to suidō*, 98–99.

The most important difference between waste disposal in Japan and in the West was that human excreta were not regarded as something that one paid to have removed, but rather as a product with a positive economic value. The night soil of Japanese cities—and Chinese as well—was long used as fertilizer. With the growth of Japan's population, the limitation of the amount of arable land and the increasingly intensified use of land to feed the growing population, combined with the relative scarcity of animal wastes and other fertilizers, meant that human waste had a value as fertilizer that far exceeded its value in the West.

Long before Edo was even established, Osaka's night soil was used as fertilizer for the surrounding farm villages. Most of it was collected, loaded onto ships, and distributed to nearby farm areas. The huge volume brought to the wharves resulted in such an unpleasant odor that there were complaints. In the Tokugawa period, the magistrates deliberated upon these complaints but concluded that "it was unavoidable for the manure boats to come into the wharves used by the tea and other ships."[11]

In the early years of the Tokugawa regime, boats were sent into Osaka loaded with vegetables and other farm produce which were exchanged for the night soil of the city. But as the price of fish and other fertilizers rose, the value of night soil rose correspondingly, and vegetables were no longer sufficient to pay for it. By the early eighteenth century, with the increase in new paddies in the Osaka area, the price of fertilizer had jumped to the point that even night soil had to be purchased with silver.

The value of human wastes was so high that rights of ownership to its components were assigned to different parties. In Osaka, the rights to fecal matter from the occupants of a dwelling belonged to the owner of the building whereas the urine belonged to the tenants. Feces were considered more valuable and hence commanded a higher price. Generally speaking, the price of fecal matter from ten households per year amounted to between two and three *bu* of silver, or over one half a *ryō* of gold. This was a considerable sum since a *ryō* during much of the Tokugawa period was sufficient to buy all the grain staple one person would eat during a year. Rent was adjusted on the basis of how many tenants there were and was raised if the number of occupants dropped.[12]

11 Wakita Osamu and Kobayashi Shigeru, *Osaka no seisan to kōtsū* (Osaka, 1973), 127.
12 Although urine is usually higher in nitrogen and potash than solid excreta and is

With the rapid growth of Osaka in the seventeenth century, the city government found by mid-century that it had to step in and form guilds to insure that waste disposal was handled properly. As the price of fertilizer rose, by the end of the century farmers from neighboring areas were forming associations for the purpose of obtaining monopsony rights to purchase night soil from various areas of Osaka. Eventually fights broke out over collection rights and prices. In the summer of 1724, two groups of villages from the Yamazaki and Takatsuki areas fought over the rights to collect night soil from various parts of the city. Other disputes arose between the guilds in the city and farmers' associations, and examples exist for the neighboring provinces of Kawachi and Settsu as well, indicating that this type of conflict was neither a localized nor an isolated event.[13]

In the three major areas of Osaka, neighboring farm villages held the rights to collect night soil from households, but they either could not or did not want to collect all of the urine. The remainder was left to be collected by *shōben nakagainin*, literally, urine jobbers. The number of jobbers gradually increased, as did jurisdictional problems. Eventually they created their own association, and in 1772 they paid a fee to the Osaka authorities to establish a *kabunakama* (guild based on ownership of shares) with the authority to enforce jurisdiction and to set prices. However, the rights to collect the urine from containers left for passersby on the street corners in Osaka were given to an outcast village named Watanabe, but even though the price of urine was lower than for fecal matter, there were constant conflicts over these collection rights. Periodically, other people tried to get these privileges away from Watanabe, but the village managed to maintain its monopoly throughout the Tokugawa period, despite sabotage of its containers, challenges by others to its collection rights, and offers to buy the rights.[14]

---

especially useful as an activator in converting crop residues to humus, it is more difficult to transport and store than solid excreta, which probably accounts for its lower price. For the price of fecal matter, see Watanabe Minoru, *Mikaihō buraku-shi no kenkyū* (Tokyo, 1965), 297. The value of a *ryō* was calculated from Yamasaki Ryūzō, "Edo chūki no bukka dōkō to keizai hendō," in Harada Toshimaru and Miyamoto Matao (eds.), *Rekishi no naka no bukka* (Tokyo, 1985), 78.

13 Wakita and Kobayashi, *Osaka*, 128.

14 Watanabe, *Mikaihō*, 292–299. See also Osaka-shi, *Osaka shishi*, I, 866–868.

In Osaka, by the mid-eighteenth century, night soil was so clearly an economic good that ownership and monopoly/monopsony rights were assigned, the formation of officially recognized associations and guilds was permitted, and the price was determined by these organizations. The price was so high that the poorer farmers had difficulty in obtaining sufficient fertilizer, and incidents of theft began to appear in the records, despite the fact that going to prison if discovered was a real risk.

In Edo, judging from official records, disputes over night soil seem not to have been the problem that they were in Osaka, but the government did have to step in to handle problems of orderly waste disposal. Edo's waste, other than night soil, can be divided into four major types: 1) household waste, probably mostly kitchen garbage; 2) trash discarded along the roads and in the waste water drains; 3) junk floating in waterways—moats, rivers, and the harbor; and 4) waste from fires. In addition, Edo had the problem of disposing of its waste water since its ample water supply meant that enormous quantities of water had to be discarded somewhere.[15]

Regulations regarding waste began to appear in Edo during the mid-seventeenth century. The focus at this time was not waste collection per se, but the growing problem of keeping the streets, open areas, and drainage ditches free from rubbish. This was clearly viewed as a problem within the purview of city government. At the same time, problems relating to the disposal of night soil came to the attention of the authorities. In 1648, city regulations required small huts and toilets along the banks of rivers to be torn down. The repeated issuance of this and other regulations over the next half century indicates that Edo residents must have been slow to comply with the new, more sanitary arrangements for waste disposal.[16]

These regulations also indicate that demand for Edo's night soil was probably not high during the early Tokugawa period and much potential fertilizer must have been wasted. However, as truck gardening developed in the area around Edo and the city

15 Hayashi Reiko, "Kinsei ni okeru jinkai shori," *Ryūtsū keizai ronshū*, VIII (1974), 72–86.
16 For information on waste disposal in Edo, see Itō, "Edo ni okeru gomi, gesui, shinyō no shori," in Toyoda, *Nihon no hōken toshi*, 431–455; Kawazoe Noboru, *Uragawa kara mita toshi* (Tokyo, 1982), 152–190.

came to rely less on a supply of daily goods from afar, the demand for night soil rose. The market for the night soil of Edo was the farm villages surrounding the city within a radius of about ten miles. By the first half of the eighteenth century, the sudden withdrawal of a particular supply of night soil could be devastating to a farmer, as alternate supplies were not easily found. A village head in the neighboring district of Tama lost his supply of fertilizer in 1725 when the main residence of the daimyo of the Owari Tokugawa burned. Before the mansion could be rebuilt, the farmer suffered major crop losses.

Contracts were given to farm villages for the night soil from specific areas in Edo. Usually each daimyo contracted out these rights, with the price determined on the basis of the market demand. For example, the Hitotsubashi daimyo sold the rights to night soil from the residence in 1742 to one Hanbei from Tanashi village in the district of Tama for the price of 1,500 large *daikon* (large white radishes), or 2,000 middle-sized *daikon*, or two *ryō* in cash, whichever Hanbei preferred, to be paid at the end of the year. Each year this daimyo house decided the price by bidding out the rights. Each daimyo made different arrangements, sometimes with the payment made twice a year, and the price as high as six *ryō* or more.

As the price of night soil rose, entrepreneurs sought rights to place containers to collect urine on busy street corners in Edo, but these petitions were denied. Since Edo was the seat of government, officials were concerned with appearance more than they seem to have been in Osaka, but they also worried about the impeding of the narrow streets and the problem of odor. One particularly innovative petition in 1789 requested permission to set out soy sauce and *sake* barrels, which would be less of an eyesore than urinals. The petitioner argued that allowing the collection of urine from passersby would add to the quantity of fertilizer, thereby reducing the price of other fertilizers, enabling farmers to use more fertilizer and produce larger harvests, and ultimately would lower price levels in general.

At the same time that the first regulations about night soil appeared, the disposal of other forms of waste was also specified. By 1655, the people of Edo were ordered to dispose of their garbage and rubbish on the island of Eitai in Edo Bay, rather than just dump it in the rivers. During the decade from 1655 to 1665, basic disposal policies were gradually put into effect: collection points for refuse collection were established in each ward; transport was contracted to specific jobbers; and the wards were ordered to bear the costs. From the ward collection points, the rubbish was loaded onto boats and transported to Eitai Island. Although the original purpose of these measures was to keep the river channels open for commerce and traffic, they resulted in the establishment of an official dump for the city located outside city limits. These policies remained in effect for the next two centuries.

The designation of Eitai Island as a dump eventually resulted in the creation of new land from the swampy ground in eastern Edo. Several other landfills also resulted in the creation of fields, so that disposing of Edo's wastes became a very profitable business. By the 1820s at least eighty contractors were involved in collecting the rubbish from Edo, encouraged in part by the creation of official organizations, the *kabunakama*. Now the townspeople had only to deposit their refuse at a collection site within the ward and pay for its collection and transportation for final disposal by a contractor. Ward fees were assessed by length of frontage and location of the property, so that, in effect, people paid a property tax. Whether renters were assessed depended on the ward.

Finally, there was the matter of drainage and disposal of waste water in Edo, which had a number of rivers and canal-like moats flowing through the city. From the number of regulations issued, the major problem seems to have been keeping the moats and river channels free from rubbish, rather than providing for drainage itself. Detailed instructions were issued: people were ordered to construct drainage channels along the fronts of their houses, under the eaves. These ditches collected runoff from the streets and roofs, as well as people's waste water. The channels, about a foot wide and a couple of feet deep, partially covered by stones to prevent people from falling in, are still to be seen in many cities, including the outskirts of modern Tokyo. Archaeological excavations in Tokyo reveal clearly the fine network of drainage ditches even within the compounds of what would be considered crowded working-class housing at best and slums at worst.[17]

Edo and Osaka were not alone among Japanese cities in their emphasis on the proper disposal of waste material and the necessity of keeping streets and waterways clean and open. Even the

17 Koizumi Hiroshi, *Edo o horu* (Tokyo, 1983), 64.

main streets in most castle towns were relatively narrow, about twenty-four feet wide, but they were "extremely well maintained and immaculately clean." The regulations regarding the maintenance of public roads were detailed and infractions were reported. In Tottori, for example, streets had to be cleared and then sprayed with water (which probably reduced the incidence of respiratory disease). In Hirado orders were issued to the effect that all bridges, gutters, and waterways should be repaired, maintained, and cleared; to make certain that this was done, officers of the town were to inspect them constantly. "No corner shall be left uncleaned." Judged by regulations alone, cleanliness and proper sanitation were of high priority among Tokugawa urban administrators.[18]

WHY JAPANESE CITIES WERE MORE HYGIENIC THAN EUROPEAN CITIES Metropolitan sanitation in Japan from the mid-seventeenth through the mid-nineteenth centuries was almost certainly better than in the West in terms of quality and quantity of the water supply and in terms of waste disposal, resulting in a healthier environment for urban populations as measured by the size of the population and mortality rates. But Japanese city life was also more sanitary than that in the West because of various customs concerning hygiene, food, and drink, and because of a lack of domestic animals. Finally, the government played a major role in setting and maintaining standards of sanitation in the cities. Evidence to support these hypotheses comes not only from descriptive material, but from comparisons made by observers from the West who visited Japan, and from the few quantitative measures we have on water quality, mortality, and life expectancy.

As already elaborated, an important difference between Japan and the West was that human excrement was an economic good in Japan, and was carefully collected for use as fertilizer, thus protecting the water supply in all phases, from source to urban pipes, and also preventing people from coming into contact with waste matter while walking on the street or in or near dumping grounds. In contrast, Westerners traditionally relied on pits in the ground, such as cesspools, for the disposal of human wastes, and

18 Murai Masuo, "Hōken-sei no seiritsu to toshi no sugata," in Morimatsu Yoshiaki et al. (eds.), *Taikei Nihon-shi sōsho* (Tokyo, 1965), XVI, 128.

the danger of polluting water supplies was ever present. Even in the 1880s, Cambridge, England, was described as "an undrained, river-polluted cesspool city." In the nineteenth century, "Leicester was typical of many towns in the way it tackled the problems of excrement removal. At mid-century it had almost 3,000 uncovered cesspits, covering 1¼ acres." Only by the end of the century had it managed to convert to a system of pails, which put an end to seepage into the sub-soil.[19]

Much has been made of the English invention of the water closet, but in the early years this system caused more problems than it solved. First, it required both a water supply and sewer system that could safely supply and remove the large quantities of water that the system used. When the water closet was first invented, Londoners flushed their wastes into the Thames, thinking that at last they were rid of a nasty problem in their houses. What they did not realize for decades was that the cause of the epidemics of infectious disease sweeping the city was the flushing of sewage into the upper Thames, since much of the city's water was taken from it downstream. Furthermore, faulty drains caused sewer gases to waft up into homes, and people with fixed basins in their bedrooms often had to cover them with towels at night, a rather primitive method of coping with this problem.[20]

Nor was the new world immune: "As late as 1849, physician John H. Griscom described the unhealthy sanitary state created on Manhattan Island by 'these thirty thousand cesspools studding it up and down, and filling the atmosphere with nauseous gases'." Stone comments that "even after the introduction of water supply systems, conditions in cities and towns remained unsanitary until properly engineered sewers replaced cesspools, beginning about 1850." Pinkney's assessment of Paris in the same year is that there was "one shockingly direct connection" between sewage disposal and the water supply. "The city drew part of its water supply from that main collector sewer, the Seine, and pumped it largely at points downstream from the mouths of sewers emptying into the river. Most of the remainder of the city's water supply came from sources little more inviting."[21]

19 Anthony S. Wohl, *Endangered Lives: Public Health in Victorian Britain* (Cambridge, Mass., 1983), 73–74, 95.
20 Thomas McKeown, *The Modern Rise of Population* (New York, 1976), 125.
21 John H. Griscom, *The Uses and Abuses of Air* (New York, 1854), 183, as quoted in

Japanese cities did not have the horrendous problems of sewage contamination of their main water supplies that London and Paris did, not only because they did not flush sewage into the rivers, but also because water in Japan tended to be purer at the source. Japan's four main islands are all dominated by mountain ranges, resulting in short, swift rivers. In addition, Japan's abundant rain, particularly during the typhoon season, helps flush out the rivers, preventing the pollution that occurs in slow, meandering water courses.

More than one scientific examination of Tokyo's water quality in the nineteenth century exists. In the mid-1870s Atkinson, an Englishman, tested Tokyo's water at various points in the system for the existence of solids, chlorine, ammonia, nitrogen, etc. At this time, it was not possible to test for bacteria content, or "germs" as they were called by Atkinson, but scientists could chemically test water for organic content which would indicate the approximate contact with raw sewage, and thus the likelihood that it would cause disease. Atkinson's survey of the Tokyo system revealed that the water was usually close to pure at the source, but the farther the samples were taken from the source, the more contaminated they proved to be. It is not surprising that his samples from surface water were contaminated; what is surprising is that early Tokyo had a water supply purer than did London. Remember that he was comparing the water supply system of a city yet to begin using modern technology with the largest city in Europe's first industrialized nation.[22]

Furthermore, Edo's system was so well designed that when it was modernized at the end of the nineteenth century, the only

May N. Stone, "The Plumbing Paradox," *Winterthur Portfolio*, XIV (1979), 292, 284. For good overviews, see Joel A. Tarr et al., "Water and Wastes: A Retrospective Assessment of Wastewater Technology in the United States, 1800–1932," *Technology and Culture*, XXV (1984), 226–263; Tarr, James McCurley, and Terry F. Yosie, "The Development and Impact of Urban Wastewater Technology: Changing Concepts of Water Quality Control, 1850–1930," in Marton V. Melosi (ed.), *Pollution and Reform in American Cities, 1870–1930* (Austin, 1980), 59–82. David H. Pinkney, *Napoleon III and the Rebuilding of Paris* (Princeton, 1958), 21.

22 R. W. Atkinson, "The Water Supply of Tokio," *Transactions of the Asiatic Society of Japan*, VI (1878), Pt. I, 96. In addition, O. Korschelt, in a paper read before the Asiatic Society of Japan on December 12, 1883, assessed the quality of wells in Tokyo and concluded that artesian wells were a suitable means of supplying water to areas of Tokyo not reached by piped in water. He was even more salutary in his assessment of Tokyo's water supply than was Atkinson.

major change was to replace the wooden pipes with impervious metal ones. Thus, the Japanese were able to use the main features of a system constructed in the seventeenth century when converting to a water supply system based on modern technology more than two centuries later. The engineering feat involved in building such a sound and large-scale system was remarkable, especially considering that dirt from the excavations for the channels and works was hauled away in baskets or straw mats.

Although London's "New River" was constructed in the same period as Edo's Kanda system, the success in bringing spring water to London in 1613 was scarcely the equivalent of the construction of the Kanda system in Edo in the same period. In London, most of the pipes were on the surface and watchmen had to be hired to deter tampering. As London expanded, the water supply became increasingly inadequate, but, unlike Edo, no ready solution was found. Pipes could be added but the supply was not increased, and so by the mid-eighteenth century Londoners could draw water only seven hours a day, three days a week. In contrast, Edo's pipes were not as strong, but they were buried and there was always a sufficient water supply twenty-four hours a day. Stoppage of water was so rare that Edo-ites made no backup arrangements for emergencies. Indeed, the Tama River system brought so much water into Edo that a waterfall in the center of the city was created from the excess, and when the Ebisu Beer Company was founded in the late nineteenth century, it was able to use the water from the Tama system.[23]

This is not to argue that the premodern Japanese water supply and waste disposal systems were without problems. When human excreta are used for fertilizer, there is always the danger of contamination—transmission of pathogens to the food supply and pollution of the water supply through runoff from fields or inadequate storage or transportation of the night soil. Although some human excreta were sold as fertilizer in the West, for the most part night soil was wasted, particularly in the largest urban areas after sewerage, or water carriage systems, were adopted. By the end of the nineteenth century, the West had some advocates of sewage farming, but public health officials, as well as the general public, had a strong bias against using human waste for

23 Sabata, *Suidō no bunka*, 32.

fertilizer. They "maintained that the raw sewage exposed farm employees to possible infection and that the vegetables grown on the farms could be the carriers of 'dangerous microbes or other parasites,' even though there was no clear evidence" of this. In fact, Asians did not merely dump raw night soil onto their fields, but they stored it at least a month in the knowledge that direct application of raw exreta was dangerous.[24]

The combination of heat and time necessary to kill various pathogens varies. Scientists also disagree or are uncertain as to the degree of contamination of water by an enteric virus that will infect a community. There are numerous documented cases of outbreaks of disease in both Asia and the West through the use of night soil or sewage for fertilizer. Thus it is difficult to determine today how safe treatments of human excreta or manure were 200 years ago. "The great majority of illnesses associated with sewage, however, appear to have been caused by application of raw or inadequately treated sewage wastewater, raw sludges, and night soil to crops which were consumed raw." And at least two studies indicate that "the predominant method of transmission of enteric viruses appears to be a direct fecal-to-oral route."[25]

It is difficult to assess the sanitation and hygiene standards of the populace in premodern times, but some information exists for elites, making possible a comparative evaluation for various nations. Although the sanitary conditions and the customs regarding personal hygiene of the elite cannot be considered representative of a society as a whole, they are indicative of what one would expect the highest standard to be. For example, in seventeenth- and eighteenth-century France, "the palaces of the Louvre, Vincennes or Fountainebleau in places became mere latrines." A house steward wrote: "In many places in the courtyard, in the upper passages, behind the doors and almost everywhere, one can see a thousand heaps of ordure, one can smell a thousand

24 Tarr, "From City to Farm: Urban Wastes and the American Farmer," *Agricultural History*, XLIX (1975), 610. F. H. King, *Farmers of Forty Centuries* (Emmaus, Pa., n.d.; orig. pub. 1911), 193–215; Reginald Reynolds, *Cleanliness and Godliness* (Garden City, 1946), 253.
25 Wylie D. Burge and Paul B. Marsh, "Infectious Hazards of Landspreading Sewage Waste," *Journal of Environmental Quality*, VII (1978), 7. Studies by G. Berg (1966) and J. W. Mosley (1972) cited in *ibid.*, 3.

unbearable stenches caused by the necessities of nature which everybody discharges there daily."[26]

In contrast, João Rodrigues, a Jesuit, who was in Japan from the late sixteenth into the early seventeenth century, noted that the Japanese

> provide their guests with very clean privies set apart in an unfrequented place far from the rooms. . . . The interior of the privies is kept extremely clean and a perfume-pan and new paper cut for use are placed there. The privy is always clean without any bad smell, for when the guests depart the man in charge cleans it out if necessary and strews clean sand so that place is left as if it had never been used. A ewer of clean water and other things needed for washing the hands are found nearby, for it is an invariable custom of both nobles and commoners to wash their hands every time after using the privy for their major and minor necessities.[27]

By the mid-nineteenth century, conditions in France were no longer so primitive, but the problems with sewage and contamination of the water supply indicated that major sanitation problems remained. In mid-nineteenth century Britain, even royalty was not immune from the effects of inadequate sewage disposal. Prince Albert, Queen Victoria's consort, is thought to have died of typhoid fever contracted from faulty drains. In contrast, in Japan in the 1870s in the privies in the "better class of private homes," an American visitor found "less annoyance and infinitely less danger . . . than are experienced in many houses of the wealthy in our great cities." His description of the privies is similar to Rodrigues' in the sixteenth century, except that attendants did not clean out the receptacle after every use, but rather it "was emptied every few days by men who have their regular routes." Morse was taken not only by the cleanliness of Japanese toilets, but also by the amount of artful carpentrywork that decorated them in homes that he visited. He was not describing the

26 Frantz Funck-Brentano, *The Old Regime in France* (London, 1929), 156. Nicholas de la Mare was house steward to the Comte de Vermandois.
27 João Rodrigues, as quoted in Michael Cooper (ed.), *They Came to Japan* (Berkeley, 1965), 221.

toilet facilities of the elite but those in the houses that he visited during his extensive stays in Japan.[28]

This is not to say that contamination from human wastes did not occur in Japan, but it was probably less frequent than in the West. And custom helped prevent Japanese from becoming ill even when their water supply was not free from impurities. The Japanese customarily drank their water boiled, usually in the form of tea, a custom remarked on by foreign visitors to Japan from the sixteenth century. With the exception of Japanese "pickles," preserved by fermentation and salt, the Japanese usually ate their food cooked, so that even if night soil was improperly applied as a fertilizer, it was less likely to make everyone sick. Within the household, each member had his own set of chopsticks, rice bowl, and teacup, which no one else used, so that it did not matter much that washing was perfunctory and in cold water. Food served outside the home was frequently finger food, and chopsticks used in restaurants were usually lacquered for easy cleaning and were not put in the mouth as were spoons in the West. By the mid-nineteenth century, disposable chopsticks had come into use.[29]

Moreover, the Japanese had strong notions about what was dirty and clean, many of which can be traced back to the Japanese native religion of Shinto and its concepts of pollution. Much of the pollution in Shinto is ritualistic, but what is considered polluting and what is purifying are related to contamination and cleanliness. Anything to do with blood, death, and illness—such as childbearing, menstruation, contact with a sick or dying person, and funerals—is considered unclean, and people used to be prohibited from participating in religious rituals, mixing with

---

28   The quotes are from Edward S. Morse, *Japanese Homes and Their Surroundings* (Rutland, 1972; orig. pub. 1887), 228, 231. See also, Wohl, *Endangered Lives*, 127; Morse, "Latrines of the East," *The American Architect and Building News*, XXXIX (18 Mar. 1893), 170–174.

29   Cooper, *They Came to Japan*, 198–199; idem, *This Island of Japon* (Tokyo, 1973), 263; Engelbert Kaempfer, *The History of Japan Together with a Description of the Kingdom of Siam, 1690–92* (Glasgow, 1906), III, 238–240. Although raw fish became popular during the Tokugawa period, particularly in large cities, it was most frequently partially preserved and fermented and not served as slices of fresh raw fish as is common today. In any case, fish came from the sea and would not have been contaminated by fertilizers. For Tokugawa dietary habits, see Watanabe, *Nihon shoku seikatsu shi* (Tokyo, 1964), 190–269; Hanley, "The Material Culture: Stability in Transition," in Jansen and Rozman (eds.), *Japan in Transition*, 454–461.

other people, and even returning home from a funeral without being purified. Salt, water, and fire were all considered purifying agents and were used both to perform religious rituals and to clean and purify. This emphasis on purification is not unique to Japan; it can be found throughout Asia, but it is particularly strong in Japan and has persisted into modern times. The strong avoidance of things dirty, while at one level almost superstitious, most certainly resulted in lack of bacterial or viral contamination for many, and impeded the spread of diseases and infections in Japan. At the everyday level, it resulted in the compulsory removal of footwear when entering a house or any other building raised from the ground, and the washing of hands after using the toilet.[30]

Japanese are known for their frequent bathing, a custom that became widespread in the Tokugawa period. Originally bathing was associated with temples, which often maintained public baths. Then, in the late sixteenth century, public baths began to appear in the largest cities, and these became so popular that by the early nineteenth century there were an estimated 600 public baths in Edo alone. The earliest baths worked on the principle of the sauna; people used relatively little hot water to steam their pores open and the dirt out. Gradually baths in which the bathers soaked in tubs of hot water began to predominate, and in time, the size of both the tubs and the bath houses increased as well. But how widespread the use of these baths was by the general public, especially women and children, is still open to question, as the bath houses had the same type of reputation as in Western cultures. Social aspects were often as important as the act of cleansing, and many of the women employed in the public baths were prostitutes. However, families that could afford them began to install baths in their homes, and the frequent mention of baths and bathing in popular literature and the depiction of them in drawings and paintings indicates how widespread the custom was. Regular laundering of clothing by the common people also began in the Tokugawa period, and the new emphasis on cleanliness must certainly have had a salutary effect on hygiene and sanitation.[31]

30 Ishige Naomichi, "Jūkyo to jū-seikatsu," in Umesao Tadao (ed.), *Nihonjin no seikatsu* (Tokyo, 1976), 29; H. Byron Earhart, *Japanese Religion* (Encino, 1974; 2nd ed.), 7; Emiko Ohnuki-Tierney, *Illness and Culture in Contemporary Japan* (Cambridge, 1984), 24.
31 Ochiai Shigeru, *Arau fūzoku-shi* (Tokyo, 1984), 71–85.

Although customs relating to hygiene within the Japanese family depended for effectiveness on individual conformity, at the public level maintenance of sanitation also depended on government. A major reason that clean streets and an adequate water supply of high quality could be maintained was the high degree of control that existed over the populace during the Tokugawa period.[32]

Government control was enhanced by two factors. First, the samurai as a class had a monopoly on government positions during the Tokugawa period. The raison d'être of this group was to govern Japan, and explicit in the neo-Confucian philosophy that the samurai adopted was the concept of rulers as benevolent, as responsible to the ruled, and as moral examples. Not only did the rulers expect such conduct from themselves, but there is evidence that the ruled expected it as well, and let the rulers know it. Second, by the mid-Tokugawa period there were more samurai than were needed to govern, and overstaffing resulted in numerous detailed regulations and sufficient officials to see that these regulations were carried out.[33]

The effect of this benevolent but thoroughgoing government can be found in the governance of Edo. The city was divided into *machi*, which were village-sized units responsible for government at the local level. This division enabled authorities to have tight control over the enormous population of the city. At large intersections in the city, the premodern equivalents of the police box were set up, not only to keep an eye out for criminal activities, but, among other things to ensure that no water pipes were leaking and that the streets were kept clear. In addition, the city authorities made use of the outcastes who lived within the city. These people not only served to keep the streets free from any dead animals, to carry away corpses, and to handle anything which ordinary residents would not touch, but also to report on anything suspicious that they found on their rounds. Thus, in the late nineteenth century, Morse could comment favorably on what

32 Hall, "Rule by Status in Tokugawa Japan," *Journal of Japanese Studies*, I (1974), 39–49.

33 Irwin Scheiner, "Benevolent Lords and Honorable Peasants: Rebellion and Peasant Consciousness in Tokugawa Japan," in Tetsuo Najita and Scheiner (eds.), *Japanese Thought in the Tokugawa Period* (Chicago, 1978), 46; Yamamura, *A Study of Samurai Income*, 47–48.

were the slums of the new city of Tokyo, less than a decade from when it had been called Edo. "In Tokio one may find streets, or narrow alleys, lined with a continuous row of the cheapest shelter; and here dwell the poorest people. Though squalid and dirty as such places appear to the Japanese, they are immaculate in comparison with the unutterable filth and misery of similar quarters in nearly all the great cities of Christendom."[34]

Finally, the Japanese did not have to cope with the density in cities that Westerners did. Tenements in Japan were one story high, not six as they commonly were in Europe. The families of the poorest daily laborers in Edo were often crammed into one-room apartments approximately nine feet square with a small entry for storing tools and footwear and for cooking. They shared toilets and access to water with other tenants in the block. But however densely these families were packed in, they were not on top of each other in multi-story buildings, nor did people live in basements. The ever-present danger from earthquakes and the light construction of Japanese housing precluded tall buildings, and the authorities forbade their construction by anyone who might be inclined to be so imprudent.[35]

Statistical evidence for the assertion that sanitation was substantially better in Japan than in Europe during the eighteenth and nineteenth centuries comes from estimates of life expectancy. Estimates for various village samples for Tokugawa Japan indicate that, by the nineteenth century, life expectancy was probably in the low forties, with five-year averages ranging from the low thirties to as high as seventy-five years. Even in the city of Takayama, for which records exist for the century from 1773 to 1871, birth and death rates were similar to the village rates: the average crude death rate for this century was 27.3 per thousand. As a metropolis, Edo probably had higher death rates than the farming villages in central Japan and certainly a lower birth rate, as the sex ratio was skewed due to the high proportion of samurai

34 Morse, *Japanese Homes*, 5–6. See Tamura Eitarō, *Chōnin no seikatsu* (Tokyo, 1966), 194–197; Harada Tomihiko, *Nihon hōken toshi kenkyū* (Tokyo, 1957), 438.

35 Robert Higgs and David Booth have found that "density effects on mortality were uniformly positive and statistically significant" in 17 American cities in 1890: "Mortality Differentials within Large American Cities in 1890," *Human Ecology*, VII (1979), 353. See also Tamura, *Chōnin no seikatsu*, 198–199; Nishikawa Kōji, *Nihon toshi-shi kenkyū* (Tokyo, 1972), 250. M. Dorothy George, *London Life in the Eighteenth Century* (New York, 1964), provides graphic descriptions of life in London.

without their families and males who migrated to the city to work. But had the death rate been significantly higher, the city would not only have had difficulty maintaining a population above a million, but contemporary Japanese would also have noted the high death rates.[36]

Tokugawa Japan and Europe in the same centuries had strikingly similar life expectancies. Life expectancy at birth in Europe in 1800 has been estimated as high as thirty-five to forty for some countries, a number higher than in the preceding centuries. Female life expectancy at birth was 42.18 in England and Wales in 1841 and 40.83 in France in 1817 to 1831. A composite figure for life expectancy for males in Western Europe in the nineteenth century, as calculated by the United Nations, is 30.6 in 1840, 41.1 in 1860, and 48.9 in 1900. Female life expectancy is estimated to have risen from 42.5 in 1840 to 52.1 by 1900. These estimates are similar to those we have for Tokugawa Japan.[37]

Although the demographic statistics available for Japan and Europe indicate a similarity in the figures, by the nineteenth century Western European nations had available modern technology and by 1850 were well into the process of industrialization with its concomitant rising standard of living. Japan, however, did not begin to use any modern technology until nearly the end of the century. Given the high proportion of Japanese who lived in cities, had sanitation been poor and the level of living low, this combination would have been reflected in high rates of morbidity and mortality.

In fact, Japan seems to have been surprisingly free from the devastating effects of epidemics. The plague never reached Japan, and cholera came only in the nineteenth century when it spread throughout the world. Intestinal worms and enteric infections—those that enter through the mouth and are spread through contamination of food and water—tended to be localized and to

36 Hanley and Yamamura, *Change in Preindustrial Japan*, 216–225; Dana Morris and Smith, "Fertility and Mortality in an Outcaste Village in Japan, 1750–1869," Hanley and Arthur P. Wolf (eds.), *Family and Population in East Asian History* (Stanford, 1985), 238–239; Yōichirō Sasaki, "Urban Migration and Fertility in Tokugawa Japan: The City of Takayama, 1773–1871," in *ibid.*, 137.

37 Joseph J. Spengler, "Demographic Factors and Early Modern Economic Development," *Daedalus* (Spring 1968), 440; United Nations, Department of Economic and Social Affairs, *The Aging of Populations and Its Economic and Social Implications* (New York, 1956), 54.

appear in endemic rather than epidemic form. This situation is what would be expected in a society which used human wastes for fertilizer. It was true for Tokugawa Japan, which would explain the relatively high death rates for children between the ages of one and four or five. Children after weaning were particularly susceptible to these diseases, but if they did not die early, they tended not to succumb to them. However, the fact that the cities with a single water source, such as Edo, Osaka, and Kyoto, did not experience rampant epidemics meant that the water supply must have been generally good.[38]

Based on the evidence available on water supply and sewage disposal systems in cities in Japan and in the West from the seventeenth through the nineteenth centuries, I argue that the level of sanitation was higher in Japanese cities than in Western ones during the same period. Not only was Japan able to provide better water and disposal systems, but Japanese customs led to better hygiene and sanitation than did Western modes of behavior. Thus Japan was able to maintain large urban populations from the sixteenth century because sanitation was better and because the Japanese had the control necessary to carry out large-scale engineering projects, to implement various systems connected with water supply and waste disposal, and to see that measures were enforced.

It might well be argued that none of the above systems, customs, or beliefs in themselves would necessarily have created more healthful conditions or been better than any sample found in the West. But the combination of them, combined with near universal application, resulted in more sanitary conditions in the city and more hygienic homes than were the norm in the West, either just prior to industrialization or in the first century of industrialization.

What has obscured the realization that the level of sanitation was higher in premodern Japanese cities than in the cities of the West in the same centuries is the fact that the situation has been the reverse in the twentieth century. In 1985, only 34 percent of Japanese communities had modern sewer systems and the resi-

38 Ann Bowman Jannetta, *Epidemics and Mortality in Early Modern Japan* (Princeton, 1987).

dents of Tamagawa Josui (Tama River Water Supply) were still without a sewer hook-up. Even after World War II, the Japanese continued to use night soil as a fertilizer and thus were seen as backward by Westerners. But it was the very success of the premodern methods for dealing with night soil that made the Japanese slow to modernize their toilet and sewage systems. In the first half of the twentieth century, the Japanese had neither the income—either private or government—nor the imminent need to spend the vast sums necessary to install flush toilets and construct water-carriage sewage systems to remove the waste water. Indeed, the very success of the premodern waste disposal system inhibited modernization in this area, for, despite the short-comings of sanitation, the Japanese today have the longest life expectancy of any major nation in the world.[39]

The rapid urbanization of the Tokugawa period and the ex-perience of the Japanese living in and administering urban centers may well have smoothed the transition of Japan from a preindus-trial to an industrial society. The Tokugawa legacy left Japan with major cities that could be easily converted into modern govern-mental and industrial centers, towns of 10,000 to 40,000 scattered throughout the country at strategic locations for governmental and economic purposes, the experience of millions of Japanese who had migrated to work in these cities under contract, and the capacity to administer large populations. This legacy meant that Japan could be transformed within decades into a modern society and could adopt modern technology more readily than if the Tokugawa experience had not occurred. It is easier to set up a modern water system if the basic system is already in place and the major task is to put in metal pipes, just as it is easier to establish universal education if education already is widespread.

The Japanese have lived in a densely populated society for nearly a millennium and have learned to live with limited re-sources on the 15 percent of the land that is not mountainous. By the Tokugawa period, the Japanese had evolved a life style that enabled them to maintain large urban populations, and this life style may well be part of the key to the success that Japan enjoys today.

39 Susan Chira, "Most Japan Houses Still Lack Comforts of Those in the U.S.," *New York Times*, 30 Oct. 1985, 1, 41.

Robert McCaa

Spanish and Nahuatl Views on Smallpox and Demographic Catastrophe in Mexico

With the 500th anniversary of European intrusion into the Americas, controversy over the demographic consequences of conquest and colonization quickened. A recent revisionist article in this journal concluded that the first old-world epidemic introduced into central Mexico, that of 1520, was "a mild attack of smallpox, such as occurred in contemporary Europe with some suffering, some deaths, and little further effect." From a cross-checking of five key sources, the author concludes that "reporting that many died of it [smallpox] must be the influence of the Franciscan myth," and "Nothing in the historical record allows us to feel confident that one-third to one-half of the Aztec population died of smallpox in 1520. No such catastrophe actually occurred."[1]

If smallpox did not contribute to demographic collapse in central Mexico in 1520, then the "catastrophe" school of contact population history is in error. If the best documented case of a "virgin soil" epidemic is wrong, the extension of the paradigm to other first encounters between Europeans and Native Ameri-

Robert McCaa is Professor of History at the University of Minnesota. He is the author of *Marriage and Fertility in Chile: Demographic Turning Points in the Petorca Valley, 1840–1976* and editor of *Latin American Population History Bulletin.*

The author thanks Ron L. McCaa for research assistance, colleagues Ward Barrett and Carla Rahn Phillips for helpful suggestions in translating sixteenth-century Spanish texts, and Ann G. Carmichael, Woodrow W. Borah, David Henige, Cecilia Rabell Romero and, especially, Francisco Guerra for their critical reading of early drafts of this article. Translations are by the author except those for which an English translation is cited. Space limitations prevent the publication of passages in the vernacular.

1   Francis J. Brooks, "Revising the Conquest of Mexico: Smallpox, Sources, and Populations," *Journal of Interdisciplinary History,* XXIV (1993), 1–29; quotations, 15, 28, 29. For informed historiographical essays on this subject, see Hanns J. Prem, "Disease in Sixteenth-Century Mexico," in Noble David Cook and W. George Lovell (eds.), *Secret Judgments of God: Old World Disease in Colonial Spanish America* (Norman, 1991), 21–48; German Somolinos d'Ardois, "Las epidemias en México Durante el siglo XVI," in Enrique Florescano and Elsa Malvido (eds.), *Ensayos sobre la historia de las epidemias en México* (Mexico City, 1982), 205; Henry F. Dobyns, "Disease Transfer at Contact," *Annual Review of Anthropology,* XXII (1993), 273–291.

cans becomes tenuous, if not untenable. Fortunately for historians, a reexamination of the Mexican case is facilitated by the many extant sources in Spanish and Nahuatl, some only recently discovered—eyewitness accounts, extensive tax records for a large number of indigenous villages and towns, many inquiries by secular and religious authorities, and chronicles by both conquerors and the conquered.

As an outsider with no stake in either the revisionist or the "High Counters" camp, I was intrigued by the radical implications of Brooks' thesis and began perusing his sources. Soon, I was lured into a rapidly escalating cross-examination of all seemingly relevant, readily available contemporary texts on the subject. Because the critique rests mainly on narratives rather than numerical evidence, I studied a wide-ranging body of sixteenth-century documents including annals, genealogies of rulers, reports, chronicles, and histories. I reexamined the five sources used by Brooks—accounts by Cortés, López de Gómara, Díaz del Castillo, and Motolinía and Sahagún, both Franciscans—and all other pertinent published sources in Spanish and Nahuatl (Table 1). I moved from a guarded sympathy for the revisionist argument to the discovery of overlooked sources, misread texts, flawed reasoning, and false analogies and, finally, to disagreement with fundamental points. I agree that an overall mortality figure of one-half for the 1520 epidemic is too high, but this fraction was discounted long ago by the principal writers on this subject. Moreover, the only source for this fraction, the *Historia de los indios de la Nueva España* (completed after 1541), is a mutilated, bastardized text attributed to, but not authored by, Motolinía.[2]

Unlike Brooks, I am confident that the impact of smallpox in New Spain was several times greater than in Europe. The alleged similarity is not corroborated by the considerable mass of evidence which has been published on this subject over the past 470 years. For the prestatistical era, precise estimates of smallpox mortality are unattainable for large regions of the world. Rather than quibble over whether the fraction of natives dying in the first smallpox epidemic was one-fifth, one-fourth, or one-third,

2 For Brooks' sources, see Table 1. Alfred W. Crosby, Jr., "Conquistador y Pestilencia: The First New World Pandemic and The Fall of the Great Indian Empires," *Hispanic American Historical Review*, XLVII (1967), 333; Toribio Motolinía, *Historia de los indios de la Nueva España* (Mexico City, 1979; 1st ed., 1858).

I canvass the sixteenth-century texts for epidemiological and demographic insights. In the end, I favor the middle ground—somewhere substantially higher than what was common to sixteenth-century Europe, but lower than the crude figure of one-half attributed to Motolinía—closer to what the Franciscan actually wrote: "in some provinces half the people died, and in others a little less."[3]

EARLY ACCOUNTS OF SMALLPOX   Brooks argued that the story of smallpox devastation originated in "Motolinía's" *Historia,* that it is the "basis (to say no more)" of subsequent descriptions of high smallpox mortality, such as those by López de Gómara and Díaz del Castillo. In Table 1, references are listed by approximate year of composition and their principal sources identified—eyewitness reports, annals, chronicles, and histories. Revisionist skepticism warns against the ready acceptance of later chronicles or histories. Yet we are faced with the reality that over the sixteenth-century many native records were destroyed by Christians in campaigns to eradicate vestiges of indigenous religion. For Spanish writers, on the other hand, there were few opportunities to publish; indeed, the important works by Cortés, López de Gómara, and Sahagún were suppressed for years, although not destroyed. Book publishing began in Mexico in the 1530s, rising to some 200 titles by the end of the century, but publication in New Spain or even Spain was an expensive and uncertain proposition. Some manuscripts on the conquest went through several copyings and enjoyed surprisingly wide circulation without being published. Others were copied by successive generations of local scribes, earlier versions having long since disappeared. Authors reworked, revised, and recopied, as new sources or interpretations appeared. Díaz del Castillo's two versions of the *Historia Verdadera* is a well-known example. The earliest copy was sent to Spain in 1576, but he continued to revise a second copy in Guatemala until

3   Toribio de Benavente o Motolinía (ed. Edmundo O'Gorman), *Memoriales o libro de las cosas de la Nueva España y de los naturales de ella* (Mexico City, 1971); idem, *Historia,* 13; in contrast to the embellished *Historia:* "in most provinces more than half died, and in others a little less." Elsewhere the text reads: "in many provinces and towns half or more of the people died, and in others less than half, or a third part." (*Memoriales,* 294). *Provincia* refers to a town or city and its surrounding villages and hamlets: "*llaman provincias los pueblos grandes, y muchas de ellas tiene poco término y no muchos vecinos*" (*Memoriales,* 245).

Table 1 The Smallpox Epidemic of 1520 in Early Colonial Accounts of the Conquest of Mexico

AUTHOR	YEARS OF COMPOSITION	YEARS OF PUBLICATION	SOURCES	SMALLPOX EPISODES CITED
Vázquez de Ayllón	1520	1866	eyewitness	Narváez' ships
Cortés[a]	1520s	1520s	eyewitness	Maxixcatzin, caciques
Martyr	1526	1520s	Cortés, reports	Cuitlahuactzin
"Historia de los mexicanos"	1530s	1882	pictographs	Cuitlahuactzin, many died
Anales de Tlatelolco I	1540s	1903	oral tradition	cocoliztli
Vázquez de Tapia	1540s	1939	eyewitness	more than one-fourth died
Motolinía Memoriales	1530–40s	1903	eyewitness	black slave, plague, half-died, some provinces
"Motolinía" Historia[a]	1540s–?	1858	Memoriales	black slave, plague, half or more died, most provinces
Sahagún[a]	1540–76	1829	native eyewitnesses	pustules, etc.
López de Gómara[a]	1540	1552	Cortés, Motolinía	two episodes: black slave, Maxixcatzin
Cervantes de Salazar	1554	1554	López de Gómara, Motolinía	little-by-little, many incidents
Díaz del Castillo[a]	1550–70s	1632	eyewitness, López de Gómara	five episodes: black slave, great mortality, Maxixcatzin, smallpox weakened warriors, Cuitlahuactzin, Chalco
Anales de Techamachalco	1564	1903	oral tradition	huey zahuatl
Aguilar	1560s	1900	eyewitness	women, soldiers
Códice Ramírez	1560	1878	oral tradition	Cuitlahuactzin
López de Velasco	1574	1894	official inquiries	never seen before
Durán	1570s	1867	Crónica X	black slave, newness
Tezozomoc	1578–98	1878	Crónica X	Cuitlahuactzin
Pomar	1580	1891	oral tradition	nursing, clothing
Muñoz Camargo	1576–85	1981	Motolinía, Sahagún	black slave; first, worst
Sahagún	1585	1840	native eyewitnesses	pustules, etc.
Anales de Tenochtitlán	1608	1902	oral tradition	totomonaliztli
Herrera	1600	1615	many, eyewitnesses	much
Chimalpahin	1620s	1889	López de Gómara, natives	many rulers died
Codex Chimalpopoca	1610–28	1945	oral tradition	many rulers died
Anales de Tlatelolco II	1700?	1948	oral tradition	bloody ears

ᵃCited by Brooks.

NOTE   For detailed discussion of sources and incidents, see text and notes.

SOURCES   Licenciado Lucas, Vázquez de Ayllón, "Relacion que hizo el Licenciado Lucas Vázquez de Ayllón, de sus diligencias para estorbar el rompimiento entre Cortés y Narváez," in Pascual de Gayangos (ed.), *Cartas y relaciones de Hernan Cortés al Emperador Carlos V* (Paris, 1866), 39, 42.

Hernando Cortés, *Cartas de Relación* (Mexico City, 1971; Biblioteca Imperial de Viena Ser. Nov. 16000).

Peter Martyr (trans. Francis August MacNutt), *De Orbe Novo: The Eight Decades of Peter Martyr D'Anghera* (New York, 1970; orig. ed., 1912).

"Historia de los mexicanos por sus pinturas," in Joaquín García Icazbalceta (ed.). *Nueva Colección de Documentos para la historia de México (siglo XVI)* (Mexico City, 1891; 2d ed., 1965), 209–240 (only the second edition contains the pictures).

Jesús Monjarás-Ruiz, Elena Limón, and María de la Cruz Paillés H. (eds.). *Obras de Robert H. Barlow, Tlatelolco: Fuentes e Historia* (Mexico City, 1989), II, 261–263.

German Vázquez (ed.), *Relación de méritos y servicios del conquistador Bernardino Vázquez de Tapia* (Madrid, 1988).

Toribio de Benavente o Motolinía (ed. Edmundo O'Gorman), *Memoriales o libro de las cosas de la Nueva España y de los naturales de ella* (Mexico City, 1971).

Toribio Motolinía, *Historia de los indios de la Nueva España* (Mexico City, 1979; orig. ed., 1858).

Bernardino de Sahagún (eds. Charles E. Dibble and Arthur J. O. Anderson), *Florentine Codex: General History of the Things of New Spain* (Santa Fe, 1955–75), XII, 81; *idem*, (trans. Howard F. Cline, ed. S. L. Cline), *The Conquest of New Spain: 1585 Revision* (Salt Lake City, 1989).

Francisco López de Gómara (ed. Carlos María de Bustamante), *Historia de las Conquistas de Hernando Cortés* (Mexico City, 1826).

Francisco Cervantes de Salazar (ed. Manuel Magallón), *Crónica de la Nueva España* (Madrid, 1971, Biblioteca de Autores Españoles vol. 245).

Bernal Díaz del Castillo, *Historia Verdadera de la Conquista de la Nueva España* (Mexico City, 1960; 5th ed.).

"Crónica local y colonial el idioma náhuatl, 1398 y 1590: Anales de Tecamachalco," in Antonio Peñafiel (ed.). *Colección de Documentos Para la Historia Mexicana* (Mexico City, 1993), 7.

Francisco (Alonso) de Aguilar, *Relación breve de la conquista de la Nueva España* (Mexico City, 1977).

Códice Ramírez manuscrito del siglo XVI intitulado: Relación del origen de los indios que habitan esta Nueva España según sus historias (Mexico City, 1975; orig. ed., 1878).

Juan Bautista Pomar, "Relación del Tezcoco," in Icazbalceta (ed.), *Nueva Colección*.

Juan López de Velasco, *Geografía y descripción universal de las Indias* (Madrid, 1971).

Diego Muñoz Camargo (ed. Rene Acuña), *Descripción de la Ciudad y Provincia de Tlaxcala de las Indias y del mar océano para el buen gobierno y enoblecimiento dellas* (Mexico City, 1981; reprint ed.).

Anales de Tenochtitlán (Codex Aubin) in James Lockhart (ed. and trans.). *We People Here: Nahuatl Accounts of the Conquest of Mexico* (Berkeley, 1993). 43, 279.

Antonio Herrera y Tordesillas, *Historia General de los Hechos de los Castellanos* (Madrid, 1936; orig. ed., 1601–15).

Chimalpahin (ed. and trans. Silvia Rendón), *Relaciones originales de Chalco Amaquemecan escritas por Don Domingo Francisco de San Antón Muñón Chimalpahin Cuauhtlehuanitzin* (Mexico City, 1965).

John Bierhorst, *History and Mythology of the Aztecs: The Codex Chimalpopoca* (Tucson, 1992).

Anales de Tlatelolco II in Lockhart *We People Here*, 37–42, 259.

his death in 1584. The first was printed in a bastardized edition almost a half-century after his death (1632); the second was not published until 1904.[4]

Representative of the annals genre is the *Anales de Tlatelolco,* two copies of which survive. The first was probably written in the 1540s and the second in the late seventeenth or early eighteenth century, but both purport to incorporate pictographs and texts created much earlier. The writings of Motolinía and Sahagún suffered similar travails. The *Historia* attributed to Motolinía was a hurried copy of his *Memoriales* (portions of which have since been lost) made, probably in Spain, by a copyeditor/publicist who lacked training in Nahuatl and also lacked Motolinía's zeal for accuracy.[5]

At issue here is the course of smallpox in a nine-month period from April 1520, when Pánfilo de Narváez landed an expeditionary force near Veracruz, to January 1521, when Cortés returned to the Central Valley of Mexico to resume his efforts to conquer the Aztec capital, Tenochtitlan.

The earliest Spanish recording of smallpox in central Mexico, dated August 30, 1520, is a report to Charles V by Vázquez de Ayllón, judge of the Real Audiencia of Santo Domingo. This report, first published in 1866, has gone unnoted by most historians. Judge Vázquez de Ayllón, writing only a few months after the event, described a voyage with the Narváez flotilla to Cozumel, an island off the east coast of the Yucatán peninsula, and then to Veracruz. On Cozumel he found very few natives and attributed their disappearance to smallpox. According to the judge, the natives had been "stuck" (*pegado*) by the disease introduced by Indians from the island of Fernandina (Cuba) who were brought to Cozumel as auxiliaries in the company of Spaniards.

4 Brooks, "Revising the Conquest," 22; Bernal Díaz del Castillo, *Historia Verdadera de la Conquista de la Nueva España* (Mexico City, 1960; 5th ed.). See also *idem* (Carmelo Saenz de Santa María), *Historia Verdadera de la Conquista de Nueva España* (Madrid, 1982), which reprints the "Remón" edition. J. Benedict Warren, "An Introductory Survey of Secular Writings in the European Tradition on Colonial Middle America, 1503–1818," in Robert Wauchope (ed.), *Handbook of Middle American Indians* (Austin, 1973), XIII, 67.

5 James Lockhart (ed. and trans.), *We People Here: Nahuatl Accounts of the Conquest of Mexico* (Berkeley, 1993), 38–42; Edmundo O'Gorman, *Incognita de la llamada 'Historia de los indios de Nueva España' atribuida a Fray Toribio Motolinía* (Mexico City, 1982), 68; Jaime González Rodríguez, "La difusión manuscrita de ideas en Nueva España (siglo XVI)," *Revista Complutense de Historia de América,* XVIII (1992), 89–116.

Vázquez de Ayllón had no theory of contagion, but his report shows that he understood how the pasty mucous of smallpox spread (*pegado* as in *pegante,* originally, fish-paste).[6]

After a deadly crossing during which a tropical storm destroyed a half-dozen ships and scattered the remainder, the flotilla regrouped to land near Veracruz and the native settlement of Cempoala. Smallpox broke out almost immediately. Vázquez de Ayllón reports that great harm had been inflicted on those lands [New Spain] because smallpox had struck the Indians there ("*porque han pegado las viruelas a los indios dellas*"). The report states unequivocally that smallpox was carried from Fernandina to the mainland by natives in the Narváez expedition. Unfortunately for the historical record, by mid-May Pánfilo de Narváez rebelled against the judge (who by this time had fallen ill also), forced him and his party onto a ship and sent them back to Cuba to be deposited in the hands of Diego Velasquez, Narváez' sponsor. Thanks to political intrigue and a second storm, the ship was carried instead to a remote corner of Hispaniola. Vázquez de Ayllón disembarked, trekked across the island on foot, and arrived safely at Santo Domingo, where he drafted a lengthy account of the affair for the emperor.[7]

This eyewitness report on events within the Narváez camp ends several weeks before the well-known confrontation with Cortés and before any large-scale effects of the introduction of smallpox could be observed. The smallpox story received only a few lines in Vázquez de Ayllón's report. Yet, the fact that disease is mentioned at all in a record detailing mutiny, subversion, and possibly the loss of a valuable colony hints at the significance of the eruption of pestilence in "those lands." The epidemic is important to the story because it reveals the recklessness of Velasquez' mutiny and his utter disregard for the prosperity both of Fernandina and of the new lands. The severity of what Vázquez de Ayllón saw with respect to smallpox is limited to the brief

6 Licenciado Lucas Vázquez de Ayllón, "Relación que hizo el licenciado Lucas Vázquez de Ayllón, de su diligencias para estorbar el rompimiento entre Cortés y Narváez," in Pascual de Gayangos (ed.), *Cartas y relaciones de Hernan Cortés al Emperador Carlos V* (Paris, 1866), 39, 42.

7 *Ibid.,* 39. For other testimony on the use of Indian auxiliaries from Fernandina, see the early account by Juan Díaz, *Provincias y regiones recientemente descubiertas en las indias occidentales, en el ultimo viaje* (Mexico City, 1972), 54; Crosby, "Conquistador y Pestilencia," 328.

phrase *"han hecho mucho daño"* (has caused great harm), but its significance required no elaboration for the emperor's advisors or others who were familiar with the demographic catastrophe unfolding in the islands.[8]

The introduction of smallpox among the Aztecs is frequently attributed to a black slave, given the name—Francisco Eguía—in one account. Hallowed by repetition, this story has become something of a trope—unlike the almost ignored tale of "Joan Garrido," also a black slave, the first to sow and harvest wheat in Mexico. The anecdote of the smallpox-infected slave occurs in most Spanish chronicles of the conquest (those by Motolinía, López de Gómara, and Díaz del Castillo—but not Cortés or Sahagún), in native-mestizo accounts such as the *Relación Geográfica* for Tlaxcala by Muñoz Camargo, the *Codex Ramírez,* Ixtlilxochitl's *Décima Tercia Relación,* and even in many modern textbook descriptions of the conquest of Mexico.[9]

According to Brooks, reciting the story undermines the credibility of all would-be chroniclers of smallpox in two ways. First, it reveals their dependence on Motolinía, the first-known written account of the tale and, second, "Motolinía's" own *Historia* is fable, an exercise in "mythopoesis," a strained allegory for the biblical account of the Ten Plagues. Brooks reasons that Motolinía needed an "Ethiopian" and that without a theory of contagion, no Spaniard would have made the connection much less remembered a source for the disease.[10]

Whether smallpox was introduced by a black slave, by Cuban Indians, or by both is important only for determining the validity of sources. No historian, not even Brooks, doubts that smallpox reached central Mexico for the first time in April or May 1520,

---

8 Vázquez de Ayllón, "Relación," 42.

9 Motolinía, *Memoriales,* 21; Francisco López de Gómara (ed. Carlos Maria de Bustamante), *Historia de las Conquistas de Hernando Cortés* Mexico City, 1826), I, 278; Díaz del Castillo, *Historia Verdadera,* I, 378; Francisco A. de Icaza, *Conquistadores y pobladores de Nueva España* (Madrid, 1923), I, 98; Andrés de Tápia, "Relacion hecha por el señor Andrés de Tápia sobre la conquista de México," in Joaquín García Icazbalceta (ed.), *Colección de documentos para la historia de México* (Mexico City, 1858), II, 593; Bernardino de Sahagún (trans. Howard F. Cline, ed. S. L. Cline), *The Conquest of New Spain: 1585 Revision* (Salt Lake City, 1989), 183; *Códice Ramírez manuscrito del siglo XVI intitulado: Relación del orígen de los indios que habitan esta Nueva España según sus historias* (Mexico City, 1975; orig. ed., 1878); D. Fernando Alva Ixtlilxochitl, *Décima tercia relación de la venida de los españoles y principio de la ley evangélica* (Mexico, 1938).

10 Brooks, "Revising the Conquest," 24–25.

with the arrival of the Narváez expedition. As to the theory of contagion, the Spanish vernacular has long provided a simple, but credible notion of how the disease was spread—in a word, *pegar* (to stick or adhere).[11]

From May to September 1520, smallpox spread slowly inland, 150 miles to Tepeaca and Tlaxcala, and then on to Tenochtitlan in September or October. A second eyewitness account of smallpox is reported in another letter to Charles V, that by Cortés dated May 15, 1522, ten months after the fall of Tenochtitlan. Cortés, seeking to justify his transgressions and to position himself to claim vast rewards from the newly conquered lands, provided an exceedingly detailed report of his actions. He described the high regard which native leaders had for him and thereby justified his usurpation of royal authority in appointing native rulers. Cortés wrote that "many chieftains were dying and they wished that by my hand and with your approval and mine others be put in their place." The many deaths of leaders were due to "the smallpox distemper *which also enveloped those of these lands like those of the islands.*" I emphasize what Brooks' paraphrase omitted: Cortés' explicit comparison of the impact in New Spain with what had happened in the islands.[12]

The guessing about how many natives peopled the islands before 1492 continues without relief (ranging for Hispaniola from 8 million to as few as 60,000), but there is widespread agreement that depredation and disease drove the native population to near extinction by 1520. Within a decade of first contact in 1492,

11 Prem, "Disease," 24. The first record of smallpox in the islands is late 1518, nearly six months after the Grijalva expedition departed from Cabo San Antón (Cuba) on May 1, 1518, and shortly before Cortés' departure for Cozumel on February 18, 1519. Narváez probably left Cuba as the epidemic peaked, arriving at Cozumel, March 4, 1520. Juan de Grijalva (trans. Henry R. Wagner), *The Discovery of New Spain in 1518 by Juan de Grijalva* (Berkeley, 1942), 26; David Henige, "When Did Smallpox Reach the New World (And Why Does It Matter)?," in Paul E. Lovejoy (ed.), *Africans in Bondage: Studies in Slavery and the Slave Trade* (Madison, 1987), 17; López de Gómara, *Historia*, I, 14; Manuel Orozco y Berra, *Historia Antigua y de la Conquista de México* (Mexico City, 1880), IV, 365–367. After three decades of historiographical infighting, Dobyns' smallpox chronology for the islands and central Mexico remains firmly in place ("An Outline of Andea Epidemic History to 1720," *Bulletin of the History of Medicine*, XXXVII (1963), 494–495.

12 Hernando Cortés, *Cartas de Relación* (Mexico City, 1971), Biblioteca Imperial de Viena Ser. Nov. 16000), 105; a modern translation is given in Crosby, "Conquistador y Pestilencia," 334. Where I translate *comprendió* as "enveloped," a popular English edition of Cortés' letters favors "raged"; see Cortés, *Five Letters* (New York, 1962), 136. Brooks, "Revising the Conquest," paraphrase, 20.

Spaniards turned to raiding nearby islands for slaves, the favored method for replenishing the labor supply. The near-demise of natives on the islands was used to justify Cortés' expedition of 1519. His license was not to conquer or settle "those lands," but to "acquire knowledge and measure the said land, and to bring captive Indians from there, from which they could serve on the island of Cuba to prospect for gold and the other things for which they are needed." Cortés chose instead to conquer, and his letters to the emperor were designed to justify his disobedience as a means of gaining a great reward.[13]

In an earlier letter to the emperor dated October 30, 1520, Cortés did not comment on smallpox or appointing chieftains to leadership. It is likely that some deaths of smallpox-infected chieftains had occurred by that date, but Cortés chose to bide his time until the wisdom of his usurpations could be made clear to the emperor. Cortés' letters, regardless of length, were not histories, but rather briefs, written to advance his cause in the eyes of Charles V. The relevance of smallpox was to warrant Cortés' actions. Otherwise disease is scarcely mentioned in his letters. From 1520 to 1526, Cortés addressed some 250 pages of correspondence to the emperor, but his account of smallpox amounts to less than a half-page of text.[14]

Cortés names only one leader who died of smallpox, Maxix-catzin, a Tlaxcalan. In 1519, Maxixcatzin was the first highland ruler to embrace Cortés' cause, and then, following the *Noche Triste* (June 30, 1520), the first to provide succor to the badly beaten cristianos. In the ensuing weeks, when the Mexica sought to press their victory by rallying all the native kingdoms against the invaders, Maxixcatzin spoke forcefully and persuasively for Tlaxcalans to remain loyal to Cortés. Fortunately for Cortés,

13 Cook, "Disease and Depopulation of Hispaniola, 1492–1518," *Colonial Latin America Review,* II (1993), 215. The governors of Hispaniola, the Heronymite Fathers, compare the devastation of the native population with the sparse fruit which remains in the orchard after harvest. Their assessment comes one year *before* smallpox struck (cited in Angel Rosenblat, *La población indígena y el mestizaje en América* (Buenos Aires, 1954; orig. ed., 1935), I, 297: *"cuanto es el redrojo que queda en los árboles después de cogida la fruta"*). Cortés, *Cartas de Relación,* 3 (letter dated July 10, 1519).
14 Gonzalo Fernández de Oviedo y Valdés relates Cortés' story in Juan Pérez de Tudela Bueso (ed.), *Historia general y natural de las Indias* (Madrid, 1959), V, 84.

Maxixcatzin's death from smallpox occurred after the loyalty of his people had been assured, but the precise date is unrecorded.[15]

CUITLAHUACTZIN AND OTHER NATIVE RULERS DIED OF SMALLPOX

Although Brooks flatly denied it, Cuitlahuactzin, the Mexican ruler, also died of smallpox, as did many other native rulers, allies and enemies alike. Within a pair of parentheses, Brooks would consign to the historian's dustbin the standard story of the Mexica hero's death from smallpox—without citing a single source or authority. The most trustworthy indigenous source, the *Anales de Tenochtitlan* (Codex Aubin), chronicled Cuitlahuatzin's death: "The tenth ruler was installed in *Ochpaniztli*, Cuitlahuatzin. He ruled for only eighty days; he died at the end of *Quecholli* of the pustules (smallpox), when the Castilians had gone to Tlaxcala." This account placed the death in the month of *Quecholli*, which in 1520 fell in late November or early December (not August or September as Brooks stated), scarcely a month before Cortés renewed the assault on the Mexican stronghold, Tenochtitlan.[16]

Some confusion about Cuitlahuatzin's death may arise because Cortés did not report the event. Indeed, Cortés' letters scarcely acknowledged the name of his most formidable opponent. On the night of June 30, the *Noche Triste*, when Cortés' troop fought their way out of Tenochtitlan, Cuitlahuactzin's forces nearly annihilated the castellanos and their Tlaxcalan auxiliaries. López de Gómara cited Cuitlahuactzin's military and diplomatic successes in rallying the natives and also reported the death as occurring from smallpox, before Christmas 1520. Díaz del Castillo remembered Cuitlahuactzin as "the lord who ejected us from Mexico" and attributed his death to smallpox as also having occurred before Christmas. Motolinía cannot be the source for these accounts because the Franciscan chronicler, like Cortés, did not mention Cuitlahuactzin. In Spain, Cuitlahuactzin's death is first chronicled by Martyr in *De Orbe Novo*, written before his own death in 1526. Martyr reported that Cuitlahuactzin (incorrectly referred to as "Hastapalappa," the name of the place he last

15 Cortés, *Cartas de Relación*, 105.
16 Brooks, "Revising the Conquest," 20; *Anales de Tenochtitlan* (Codex Aubin) in James Lockhart (ed. and trans.), *We People Here: Nahuatl Accounts of the Conquest of Mexico* (Berkeley, 1993), 279.

ruled) "had been named king at Temistitan [Tenochtitlan], but after a reign of four months had died of smallpox and had been succeeded by his sister's son, Catamazin [Cuauhtémoc]." Martyr did not reveal his sources, but he was not following any of Cortés' extant *Cartas*.[17]

Sixteenth-century indigenous annals told the same story: "Upon the death of Mutezuma those of Mexico made Cuitlavazi from Estapalapa, brother of Mutezuma, their leader. He was lord for eighty days: smallpox was given to all the Indians and many died, before they [the Castilians] returned to conquer the city." The *Crónica Mexicayotl*, written down in 1609, interpreted "*Quecholli*" as December 3 and noted as well the death of Axayacatzin, Cuitlahuactzin's son, also from smallpox (*totomonalliztli*). Sahagún's personal history of the conquest, completed in 1585, confirmed these accounts and tersely assessed the military significance of the epidemic: "Among the Mexicans who fell victim to this pestilence was the lord Cuitlahuactzin, who they had elected a little earlier. Many leaders, many veteran soldiers, and valiant men who were their defense in time of war, also died." Orozco y Berra, a meticulous nineteenth-century Mexican historian, ascribed Cuitlahuactzin's death to smallpox, dated about November 25.[18]

The Nahuatl sources that report "cause of death" agree that Cuitlahuactzin succumbed to an unusual, terrible pestilence—reported variously as *cocoliztli* (illness, great plague or pestilence, smallpox), *huey zahuatl* (great pestilence of smallpox, great ulcerous leprosy), or *totomonaliztli* (blisters, smallpox). These generic terms describe visible symptoms. A precise translation is impossible because there was nothing like smallpox in the Nahuatl lexicon. Barlow interpreted *totomonaliztli* as *calenturas* (fevers) and Lockhart favored "pustules." A sixteenth-century *mexicana-castellana* dictionary defined the root term *totomonaltia* as *hazer a otro bexigas o ampollas* (to make blisters or pustules [of smallpox] under the skin of another). The *Anales de Tenochtitlan* recorded Cuitla-

17 Sahagún, *Conquest*, 103; López de Gómara, *Historia*, II, 14; Díaz del Castillo, *Historia Verdadera*, I, 414; Peter Martyr (trans. Francis August MacNutt), *De Orbe Novo:* The Eight Decades of Peter Martyr D'Anghera (New York, 1970; orig. ed., 1912), II, 149.
18 "Historia de los mexicanos por sus pinturas," in Icazbalceta (ed.), *Nueva Colección de Documentos para la historia de México (siglo XVI)* (Mexico City, 1891; 2d. ed., 1965), 233 (only the 2d ed. contains the pictures); Hernando Alvarado Tezozomoc (ed. Adrián León), *Crónica Mexicayotl* (Mexico City, 1949), 160. I follow Manuel Orozco y Berra's chronology in *Historia Antigua* (Mexico City, 1880), IV, 364–372. Sahagún, *Conquest*, 103.

huatzin's reign and death. The accompanying pictograph showed his enshrouded corpse encircled with tiny globes (*ampollas*), the symbol for smallpox according to Orozco y Berra. Chimalpahin, the historian of Chalco, also attributed the death to "pustules and ulcers from smallpox" (*ampollas y llagas de viruelas* [*çahuatl*]).[19]

The evidence that smallpox ravaged the native elites pervades the historical record. The story is significant because the epidemic devastated native diplomatic and military capabilities precisely as Cortes prepared to renew his assault on Tenochtitlan. Chimalpahin, a native historian, reported the smallpox-inflicted deaths of some of the lords of Chalco, using the word *çahuatl* four times in a brief passage. A Nahuatl-French edition of Chimalpahin's *Séptima Relación* first published a century ago, invariably translated *çahuatl* as "*variole*" (smallpox). Chimalpahin reported:

Year 2-flint, 1520. Then there was the plague [*çahuatl*] which caused great mortality. From it died the Huehue Yotzintli Tlayllótlac Teuhctli, Señor of Tzacualtitlan Tenanco Amaquemecan. He ruled thirty-three years.

19 All of the most important sources which mention Cuitlahuatzin's death agree on the essentials, although none in the same words. Consider the following: Jesús Monjarás-Ruiz, Elena Limón, and María de la Cruz Paillés H. (eds.), *Obras de Robert H. Barlow, Tlatelolco: Fuentes e Historia* (Mexico City, 1989), II, 263; Tezozomoc, *Crónica mexicayotl*, 160; Bernardino de Sahagún (eds. Charles E. Dibble and Arthur J. O. Anderson), *Florentine Codex: General History of the Things of New Spain* (Santa Fe, 1955–75), VIII, 4, 22; *idem, Conquest*, 103; López de Gómara, *Historia*, II, 14; Díaz del Castillo, *Historia Verdadera*, I, 414; "Historia de los mexicanos," in Icazbalceta (ed.), *Nueva Colección*, 233; Ixtlilxochitl, *Décima tercia relación*, 13; *Anales de Tenochtitlan* in Lockhart, *We People Here*, 279; Chimalpahin (ed. and trans. Silvia Rendón), *Relaciones originales de Chalco Amaquemecan escritas por Don Domingo Francisco de San Antón Muñón Chimalpahin Cuauhtlehuanitzin* (Mexico City, 1965), 236.

Notwithstanding the relative late recording of the Tenochtitlan annals, Lockhart concluded that "in all likelihood he [the writer] has given us quite untouched and authentic elements of Tenochca oral and written tradition." Most authorities think the Annals were written in 1528, but Lockhart argued that internal linguistic evidence suggests the 1540s as a more likely date of composition (Ibid., 39). In any case, this is an early indigenous source based on oral tradition.

The Spanish loan word for smallpox, viruelas, does not enter written Nahuatl until the late sixteenth-century. The imputation of smallpox in this translation is by Lockhart; see also Alonso de Molina, *Vocabulario en lengua castellana y mexicana y mexicana y castellana* (Mexico City, 1970; orig. ed., 1571), 150v. Other episodes of smallpox in 1520 are discussed in Chimalpahin, *Relaciones originales*, 158. Although written in Nahuatl after 1620, these *relaciones* were based on pictographs and oral traditions (Lockhart, *We People Here*, 39). The interpretation of the pictographic evidence is Orozco y Berra, *Historia Antigua*, IV, 493, n. 1.

And from this same thing died his adviser . . . Also of smallpox [*çahuatl*] died Señora Tlacocihuatzin . . . From the same cause died Itzcahuatzin y Tlatquic, from Itzcahuacan, who succeeded in governing thirty-five years and his own son, the said Necuametzin [also died of smallpox] . . .

Díaz del Castillo attested as well that the lord of Chalco died of smallpox, but López de Gómara only noted the death without stating the cause. Cortés scarcely mentioned the Chalco incident, and Motolinía ignored it entirely. The absence of comments by Cortés or Motolinía is insignificant because there is ample independent evidence of smallpox striking down many of the native elite.[20]

Other Nahuatl sources related the epidemic in a single sentence, such as the *Anales de Tlatelolco,* where some 4,000 words were allotted to the conquest but only two lines to the epidemic: "Then a plague [*cocoliztli*] broke out of coughing, fever, and pox [*çahuatl*]. When the plague [*cocoliztli*] lessened somewhat, (the Spaniards) came back." In Cuauhtitlan, the entry for 1520 reads: "Then Yohualtonatiuh was inaugurated. It was in his time that the Spaniards arrived. Both Citlalcoatl and Yohualtonatiuh died of the smallpox." Outside the central basin and fifty miles southeast of Puebla in the district of Tepeaca, the surviving copy of the *Annals of Tecamachalco,* which dates from the 1590s, chronicled the event-of-the-year for 1520 as "very frightful great smallpox" ("*cenca temahmauhti ynic mo chiuh huey zahuatl*"). This chronicle omitted any mention of conquest or deaths due to war. Smallpox was the event for 1520.[21]

The best test would be to tally all the Nahuatl annals by whether smallpox is or is not mentioned for 1520. Pending that exercise, it is evident that any survey of native annals and picto-

20 Chimalpahin wrote that many regional native leaders died of disease within a year of paying homage to the Spaniards in Tenochtitlan. See Susan Schroeder, *Chimalpahin & the Kingdoms of Chalco* (Tucson, 1991), 34. Chimalpahin (trans. Rémi Siméon), *Annales de Domingo Francisco de San Antón Muñón Chimalpahin Quauhtlehuanitzin: Sixième et Septième Relations (1258–1612)* (Paris, 1889); Díaz del Castillo, *Historia Verdadera,* I, 414; López de Gómara, *Historia,* II, 23.
21 *Anales de Tlatelolco II* in Lockhart, *We People Here,* 259; John Bierhorst, *History and Mythology of the Aztecs: The Codex Chimalpopoca* (Tucson, 1992), 79; "Crónica local y colonial en idioma náhuatl, 1398 y 1590: Anales de Tecamachalco," in Antonio Peñafiel (ed.), *Colección de Documentos Para la Historica Mexicana* (Mexico City, 1903), 7.

graphs will show widespread, almost universal reference to the epidemic and its devastation of the native elite.

The military significance of the pestilence was enormous. Upon accession Mexica rulers quickly sought to establish hegemony and legitimacy through force, by raiding subject towns. In 1520, with the sudden death of Cuitlahuatzin and the ascent of the youthful Cuauhtémoc, there was no opportunity to impose allegiance through war. Instead, Cortés proceeded to pick off subject-towns, often through diplomacy, one-by-one. An authoritative military history contended that ultimately: "Cortés' victory was more political than military, . . . With the fall of Tenochtitlan, the rest of Mesoamerica fell to Spanish domination with little or no struggle."[22]

MOTOLINIA AND OTHER CONTEMPORARY SOURCES Brooks questioned the veracity of supposed eyewitness accounts of the epidemic claiming that they were derived from a "Franciscan myth," a history authored by Motolinía and tailored to fit biblical prophecy. Brooks saw "Motolinía's" Historia as the keystone in the argument that smallpox devastated Mexico in 1520. The commonalties among the texts were seen as weakening their credibility, but common threads may strengthen the fabric, reenforcing agreement on key themes. Brooks suggested that López de Gómara copied from the Historia and, in turn, Díaz del Castillo from López de Gómara, yet their descriptions differ, as shown in Table 2. López de Gómara repeatedly acknowledged his dependence upon Motolinía—a fact long recognized by Mexicanists—but Cortés' secretary also used a variety of other sources, some of which are no longer available. In turn, Díaz del Castillo's "True History" was written, in part, to correct the excesses of López de Gómara's "Conquistas de Cortés." I was surprised to discover that Motolinía reported only one anecdote regarding smallpox, whereas López de Gómara recounts three, and Díaz del Castillo, five.[23]

Motolinía's uniqueness lies in his use of biblical allegory and the observation that natives did not know how to deal with

22 Ross Hassig, War and Society in Ancient Mesoamerica (Berkeley, 1992), 164.
23 Brooks, "Revising the Conquest," 21–23; López de Gómara, Historia, I, 278; Motolinía, Memoriales, xcviii, n. 32, 21.

Table 2 Smallpox Anecodotes in Motolinía, Gómara, and Díaz del Castillo

DESCRIPTIONS	MOTOLINÍA	GÓMARA	DÍAZ DEL CASTILLO
Cempoala ("esta tierra")			
plague	yes	–	–
black slave as source	yes	yes	yes
"pegar" (Indians)	yes	yes	yes
slept and ate together	–	yes	–
great sickness	yes	yes	–
great mortality	–	–	yes
some province, half	yes	yes	–
did not know the remedy	yes	–	–
bathe often	yes	yes	yes
no one to make bread	yes	yes	–
everyone in a house	yes	yes	–
pulled the houses down on them	yes	yes	–
covered with the pox	yes	–	yes
leprous	yes	yes	–
filled with holes	yes	yes	–
Tlaxcala: Cortés' appointing leaders (Maxixcatzin)			
Maxixcatzin	–	yes	yes
many leaders died of smallpox	–	yes	yes
pox so common	–	–	yes
Indians from distant lands	–	–	yes
Entry to the Valley of Mexico			
smallpox weakened warriors	–	–	yes
Tenochtitlan			
Cuitlahuatzin died from smallpox	–	yes	yes
Chalco			
leader died of smallpox	–	–	yes

NOTE   "–" signifies not mentioned.

SOURCES   López de Gómara, *Historia,* I, 278; Motolinía, *Memoriales,* 21; Díaz del Castillo, *Historia Verdadera,* I, 373, 378, 425, 438, II, 379.

smallpox. López de Gómara, unlike other chroniclers, described pox as hitting (*pegó*) a single house in "Zempóalam" (implied, but not stated in Motolinía) and then spreading "from one Indian to another and because the Indians were many and slept and ate together, spreading widely and quickly, killing as it went throughout that land"—other details which went unreported by Motolinía. Díaz del Castillo was present in Cempoala before the smallpox attack had subsided. He related its spread in terms of "striking and filling all the land with it [smallpox]", "from which there was great carnage and according to what the Indians said they had never had this illness before." These authors agreed on the severity of the attack, but they never cited the same set of episodes to prove their points.[24]

Any assertion that Díaz del Castillo never saw smallpox in Mexico is simply false. Díaz del Castillo arrived in Cempoala in May 1520 and was present later in Tlaxcala, when Cortés was appointing leaders to replace those felled by the disease. For January 1521, Díaz remarked that, upon beginning the final campaign against Tenochtitlan, he and his companions reentered Texcoco, a twin city of the Aztec capital, without opposition, in part due to the fact that many warriors were still recovering from smallpox and were too weak to fight as a result of the illness which hit and spread throughout the land. Abridged English translations of the *Historica Verdadera* often omit this and other episodes dealing with smallpox.[25]

Brooks insisted that Motolinía's account of the spread of illness came from biblical notions of the clean and the unclean, but it is telling that Motolinía and most sixteenth-century Spanish writers, secular as well as religious, uniformly relied on the word *pegar* to convey, somewhat metaphorically, the means of transmission of smallpox. The word is used to describe the spread of *matlazahuatl* (typhus), plague, and other diseases which are now considered contagious. Indeed, Nebrija's Spanish-Latin vocabulary defined "contagion" as "an illness which sticks" (*dolencia que*

24 Motolinía, *Historia;* Díaz del Castillo, *Historia Verdadera,* I, 373, 378, 425, 438, II, 379. Maurice Keatinge reduces the account to: "a Negro who was in smallpox, an unfortunate importation for that country for the disease spread with inconceivable rapidity, and the Indians died by the thousands" (*The True History of the Conquest of Mexico by Capitan Bernal Diaz del Castillo, One of the Conquerors, Written in the Year 1568* [London, 1800], 206). Alfred Percival Maudslay, who based his translation (*The Discovery and Conquest of Mexico, 1517–1521* [London, 1928], 399) on the Hakluyt Society's publication of the Guatemala text, offers a literal phrasing of "*pegase e hinchiese toda la tierra de ellas, de lo cual hubo gran mortandad*": "the whole country was stricken and filled with it [smallpox] and from which there was great mortality." No translator made much of the chronicler's use of the subjunctive. Hugh Thomas, relying on a seventeenth-century source (Fernando Alva de Ixtlilochitl), placed the Cempoala outbreak before the expulsion of Spaniards from Tenochtitlan (*The Conquest of Mexico* [London, 1993], 741, n. 63).

25 The passage paraphrased here is rarely translated in English editions (Díaz del Castillo, *Historia Verdadera,* I, 438). Alone among the Romance languages, sixteenth-century Spanish used *cundir* to denote the propagation of pestilence; see Joan Corominas, *Diccionario crítico etimológico castellano e hispánico* (Madrid, 1980) I, 982; Elio Antonio de Nebrija, *Vocabulario de Romance en Latin* (Madrid, 1973; orig. ed., 1516) defined *cundir* as "to spread little-by-little" (this revised version supersedes the 1495 edition).

se pega). *Pegar* also describes how fire is spread and the means by which one gets vices, customs, opinions, knowledge and, even, jokes. Thanks to the word *pegar,* by the seventeenth-century, as the theory of communicable disease became respectable among educated Europeans, Spanish folk discourse required little adjustment to explain the transmission of contagious diseases (*"Vale tambien comunicar una cosa a otra. Comunmente se dice de las enfermedádes contagiósas."*).[26]

Motolinía, like Vázquez de Ayllón and many other eyewitness chroniclers, used *pegar* to describe the spread of smallpox. To explain transmission from the natives of Fernandina to those of Cempoala, *han pegado* was chosen. Two decades later, Motolinía's *Memoriales* employed the same imagery: smallpox spread to the Indians (*"pegar a los indios"*). Sahagún and his assistants, translating from the Nahuatl, described death from smallpox as "the sticky [spreading?] disease" (*"la muerte pegajosa"*) "of which many died, but others died only of hunger because no one cared for anyone else." When the first measles epidemic struck in 1531, Motolinía described it as "jumping" (*saltar*) from a Spaniard:

> . . . and from him it jumped to the Indians, and if there had not been much advance warning so that they could be told, prepared and even preached that they not bathe or take other remedies contrary to the illness; and with this pleased the Lord so that not as many died as from smallpox; and they called this the year of the small leprosy (*lepra*) and for the first, the year of the great leprosy.[27]

The notion of the communicability of disease might not enter formal European discourse until the middle of the sixteenth-century, but, as early as 1431, the imagery was circulating in a Spanish medical manual written in the vernacular to facilitate its dissemination. Later, *pegar* appears frequently in the writings of the first *conquistadores* of New Spain.[28]

26 Brooks, "Revising the Conquest," 26. Nebrija, *Vocabulario de Romance,* s.v. *"contagion"*; Real Academia Española, *Diccionario de la lengua castellana* (Madrid, 1726–39), s.v. *"pegar."* Cortés used *se pegó* to describe how pestilence was inflicted upon Spanish judges who were sent in 1530 to inquire about his conduct and thus was spread to New Spain (*Cartas,* 276).

27 Motolinía, *Memoriales,* 30.

28 Alonso de Chirino (ed. Maria Teresa Herrera), *Menor Daño de la medicina de Alonso de Chirino, edición crítica y glosario* (Salamanca, 1973); completed before 1431, Chirino's work

Also mistaken is the argument that Motolinía simply wrote to emphasize parallels between the suffering of the chosen people in Egypt and the natives in New Spain. Motolinía recounted the Ten Plagues, but then, in a passage expunged from the *Historia,* challenged popular Spanish beliefs by contrasting the plagues of biblical Egypt with those of contemporary New Spain:

> Well considered, there are differences, great differences, between these plagues and those of Egypt. First, in only one of those [of Egypt], and that in the last, were there deaths of people; but here, in each of these there have been many deaths. Second, in each one of the houses there remained someone to mourn the dead, and here, of the plagues already described, many houses were left abandoned, because all their occupants died. Third, in Egypt, all the plagues lasted only a few days, and here, some a very long time. Those, by the commandment of God: most of these by the cruelty and depravity of men, although God permitted it.[29]

The Franciscan was not guilty of mythopoesis, as Brooks suggested. Motolinía engaged his Catholic readers' religious beliefs—that the natives' afflictions were due to God's wrath—then he disputed the commonplace thesis of conquest as fulfillment of biblical prophesy by emphasizing the vast differences between the plagues of Egypt and those of New Spain. Historians who traffic in English translations miss the subtlety of Motolinía's argument because they, like Brooks, favor the *Historia* (first published in 1858; first English edition 1949) over the *Memoriales* (first published in 1903; no English translation). Confusion reigns because

---

survives in six slightly varying copies. Chapter VII examines diseases that stick ("*De las enfermedades que se pegan*") and places smallpox among them, 34. Vázquez de Ayllón, "Relacion," 42. Translated as "*muerte pegajosa*" by Alejandra Moreno Tosanco in Daniel Cosío Villegas (ed.), *Historia General de México* (Mexico City, 1976), II, 9–10. Other sixteenth-century writers who used *pegar* are: Díaz del Castillo to describe the transmission of *modorra* (*Historia Verdadera*, II, 263); Diego Muñoz Camargo (ed. Rene Acuña), *Descripción de la Ciudad y Provincia de Tlaxcala de las Indias y del mar océano para el buen gobierno y enoblecimiento dellas* (Mexico City, 1981; reprint ed.), 35v: "*las viruelas que truxo y pego*"; Herrera y Tordesillas, *Historia General*, Decada II, libro 10, cap. IV (398): "*las viruelas pegándose con los indios*"; *Códice Ramírez;* Francisco Cervantes de Salazar (ed. Manuel Magallón), *Crónica de la Nueva España* (Madrid, 1971, Biblioteca de Autores Españoles vol. 245), II, 98; Juan López de Velasco, *Geografía y descripción universal de las Indias* (Madrid, 1971), 14.
29 Motolinía, *Memoriales*, 30.

the original manuscripts of both are missing, and the extant copies are incomplete.

Since 1982 scholars have known that the *Historia* is an abridged version, rather "an atrocious mutilation," of the *Memoriales*. The *Historia* was extracted from the *Memoriales,* hastily edited and transcribed, perhaps dictated, and certainly altered, probably in Spain by someone poorly informed of conditions in New Spain, wholly ignorant of Nahuatl, unclear about the making of tortillas, and even wrong about the year the Franciscans first arrived in New Spain. Brooks compounded the folly by imagining the *Memoriales* to be a derivative of the *Historia*. Motolinía, an informed, sympathetic observer who entered New Spain in 1524, quickly became a skilled Nahuatl linguist and continued his ecclessiastical work in Mexico for almost forty-five years. He would not have committed the factual and linguistic errors unique to the *Historia*. O'Gorman argued that the *Historia* was constructed in Spain from Motolinía's *Memoriales* to provide testimony for revoking the New Laws. The mutilation of the text is so extensive that O'Gorman maintained that the *Historia* should no longer be attributed to Motolinía.[30]

Sixteenth-century chroniclers—López de Gómara, Zorita, Cervantes de Salazar, Mendieta, and Torquemada among others—favored the *Memoriales,* often quoting long passages from it. Brooks argued that Mendieta "simply copied" Motolinía, which he did (a fact widely recognized by modern historians who rarely cite Mendieta's account of the conquest), but it is the *Memoriales* that he relied upon, not the *Historia*. Twentieth-century historians and translators, unfortunately, favor the *Historia*. This choice is a double misfortune, because the smallpox story in the *Historia* is an exaggeration of the *Memoriales*. The *Historia* subverts Motolinía's intentions by excising the contrasts present in the *Memoriales*. The *Historia* compounds the offense by heightening the argument of divine punishment through the insertion of the phrase "*y castigo esta tierra y a los que en ella se hallaron.*" The greatest distortion is inflating the proportion dying from "half" to "more than half"

---

30 *Ibid.,* viii, ix, lvii-lviii; Brooks, "Revising the Conquest," 22; O'Gorman, *Incognita,* 68, 73–74. The cover letter which accompanied the manuscript copy of *Historia* was used to establish the authorship of the opus. Yet, the document, which is undated and unsigned, reported events occurring as many as two years after the letter bearing Motolinía's dated signature. See O'Gorman, introduction, *Memoriales,* lxxxiv-lxxxvi.

and the number of provinces where this was the rule from "some" to "most." O'Gorman detailed many of the mutilations present in Motolinía's *Historia,* although the embellishment of the fraction dying from smallpox is not among them.[31]

Taken as a whole, the more restrained account in the *Memoriales* bolsters the credibility of Motolinía's work. Motolinía did not distort his text to pander to the religious sensibilities of his readers or his own. He had no means of ascertaining the precise fraction of natives who died, but the order of magnitude which he chose ("one-half") did not come from Revelations, where "one-third" is the constant refrain.[32] By using the fraction "one-half," his Spanish readers would have inferred that the force of the epidemic was enormous, of much greater magnitude than in Spain.

SPAIN AND NEW SPAIN   Since Brooks reduced the epidemic of 1520 to a "mild attack of smallpox, such as occurred in contemporary Europe," a comparison with Europe and with Spain, provides much needed perspective. For the period prior to 1492, Guerra identified the most reliable sources of Iberian epidemiological history as book-length manuscripts by Samuel ben Waqar, Juan de Aviñón, and Alonso de Chirino, three Jewish doctors. All of them ranked smallpox among the most common, but not the most deadly, diseases of their time. Plague, on the other hand, was a different matter. For plague, Chirino's practical guide for the layperson, which he completed before 1431, offered two bits of advice—first, pray, then flee. For smallpox he recommended deliberate care. Chirino's manual classified smallpox with diseases that stick (*enfermedades que se pegan*) and warned that the healthy should not go near, sleep with, nor be in close quarters with anyone ill with these diseases. He did not advise prayer (the victims, being young children, were innocent) or flight (uncalled for given the low levels of mortality).[33]

31 Motolinía, *Memoriales,* vii, 21; Ernest J. Burrus, "Religious Chroniclers and Historians: A Summary with Annotated Bibliography," *Handbook of Middle American Indians,* XIII, 144; Jerónimo de Mendieta, *Historia eclesiástica indiana* (Mexico City, 1945; 2d ed.); Juan de Torquemada, *Monarquía indiana* (Madrid, 1723; orig. ed., 1615), I, 512; Crosby, "Conquistador y Pestilencia," 333.
32 Rev. 8:7–13.
33 Brooks, "Revising the Conquest," 16–17, 29; Francisco Guerra, "Origen de las

Aviñón's manual described three smallpox epidemics striking Seville at intervals of some thirteen years, in 1393, 1407, and 1420. For 1420, he wrote: "smallpox raged among the children, and many of them died; and it was a good year for bread and for wine." Raging smallpox had no effect on the agrarian economy of Seville.[34]

For sixteenth-century Spain, Villalba's classic *Epidemiología* listed forty-nine epidemics, half attributed to plague (*peste*) but only six to smallpox. From the brevity of the passages on smallpox, Villalba did not seem to be greatly concerned with the disease. Likewise, Pérez Moreda's recent, comprehensive history of mortality crises in early modern Spain disposed of smallpox in a few pages. The period of greatest concern was the eighteenth-century, when efforts were being made to limit virulence. Two centuries earlier, smallpox was ubiquitous, but mortality crises due to the disease uncommon. Ashburn reported that "so common was smallpox in Spanish children that Ruy Díaz de Isla cited as remarkable the fact that he knew a man who had not had it until after his twentieth year."[35]

Fracastoro classified smallpox with mild diseases of childhood such as chicken pox and measles that "attack children especially, adults rarely, the elderly hardly ever. But they seem to attack everyone once in life." Fracastoro's translator noted that "since small-pox, under variolae, is so lightly treated by Fracastorius, as a malady to which practically everyone was then subject, it must have been a mild and rarely fatal strain." According to the most authoritative modern study the strain or strains of smallpox common to that era were exceedingly benign throughout sixteenth-century Europe. Only in the following century and later did it become a virulent killer.[36]

epidemias en la conquista de América," *Quinto centenario*, XIV (1988), 44; Chirino, *Menor Daño*, 39–40, 84–85, 34.

34 Juan de Aviñón, *Sevillana Medicina Que trata el modo conservativo y curativo de los que habitan en la muy insigne ciudad de Sevilla, la cual sirve y aprovecha para cualquier otro lugar de estos reinos* (Seville, 1885; orig. ed., 1545; manuscript completed 1420), 33–34, 38.

35 Vicente Pérez Moreda, *La crisis de mortalidad en la España interior (siglos XVI-XIX)* (Madrid, 1980), 351; Joaquin Villalba, *Epidemiología Española: o Historia cronológica de los pestes, contagios, epidemias y epizootias que han acaecido en España desde la venida de los cartagineses, hasta el año 1801* (Madrid, 1802); Percy Moreau Ashburn, *The Ranks of Death: A Medical History of the Conquest of America* (New York, 1947), 86, citing the *Tratado contra el mal serpentino . . .* (Seville, 1539).

36 Girolamo Fracastoro (trans. Wilmer Cave Wright), *De Contagione et Contagiosis Morbis*

In contrast, the smallpox which struck Amerindians, adults as well as children, was severe and often fatal. The impact of smallpox in New Spain was wholly unlike that in Spain. In Spain, it was a disease of childhood, whereas in New Spain the attack of 1520 struck all ages, including many native leaders. Spanish eyewitnesses compared the outbreak with what had happened in the islands, not with anything in Spain or Europe. In New Spain, unlike Spain, smallpox was a lethal pestilence. If we assume that children made up one-third of the native population, then the crude rate of smallpox mortality among the natives would start at three times the rate for European populations that were subject to regular outbreaks of the disease. Among Amerindians, the absence of care and caretakers propelled smallpox mortality to catastrophic levels, but genetic factors probably played a role as well.

SMALLPOX MORBIDITY AND GENETIC DIVERSITY   Genetic immunity is a common explanation for the enormous difference in death rates between Europeans and Amerindians, but there is no proof for this hypothesis. Few genetic differences distinguish new-world populations from the old, and none has a demonstrated advantage against the smallpox virus. Genetic diversity, rather than immunity, may be the key, as Francis Black, a viral epidemiologist, recently argued. Human geneticists reported that Amerindians (along with Polynesians and New Guineans) are unusually homogeneous genetically. The smallpox virus adapts quickly to a host's immunological response—not mutating into a new strain, but rather preparing for battle with other hosts of nearly identical genetic makeup.

---

et Eurum Curatione, Libri III (New York, 1930), 73, 307; my translation retains the gender-neutral tone of Fracastoro's Latin: "Contingit igitur ejusmodi febres praecipue pueris, raro viris, rarissime senibus: videntur autem et omnibus semel in vita aut accidere." Ann G. Carmichael and Arthur M. Silverstein, "Smallpox in Europe before the Seventeenth-century: Virulent Killer or Benign Disease?," Journal of the History of Medicine and Allied Sciences, XLII (1987), 168. The thesis of increasing virulence of smallpox in the seventeenth-century has since been confirmed for England by a sophisticated demographic study which relies on parish records instead of the narrative sources used by Carmichael and Silverstein: S. R. Duncan, Susan Scott, and C. J. Duncan, "An Hypothesis for the Periodicity of Smallpox Epidemics as Revealed by Time Series Analysis," Journal of Theoretical Biology, CLX (1993), 234. Nevertheless, the fifteenth-century Spanish medical sources cited above suggest caution. The absence of reliable parish registers for late medieval and early modern times makes it difficult to resolve the question of the intensity of smallpox mortality for that era.

Field research on measles is the most convincing. Measles acquired from a member of one's family tends to be more virulent than that acquired from a stranger. According to Black, "virus grown in one host is preadapted to a genetically like host and thereby gains virulence." The genetic key to successfully defending against an attack of virulent smallpox is the production of histocompatibility antigens. Unfortunately, in this regard, Amerindians show only one-sixty-fourth the genetic diversity of Africans or Europeans. The odds worsen when exposure is simultaneous and from multiple sources, particularly from members of one's own family. The close living quarters, described by López de Gómara and Sahagún, would heighten virulence as the smallpox spread through families and compactly settled communities.[37]

CARE Whatever geneticists ultimately teach historians about immunity or diversity in explaining the virulence of the disease, the role of social agency is also important. We know, and the Spaniards knew, as Chirino's medical manual made clear, that nursing reduces smallpox mortality. Whereas Europeans possessed no herbs, antibiotics, or prophylaxes, they, unlike the natives, understood that chances of recovery improved with care—water, food, and clean, warm clothing. What astonished Spanish eyewitnesses of this first epidemic was that it struck adults as well as children. In reaching everyone, the attack left the population without caregivers or nurturers, a fact frequently noted in both Spanish and Nahuatl chronicles. Motolinía's *Memoriales* recounted the lethal effects of this horror: "because they all fell ill at a stroke, [the Indians] could not nurse one another, nor was there anyone

---

37 Francis L. Black, "Why Did They Die?," *Science*, CCLVIII (1992), 1739. Black emphasized that the issue is genetic diversity, not inferiority. The data which he reported are for Amerindians in South America. Robert Larocque, "Le rôle de la contagion dans la conquête des Amériques: Importance exagérée atribuée aux agents infectieux," *Recerches amérindiennes au Quebéc*, XVIII (1988), 11. The genetic immunity hypothesis appears widely in the literature, from monographs to textbooks. See Miguel E. Bustamante, "Cuatrocientos años de viruela en México," in *idem* (ed.), *Cinco personajes de la salud en México* (Mexico City, 1986), 21; Peter Gerhard, *Geografía Histórica de la Nueva España 1519–1821* (Mexico City, 1986), 20; Mark A. Burkholder and Lyman L. Johnson, *Colonial Latin America* (Oxford, 1994), 101. Lifetime immunity is factored into Whitmore's simulations: Thomas M. Whitmore, *Disease and Death in Early Colonial Mexico: Simulating Amerindian Depopulation* (Boulder, 1992), 54–58. López de Gómara, *Historia*, I, 278.

to make bread, and in many parts it happened that all the residents of a house died and in others almost no one was left."[38]

Subsequent smallpox epidemics were less deadly because, on the one hand, lifetime immunity meant that survivors of an earlier epidemic were available to provide nursing and, on the other, Indians quickly adopted more appropriate methods of care. This change so impressed Pomar that his *Relación del Texcoco* (written in the 1580s) attributed better survival to improved care (however mistaken in his remedy): "until they understood and became accustomed to wrap themselves and to sweat and to do other remedies that necessity and experience taught them with which afterwards here in other times when it [smallpox] has hit them, they have cured themselves." Muñoz Camargo, in trying to account for the enormous mortality among the Tlaxcalans as a result of the new diseases, offered fatalism as an explanation: "they do not protect themselves from contagious illnesses; upon falling ill they are fatalistic and they permit themselves to die like beasts." His account is distinct from others in that it looked at the conquest from beyond the Central Basin, at a people who collaborated with the Spanish against the ancestral enemy, the Mexica, but who suffered the catastrophe anyway.[39]

Brooks chided Spanish writers for alleged patronizing cultural chauvinism—that the Indians had no cure for smallpox—but he wrongly imposed on their texts an anachronistic, late twentieth-century meaning for "cure," as in the elusive "cure for cancer." Among Spaniards in the sixteenth-century, the most common meaning of *curar* was simply to care for or nurse the sick (which was precisely the point of Chirino's manual—to debunk the life-threatening cures of surgeons, physics, and phlebotomists and provide the least damaging care), including the

---

38 Motolinía, *Memoriales*, 21.
39 Juan Bautista Pomar, "Relación del Texcoco," in Icazbalceta (ed.), *Nueva Colección*, 52; Muñoz Camargo, *Descripción de la Ciudad*, 77v, 78. Henige insinuated that bathing as a cure should be discounted as a trope (Henige, "When Did Smallpox," 24), but consider that Sahagun's Nahuatl informants recommended bathing for a variety of skin-related and other maladies (*Florentine Codex*, X, 149–157), such as pustules ("*nanaoatl*"), skin sores, hemorrhoids, stiff neck, coughing, breast tumor, jigger fleas, broken bones, divine sickness ("*la lepra*" or "*Teucoculiztli inamjc*"), and benumbed feet—but not for pus or blood in the urine, swelling of the throat, cysts, abscesses of the neck, chest ailments or shortness of breath, swelling from sprains, constant coughing, spitting of blood, stomach pains, colic, bloody flux, diarrhea, tumors, swellings (leg, knee), urinary obstruction, fevers, festering, burns, or cuts.

payment for care (*gasto de la cura*) and assistance (*la assistencia del enfermo*). Likewise, for the Spanish *remedio,* the modern English cognate may be deceptive. *Remedio* was defined broadly in the early modern era to include "medicine, or anything else, which serves to recover or maintain health."[40]

The potency of nursing in reducing smallpox mortality is revealed by Frost, who reexamined an epidemic among the Hopi and Pueblo at the end of the nineteenth century. The shockingly high death rates among the Pueblo are well known, but the remedial effect of nursing is not given its due in scholarly histories, even though Crosby stressed its importance in his widely cited essay.[41]

Frost's reanalysis of the notorious epidemic of 1898–99 confirmed an account by a Bureau of Indian Affairs administrator made almost a century ago. The report showed that among 421 Hopis who were infected by smallpox and elected to receive care, only 24 died compared with 163 deaths in a settlement only half as large, but which declined care. These figures yield crude death rates of 6 percent and 74 percent. Mortality was more than twelve times greater for those without care. Nursing thus reduced smallpox mortality from catastrophic to tolerable levels. Those who were experienced with smallpox recognized the importance of nursing and often tried to alleviate suffering and thereby reduce the death toll. Whether Cortés or his soldiers provided care for their Tlaxcalan allies is unknown, but it is certain that their Mexica enemies received none because as the epidemic enveloped Tenochtitlan the only Spaniards remaining in the city were dead ones.[42]

40 Brooks, "Revising the Conquest," 26. Motolinía wrote (*Memoriales,* 21): "*porque como todos enfermaron de golpe, no podían curar unos de otros.*" *Diccionario de la lengua castellana,* s.v. "*curar*" ("*Se toma tambien por Cuidar: y en este sentido se usó mucho esta voz en lo antiguo*") and "*remedio*" ("*por lo mismo que medicamento, ú por qualquiera cosa, que sirve para recobrar ó conservar la salúd*"). Chirino, *Menor daño,* 80r: "*vos guardedes quanto pudierdes de la maldat de çerugianos que son muy malos omenes e peores que físicos si peores se pueden aver.*"
41 Richard H. Frost, "The Pueblo Indian Smallpox Epidemic in New Mexico, 1898–1899," *Bulletin of the History of Medicine,* LXIV (1990), 435; Dobyns cited this evidence in *From Fire to Flood: Historic Human Destruction of Sonoran Desert Riverine Oases* (Socorro, Ariz., 1981). Another well-documented case of the success of basic care in reducing mortality from viral infection is Robert J. Wolfe, "Alaska's Great Sickness, 1900: Epidemic of Measles and Influenza in a Virgin Soil Population," *Proceedings of the American Philosophical Society,* CXXVI (1982), 91–121.
42 Frost, "Pueblo Indian Smallpox Epidemic," 437. For the epidemic of 1520 in Ten-

SEVERITY   A quantitative assessment of the severity of the 1520 epidemic is impossible. At best a consensus on the order of magnitude may emerge from close analysis of a wide range of contemporary sources: early Spanish accounts, native annals, texts, and sixteenth-century histories which compare the relative devastation of war and the early epidemics.

Contemporary Spanish texts reveal that their authors were familiar with smallpox and smallpox mortality. The fact that chroniclers described the epidemic of 1520 in detail suggests unusual severity. Vázquez de Ayllón, Cortés, and others compared the attack with epidemics in the islands, and never with Spain. Motolinía, in the *Memoriales* but not in the *Historia,* contrasted smallpox mortality with deaths from the siege of Tenochtitlan, stating that for the former the principal victims were the poor and the children (*pobres y pequeños*), and in the latter it was the lords and the leaders (*señores y principales*). Most of the *castellanos* who accompanied Cortés did not say or write much about the conquest, but those who did commented extensively on the devastation of the pestilence. Vázquez de Tapia, in a claim to the crown for compensation as a participant in the siege of Tenochtitlan, testified:

> The pestilence of measles and smallpox was so severe and cruel that more than one-fourth of the Indian people in all the land died— and this loss had the effect of hastening the end of the fighting because there died a great quantity of men and warriors and many lords and captains and valiant men against whom we would have had to fight and deal with as enemies, and miraculously Our Lord killed them and removed them from before us.[43]

---

ochtitlan, the *Florentine Codex* depicted pustules distinctly visible on five smallpox-infected adults. All were wrapped in blankets. Pain could be discerned in faces and body positions. One victim was crying out while another received care from a woman who was touching and consoling the patient. Note that this scene is contradicted by the Nahuatl text, which stated that "no one took care of others." As generalizations, I trust the text over the pictures. According to Lockhart, Sahagún conceived the pictures as filler, so that the columns of Nahuatl text and Spanish translation could be kept running side-by-side. Illustrations were hastily drawn once the transcriptions of texts were finished. Some illustrations went uncolored, and others were never drawn, their panels left completely blank (Lockhart, *We People Here,* 11, 185). This important document is widely available in a magnificent facsimile edition: Secretaría de Gobernación, *Códice florentino* (Mexico, 1979), III, book 12, chap. 29, fol. 53.
43 Vázquez de Ayllón, "Relacion," 42; Cortés, *Cartas de relación,* 105; Motolinía, *Me-*

Native annals, unlike Spanish chronicles, recorded the most important events for each year. Before 1519 native annals reported pestilence or famine only when devastation was prolonged, often for a year or more. In the century before European instrusion (1420–1519), the *Annals of Cuauhtitlan* reported seven famines and two epidemics—all multiyear phenomena. Then, for 1520, the most notable event was smallpox, when the death of two leaders from the disease was chronicled. Since smallpox outbreaks remain in any one place only for a couple of months, it should be surprising to find smallpox recorded. Yet, 1520 is often named the year-of-the-pox in native annals, such as the *Annals of Tlatelolco* and the *Annals of Tenochtitlan*. One of the most interesting annals, the *Códice Telleriano Remensis,* is rendered useless by the loss of pictographs for 1516 through 1527. Of the surviving pictographs for the postconquest period, 1528–60, this *Códice* recorded four epidemics: measles (1531), smallpox (1538), a great mortality ("*una gran mortandad,*" 1544–45), and mumps (1550).[44]

In Nahuatl texts written in the Roman alphabet, the horror of smallpox is told again and again. The longest native account is in Sahagún's monumental ethnohistorical treatise, the *General History of the Things of New Spain*. A distillation of testimony of Nahua leaders and informants in three towns, the clinical, yet melancholic descriptions have made this one of the most widely cited Nahautl texts on the conquest. English translations are available in three editions. The first, published in 1955 by Dibble and Anderson, is often cited in extenso. Brooks used the second translation, published in 1975. I favor a third by Lockhart (1993), the first to offer English translations of both the original Nahuatl (probably completed in 1555) and the accompanying Spanish gloss (written before 1586). The most informed, comprehensive account of smallpox epidemic is in the

> Twenty-ninth chapter, where it is said how, at the time the Spaniards left Mexico, there came an illness of pustules of which many local people died; it was called 'the great rash' (smallpox).

moriales, 41; Vázquez (ed.), *Relación de meritos y servicios del conquistador Bernardino Vázquez de Tapia* (Madrid, 1988), 148.

44 Lockhart, *We People Here,* 259, 279; José Corona Nuñez (ed.), *Antiguedades de Mexico: Basadas en la recopilación de Lord Kingsborough* (Mexico City, 1964–67), I, 42–43; Bierhorst, *History and Mythology,* 79.

Before the Spaniards appeared to us [again], first an epidemic broke out, a sickness of pustules. It began in Tepeilhuitl ['which is at the end of September,' according to the accompanying Spanish gloss]. Large bumps spread on people, some were entirely covered. They spread everywhere, on the face, the head, the chest, etc. (The disease) brought great desolation; a great many died of it. They could no longer walk about, but lay in their dwellings and sleeping places, no longer able to move or stir. They were unable to change position, to stretch out on their sides or face down, or raise their heads. And when they made a motion, they called out loudly. The pustules that covered people caused great desolation; very many people died of them, and many just starved to death; starvation reigned, and no one took care of others any longer.

On some people, the pustules appeared only far apart, and they did not suffer greatly, nor did many of them die of it. But many people's faces were spoiled by it, their faces and noses were made rough. Some lost an eye or were blinded.

The disease of the pustules lasted a full sixty days; after sixty days it abated and ended. When people were convalescing and reviving, the pustules disease began to move in the direction of Chalco. And many were disabled or paralyzed by it, but they were not disabled forever. It broke out in Teotleco, and it abated in Panquetzaliztli. The Mexica warriors were greatly weakened by it.[45]

45 Lockhart, *We People Here*, 180, 182; Sahagún (eds. Dibble and Anderson), *Florentine Codex*, XII, chap. 29 (1st and 2d eds.). The fact that Brooks "cannot recall one [historian] who quotes the qualifications in the second paragraph" is due to faulty memory and flawed transcription ("Revising the Conquest," 28, n. 40). He omitted text and erased the division between paragraphs two and three. Crosby and Padden quoted paragraphs one and two in their entirety. They omitted paragraph three, perhaps because it seemed less important in the translation from which they worked, but they are in good company. The sixteenth-century Spanish digest of the Nahuatl text omitted all but the first sentence of paragraph three (*Códice florentino*, III, book 12, chap. 29, fol. 53). See Crosby, "Conquistador y Pestilencia," 336; Robert C. Padden, *The Hummingbird and the Hawk: Conquest and Sovereignty in the Valley of Mexico, 1503–1541* (New York, 1970), 206; Miguel León-Portilla (ed.), *The Broken Spears: The Aztec Account of the Conquest of Mexico* (Boston, 1962), 93. Both the English and Spanish translation of the last line of paragraph three changed greatly over the years and with it the significance of the passage for understanding the impact of smallpox. The 1955 edition by Dibble and Anderson (XII, 81) reads: "Then the Mexicans, the chieftains, could revive." A second edition published in 1975 (cited by Brooks) favors a translation with broader demographic implications (XII, 83): "At that time the Mexicans, the brave warriors were able to recover from the pestilence." Then, in 1993, Lockhart's translation elicits nuances unnoted by earlier philologists: "The Mexica warriors were greatly weakened by it." This reading fits neatly with Díaz del Castillo's account of smallpox-weakened warriors encountered on the Spaniards' return to Texcoco in January 1521 (*Historia Verdadera*, I, 438). Likewise, Muñoz Camargo (*Descripción de la*

Brooks interpreted the 1975 translation of this passage as evidence that "it is reasonable to credit their collective memory with knowledge that not many died" even though the text itself stated unequivocally that the pustules brought "great desolation," that "very many died," and "many just starved to death." His revisionist zeal divined the ever-present hand of Motolinía in this passage, but consider Sahagún's own explanation of how the manuscript was composed:

> When this manuscript was written (which is now over thirty years ago [that is, 1555]) everything was written in the Mexican language and was afterwards put into Spanish. Those who helped me write it were prominent elders, well versed in all matters, relating not only to idolatry but also to government and its offices, who were present in the war when this city was conquered.[46]

Chapter 29, unlike the Spanish chronicles, reads like a pictorial history of the Nahuas' suffering, rendered in their own words. Lockhart characterized the entire book as "authentic oral

---

Ciudad, 35v) attributes the brevity of the reconquest to the fact that the Mexican warriors were emaciated and sick, recently recovered from the illness [smallpox] ("*la qual fue parte para qe mas ayna se acabasse la Guerra de Mexico por que los cogio flacos y enfermos recien salidos de la enfermedad*").

The three renderings of the last sentence of paragraph three (in the Nahuatl: *vncan vel caxavaque in Mexica, in tiacaoan*) reflect the ambiguities of "*tiacauh*." An authoritative Spanish translation of the *Historia general de las cosas de Nueva España* by Wigberto Jiménez Moreno—(Mexico City, 1938), IV, 192—translated the word as "*caudillo*" (chief), whereas Angel Maria Garibay Kintana, in his translation (Mexico, 1956, IV, 137), elected "*guerreros*" (warriors). Lockhart reasoned that the term, which occurred many times in book 12, meant something like "our men," but he "uniformly translated it simply as 'warriors'" (*We People Here,* 23). Molina defined *tiacaoan* as valiant men, brave soldiers, and *caxauhqui* as weakened, sickly, or enfeebled (*Vocabulario,* 112v, 13).

The entire English text, based on Garibay Kintana's Spanish translation but without his extensive bibliographical notes, is available in a paperback edition first published in 1962 and now in its ninth printing (León-Portilla, *Broken Spears* [Boston, 1993]). José Luís Martínez, *El "Códice Florentino" y la "Historia General" de Sahagún* (Mexico City, 1989), 93–153.

46 Brooks, "Revising the Conquest," 28. Sahagún, *Conquest,* 2; Luís Leal, "El libro XII de Sahagún," *Historia Mexicana,* V (1955), 186–204. For an informed, nuanced discussion of Sahagún's methods, see Ellen T. Baird, *The Drawings of Sahagún's Primeros Memoriales: Structure and Style* (Norman, 1993), 14. Few modern ethnohistorians have achieved the methodological sophistication of Sahagún's work. His method is explained in *Florentine Codex,* I, 53–54. Lockhart (*We People Here,* 31) concluded that ". . . I for one have failed to find anything Spanish about the syntax, usage, or general vocabulary [of book XII]."

tradition with an emphasis on visuality" and "an authentic expression of indigenous people." "Signs of active intervention by Sahagún are minimal." Motolinía's influence was nil. Sahagún thought the Nahua conquest narrative to be so one-sided and anti-Spanish that, to redress the balance, he wrote his own history, which he completed in 1585. The comparable passage of Sahagún's *Conquest* offers the Spanish view. Note the shift from visual description to interpretive synthesis:

> During this epidemic, the Spaniards, rested and recovered, were already in Tlaxcala. Having taken courage and energy because of reinforcements who had come to them and because of the ravages of the [Mexican] people that the pestilence was causing, firmly believing that God was on their side, being again allied with the Tlaxcalans, and attending to all the necessary preparations to return against the Mexicans, they began to construct the brigantines.[47]

Historians and chroniclers began to compare the severity of the various epidemics toward the middle of the sixteenth-century. Motolinía, writing in 1542, saw three great devastations, which he sought to fit to years ending in "one," the most important being the war, pestilence, and famine of "1521." Several years after his manuscript was shipped to Spain (and while its author was in Guatemala), the great devastation of 1545 broke out so we cannot know how his numerology would have taken this into account.[48]

On November 8, 1576, as the third great epidemic of the century unfolded, Sahagún, in a rare direct intervention in the *General History* and for which there is no corresponding Nahuatl text, mused whether the present plague would exterminate the native people. He addressed the question directly and forcefully, leaving no doubt that the smallpox attack of 1520 was exceedingly lethal (*murio casi infinita gente*)—more deadly even than the war—but the deadliest was the *matlazahuatl* epidemic of 1545, "a very great and universal pestilence where, in all of New Spain, the greater part of the people who lived therein died." In Tlatelolco

---

47 Sahagún, *Conquest*, 103; for Cline's analysis of the Spanish perspective in Sahagún's *Conquest*, see 2–15. Leal argued that book 12 has an authentically native viewpoint which presents the conquistadores in much more negative tones than the Spanish chroniclers, including Sahagún himself ("El libro," 202). Lockhart, *We People Here*, 10–11, 34–35.
48 Motolinía, *Memoriales*, 292–295.

alone, Sahagún claimed to have buried 10,000 and fell ill to the disease himself. As he wrote in November 1576, the number of deaths mounted daily. According to Sahagún, many were dying of hunger, without care, and with no one even to provide a jar of water—charitable relief having been exhausted. He feared that if the contagion continued for another three or four months that no natives would be left, that the land would revert to wild beasts and wilderness. He reasoned that Spaniards were too few to settle the land, and the Indians were becoming extinct.[49]

Pomar, the historian of the city of Texcoco, also singled out three great epidemics of the century—1520, 1545, and 1576—but characterized that of 1520 as the worst. He reported that Texcoco, which surrendered to Cortés without a struggle, used to number some 15,000 citizens (*vecinos*) but did not have 600 as he wrote in the 1580s. Many smaller subject villages had disappeared entirely.[50]

I prefer the most explicitly quantitatively reasoned assessment, by Muñoz Camargo for the province of Tlaxcala, also drafted in the 1580s but only published in 1981:

> I say that the first [1520] ought to be the greatest because there were more people, and the second [1545] was also very great because the land was very full [of people], and this last one [1576] was not as great as the first two because although many people died many escaped with the remedies that the Spaniards and the religious people provided.[51]

Evidence from a wide variety of sixteenth-century Spanish and Nahuatl sources point to a single conclusion: the smallpox epidemic of 1520 ranked among the three worst demographic crises of the century. The death rate from smallpox and starvation in 1520–21 was probably less than for the *matlazahuatl* epidemics of 1545–46 and 1576–77. Nonetheless, if we accept the intelligence offered by one of the most celebrated native chroniclers of the colonial era, the smallpox epidemic of 1520 was the greatest

49 Moreno Jiménez, *Historia general,* III, 355–361.
50 Pomar, "Relación del Texcoco," 49.
51 Muñoz Camargo, *Descripción de la Ciudad,* 36.

demographic catastrophe of the century for the Nahuatl-speaking people of central Mexico.[52]

Consensus is emerging on the scale, causes, and consequences of the demographic disaster which struck sixteenth-century Mexico. There is agreement that a demographic catastrophe occurred and that epidemic disease was a dominant factor in initiating a die-off, beginning, in Mexico, with smallpox in 1520. But the role of disease cannot be understood without taking into account the harsh treatment (forced migration, enslavement, abusive labor demands, and exorbitant tribute payments) and ecological devastation that accompanied Spanish colonization. Killing associated with war and conquest was clearly a secondary factor, except in isolated cases, such as the deliberate destruction of Cholula or the leveling of Tenochtitlan.

A fair-minded cross-examination of the broad range of primary sources for the epidemic of 1520 leaves little doubt that smallpox swept throughout the central Mexican basin, causing enormous mortality. The epidemic ranked with the deadliest disasters that native annals customarily recorded. Whether the fraction of smallpox deaths was one-tenth or one-half, we have no way of knowing, but from my reading of the texts discussed here, the true fraction must fall within these extremes, perhaps near the midpoint.

If we leave aside the controversy over the size of Amerindian populations at contact, there emerges a broad agreement in the Spanish and Nahuatl narratives and in the patterns of decline sketched by historians.

For historians who abide quantification, expert estimates point to overall levels of demographic destruction in sixteenth-

52 For accounts of other regions see Antonio de Ciudad Real, *Tratado curioso y docto de las grandezas de la Nueva España* (Mexico City, 1976; orig. ed., 1872), I, 70, 95, II, 73. Alonso de Aguilar, *Relación breve de la conquista de la Nueva España* (Mexico City, 1954), 97; Nicolás León (trans.), *Códice Sierra* (Mexico City, 1933), 9; Díaz del Castillo, *Historia Verdadera*, II, 292. Gerhard (*Geografía Histórica*) provided a comprehensive town-by-town survey of population figures, which he laboriously extracted from geographical treatises (*Relaciones Geográficas*), tribute counts, censuses, and other available sources. Sanders saw only two major epidemics in the sixteenth-century, but he did not consider any evidence for 1520: William T. Sanders, "The Population of the Central Mexican Symbiotic Region, the Basin of Mexico, and the Teotihuacan Valley in the Sixteenth-century," in William M. Denevan (ed.), *The Native Population of the Americas in 1492* (Madison, 1976), 129.

century central Mexico exceeding 50 percent, probably ranging beyond 75 percent, and even topping 90 percent in some large regions such as the tropical lowlands. Vociferous debates over population sizes often overlook similarities in the scale of demographic collapse. To reduce historiographical uncertainty further will require much additional, careful sifting of archival and archaeological evidence—tasks which, in recent decades, few seem inclined to undertake.[53]

In the meantime, I find convincing the testimony of Licenciado Francisco Ceynos, who sums up the opinion of many enlightened sixteenth-century Spanish observers. Ceynos, after five years as fiscal on the Royal Council of the Indies, arrived in Mexico in 1530 to sit on the Real Audiencia of Mexico City. A royal judge (*oidor*) for more than thirty years, he fought against the widespread practice of enslaving Indians and against the extreme labor and tribute burdens common in that era. On March 1, 1565, he completed a lengthy recommendation on colonization policies suitable for newly conquered regions. As preamble he reviewed briefly the demographic tragedy of Spanish colonization in Mexico:

> . . . and it is certain that from the day that D. Hernando Cortés, the Marquis del Valle, entered this land, in the seven years, more or less, that he conquered and governed it, the natives suffered many deaths, and many terrible dealings, robberies and oppressions were inflicted on them, taking advantage of their persons and their lands, without order, weight nor measure; . . . the people diminished in great number, as much due to excessive taxes and mistreatment, as to illness and smallpox, such that now a very great and notable fraction of the people are gone, and especially in the hot country.[54]

We do not know what number, percentage, or ratio that Ceynos had in mind for "*grandes muertes,*" "*gran cantidad,*" or "*faltó*

---

53 Michael E. Smith, Cynthia Heath-Smith, Ronald Kohler, Joan Odess, Sharon Spanogle, and Timothy Sullivan, "The Size of the Aztec City of Yautepec: Urban Survey in Central Mexico," *Ancient Mesoamerica*, V (1994), 1–11; Henige, "Native American Population at Contact: Standards of Proof and Styles of Discourse in the Debate," *Latin American Population History Bulletin*, XXII (1992), 22.

54 Francisco Ceynos, "Carta del doctor Francisco Ceynos," in Icazbalceta (ed.), *Colección de documentos*, II, 237.

muy grande y notable parte de la gente," but what he wrote has the ring of truth. He reported a disaster on a scale unimaginable to contemporary Europeans. If five centuries later this thesis remains beyond the domain of "reasonable probability" for some historians, their number, too, is diminishing as the evidence of demographic catastrophe accumulates.

Dauril Alden and Joseph C. Miller

Out of Africa: The Slave Trade and the Transmission of Smallpox to Brazil, 1560–1831

Among the "shock troops of the conquest" of the Americas—the variety of infectious diseases introduced to the New World from Europe and Africa—smallpox was undoubtedly the leading killer. Certainly that was the case in colonial Brazil. We suggest that for much of the period between the beginning of European contact (1500) and about 1831, when legal forms of the slave trade were ended, the primary source of smallpox contagion in Brazil was tropical Africa.

Our argument may be summarized as follows:

(1) Prior to the arrival of the first Europeans, smallpox (*Variola major,* the only one of three modern species of the virus then existing) was unknown in the future Portuguese colony, or in any other part of the Americas.

(2) Because the pox survived in a community only as long as sufficient susceptibles existed to sustain the disease, and because of Brazil's persisting low population densities, *Variola* probably did not become endemic there until the nineteenth century. New outbreaks of the sickness, at least massive ones, therefore followed reintroductions from external sources, initially European but subsequently African.

(3) As a prime New World importer of slaves, Brazil received regular infusions of potential African carriers of the disease, mainly from the Upper Guinea Coast (Senegambia) in the six-

Dauril Alden is Professor of History at the University of Washington. He is the author of *Royal Government in Colonial Brazil* (Berkeley, 1968). Joseph C. Miller is Professor of History at the University of Virginia. He is the author of *Slavery: A Worldwide Bibliography, 1900–1982* (White Plains, N.Y., 1985).

The authors gratefully acknowledge the stimulation and encouragement from panelists and members of the audience at the initial presentation of this research at the 1982 meeting of the American Historical Association. Ann C. Carmichael and Donald R. Hopkins made informed critiques of earlier drafts. Miller is grateful to the National Library of Medicine for financial and skilled staff support, and to the University of Virginia. Alden joins his thanks, especially to Dorothy Hanks at the National Library of Medicine, Dorothy Welker, and the John Simon Guggenheim Memorial Foundation.

teenth century, from the southwestern littoral between 4° and 18° S. lat. (known as Angola) beginning in the early seventeenth century, from the Mina (or Lower Guinea) Coast of what is today Togo, Bénin, and southwestern Nigeria after about 1700, and by the end of the eighteenth century also from southeastern Africa (or Mozambique).

(4) Periodic drought, famine, and epidemic smallpox in the parts of Africa that contributed significant numbers of slaves to Brazil corresponded reasonably well with the timing of major smallpox eruptions in the Portuguese colony from the seventeenth through the early nineteenth centuries.

(5) Conditions in Africa and on the middle passage favored transmission of the infection in the bodies of the unfortunates sent as slaves to Brazil. Normally dispersed African populations became compressed in relatively moist regions during droughts, when infections quickly spread among non-immunes. Transmission of such diseases intensified further among slaves awaiting shipment in maritime barracoons and among undernourished, sick captives crowded closely together on the decks of slave ships. The thirty- to fifty-day Atlantic crossing permitted more than one cycle of infection among the several hundred chattels aboard the typical slaver.

(6) Demographic patterns in Brazil explain the subsequent spread of the disease in epidemic form among American populations. When the slaves reached one of the major Brazilian ports—Recife de Pernambuco, Salvador da Bahia, and Rio de Janeiro on the east coast, and São Luis do Maranhão and Belém do Pará on the northern coast—they spread contagion rapidly from the waterside sheds in which they waited to be auctioned off throughout the commercial quarters of those towns. As they moved inland to plantations, mines, and settlements, the African newcomers transmitted the virus to virgin Amerindian populations and to previously unexposed individuals of African origin with whom they came into close contact.

ORIGINS AND IMPLANTATION OF SMALLPOX IN THE NEW WORLD
Smallpox is an orthopoxvirus, a genus that includes, among others, camelpox, cowpox, monkeypox, and vaccinia. The most common means of transmission was via virus-bearing moisture droplets exhaled by afflicted persons and inhaled by those with

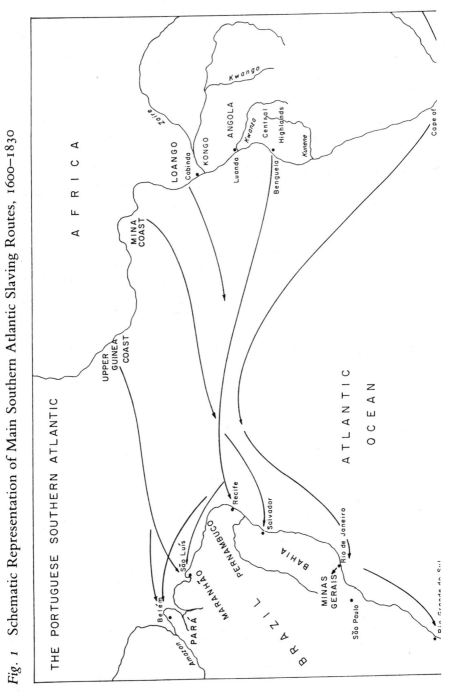

Fig. 1 Schematic Representation of Main Southern Atlantic Slaving Routes, 1600–1830

whom they came into close contact. Although not everyone exposed became ill, as many as one out of two within the same household was likely to catch the infection. Once infected, the victim confronted his or her destiny, for there was no effective treatment for the malady. The disease characteristically announced itself by provoking headaches, fevers, chills, and nausea. After those signs subsided, a rash appeared, first and most intensively on the face, throat, arms, and hands, and subsequently but with diminishing densities throughout the entire torso. More damaging than these visible manifestations were the attacks of the virus on internal organs, whose eventual failure brought death to as many as one out of four sufferers. Survivors were often left disfigured with pockmarks and sometimes suffered blindness. Although generally granted lifelong immunity from reinfection, they not infrequently succumbed to secondary bacterial infections introduced through unhealed lesions or fell to the malnutrition that often succeeded disruptions of agriculture and trade during epidemics.[1]

The origins of smallpox are unknown. It presumably mutated from one of the non-lethal animal poxes into some early agricultural settlement in Asia or Africa about 10,000 BC. Although smallpox was certainly present in Egypt by c 1570 BC, the earliest specific reports of it in sub-Saharan Africa date from 1589 (southeast Africa) and c 1620 in Angola. However, it is thought to have been active several centuries earlier in West Africa.[2]

Smallpox generally arrived in the New World during or immediately after the European conquests, often via Africans. Hispaniola, Spain's only American settlement from 1493 to 1509, is reported to have experienced two smallpox epidemics between 1507 and 1517, possibly from illicitly landed slaves from West Africa, although the disease was then epidemic in the Iberian

---

1 The appearance of Donald R. Hopkins' *Princes and Peasants: Smallpox in History* (Chicago, 1983), has saved us much discussion of the pathology and epidemiology of the disease and numerous references to the older literature. In general, these notes represent a substantial condensation of the literature consulted and the documentation that supports our argument. Interested readers are invited to contact the authors for much longer and more fully documented versions of this essay. The appendix summarizes the full set of events in Africa and Brazil on which we base the case argued in the text.

2 *Ibid.*; Eugenia W. Herbert, "Smallpox Inoculation in Africa," *Journal of African History*, XVI (1975), 539–559.

peninsula. The contagion spread quickly to the adjacent islands of Puerto Rico and Cuba during the early months of 1519 and then to Yucatán and Veracruz on the American mainland. According to contemporary chroniclers, the vector was an African slave who landed at both places, but it is uncertain whether he acquired the malady in Africa, Iberia, or one of the Greater Antilles. A year or so later the pox raced south through Central America, and by the mid-1520s it had jumped to the Inca empire. Between 1558 and 1560, *Variola* of undetermined provenance reached the Rio de la Plata.[3]

The Brazilian Indians became its next victims in the first smallpox pandemic to sweep Portugal's New World possessions from 1562 to 1565. This initial infection came from Portugal rather than Africa, beginning in the colonial capital at Salvador (or Bahia) after a disease-laden ship arrived from Lisbon. The virus assaulted nascent Jesuit missions near All Saints Bay, wiping out an estimated 30,000 Indians within three or four months. It then leapfrogged up and down the coast, attacking virgin Amerindian populations wherever there were Portuguese settlements or mission stations from Pernambuco in the North to São Vicente in the South. From the seacoast of the latter it ascended to the inland plateau at the Jesuit mission at Piratininga near the fledgling town of São Paulo. The eruption was a classic virgin-soil epidemic which attacked only the indigenous peoples, usually causing death within three or four days, especially among young children.[4]

By the following decade, Brazil was booming as the world's leading producer of cane sugar, and planters shifted from Amerindian labor to African slaves to sustain the rapid rate of economic growth. The increasing numbers of Africans—perhaps 40,000 between 1576 and 1600—do not seem to have touched off major

---

3 Hopkins, *Princes and Peasants*, 204–226; Henry F. Dobyns, "An Outline of Andean Epidemic History to 1720," *Bulletin of the History of Medicine*, XVIII (1963), 493–515. For a critical examination of the evidence on the introduction of smallpox to the New World, David Henige, "When Did Smallpox Reach the New World (And Why Does It Matter)?" in Paul E. Lovejoy (ed.), *Africans in Bondage: Studies in Slavery and the Slave Trade* (Madison, 1986), 11–26.

4 In general, see the pioneering work of Octávio de Freitas, *Doenças africanas no Brasil* (São Paulo, 1935), who did not have the advantage of documentation available to us. The key contemporary reports of the first pandemic come from Jesuit accounts: e.g., Serafim Leite (ed.), *Monumenta brasiliae* (Rome, 1960), IV, 9–22, 178–181; Alfredo do Valle Cabral (ed.), *Cartas avulsas (1550–1568)* (Rio de Janeiro, 1931), 207, 258, 458, 462.

smallpox epidemics during the remainder of the sixteenth century, although the disease broke out locally on at least three occasions in 1585, 1597, and 1599. The second of these minor epidemics, which forced a Portuguese commander to abandon a military campaign to occupy the coast of Rio Grande do Norte, in north-easternmost Brazil, may represent the first introduction of the pox from West Africa to Brazil. French ships frequented that part of the coast in search of brazilwood, and in that same year a French vessel that had earlier raided the Portuguese factory at Arguin island off the Saharan coast arrived in Bahia bearing small-pox. Droughts had struck the Cape Verde Islands off the West African mainland between 1580 and 1582 and again in 1594, and the years 1574 to 1587 witnessed a succession of failed rains, famine, and sickness in Angola.[5]

THE SPREAD OF SMALLPOX IN THE SEVENTEENTH CENTURY   Slaves reached Brazil in increasing numbers—from around 4,000 a year to as many as 6,000 to 7,000—throughout the seventeenth cen-tury, and smallpox epidemics increased apace. Their African provenance also became more clearly established. The next out-break of smallpox occurred in 1613, when extensive mortality depleted the slaves on the sugar estates in Rio de Janeiro. It was attributed explicitly by contemporaries to blacks. Three years later, what was termed *sarampo e bexigas*—measles (then difficult to distinguish from smallpox and several other rash-provoking maladies) and smallpox—attacked the northeast. Its source was identified as slaves from the Kongo in central Africa and from Allada on the Lower Guinea Coast.[6]

5   Stuart B. Schwartz, "Indian Labor and New World Plantations: European Demands and Indian Responses in Northeastern Brazil," *American Historical Review*, LXXXVIII (1978), 43–79, and a personal communication from Schwartz to Alden. For slave import data, we rely throughout on Philip D. Curtin, *The Atlantic Slave Trade: A Census* (Madison, 1969), as modified by Paul E. Lovejoy, "The Volume of the Atlantic Slave Trade: A Synthesis," *Journal of African History*, XXIII (1982), 473–502. The data on West African climate come from Curtin, *Economic Change in Pre-Colonial Africa: Senegambia in the Era of the Slave Trade* (Madison, 1975), II, 3–7; and from many works by Sharon Nicholson (most recently, an NSF Final Report, ATM 77-21547, "Study of Environmental and Cli-matic Changes in Africa during the Last Five Centuries") and António Carreira (e.g., "Crises em Cabo Verde nos séculos xvi e xvii," *Geográphica*, VI [1966], 35–45). Vicente do Salvador (eds. João Capistrano de Abreu and Rodolfo Garcia), *História do Brasil 1500–1627* (São Paulo, 1954; 4th ed.).
6   Vivaldo Coaracy, *O Rio de Janeiro no século 17* (Rio de Janeiro, 1965), 38; Ambrosio

Two further outbreaks of pox occurred at the beginning of the 1620s. The first, another visitation upon the north coast, came via a ship from Pernambuco that brought the scourge to São Luis do Maranhão in 1621. The same epidemic swept on through Pernambuco and three other northeastern captaincies between 1621 and 1623. Although the extent of casualties is unknown, the contagion was sufficiently severe to provoke municipal authorities in Pernambuco to impose the first recorded quarantine for slaves arriving in Brazil.[7]

The simultaneous reappearance of smallpox in both northern and southern Brazil at this time coincided with new cycles of drought, attendant famine, and disease in both sahelian West Africa and Angola. The usually populous southern margins of the Sahara Desert appear to have enjoyed favorable rainfall during the fifteenth and sixteenth centuries, but they became increasingly arid during the next 200 years or so. As the dryness spread, numerous populations along the desert margins fell into conflict over shrinking living space. Their wars contributed captives to the streams of refugees that supplied slaves to Europeans buying labor along the West African coast. The populous interior delta of the Niger River experienced drought by 1617, and the Cape Verde Islands were beset by famine and sickness in 1620. Angola experienced a major smallpox epidemic, exacerbated by drought, from 1625 to 1628. In the mid-1620s, several slave ships from Luanda, the main port on the Angolan coast, reached Salvador after suffering extraordinarily high losses among their human cargoes. Nevertheless, smallpox-afflicted survivors were landed.[8]

Despite intensive fighting and population dislocations from the Dutch seizure of Brazil between 1630 and 1654, and the efforts of the Dutch to resupply the Northeast with fresh slaves from parallel conquests in Africa, the American colony appears to have

Fernandes Brandão (ed. Garcia), *Diálogos das grandezas do Brasil* (1618) (Salvador, 1956), 124–125; António de Santa Maria Jaboatão, *Novo orbe seráfico brasilico* (Rio de Janeiro, 1858), I, 191–192.

7 Bernardo Pereira Berredo, *Annaes historicos* (1749) (Florence, 1905; 3rd ed.), I, 192, par. 487; Gilberto Osório de Andrade, "As bexigas em Pernambuco," in Simão Pinheiro Morão, João Ferreyra da Rosa, and Miguel Dias Pimenta, *Notícia dos três primeiros livros em vernáculo sobre a medicina no Brasil* (Pernambuco, 1956), 13.

8 Sources for climate history in Angola are nearly all cited in Miller, "The Significance of Drought, Disease, and Famine in the Agriculturally Marginal Zones of West-Central Africa," *Journal of African History*, XXIII (1982), 17–61.

escaped a serious encounter with the pox until 1641. That year excessively heavy rains fell in the Northeast, and a virulent pandemic of smallpox swept throughout Dutch-held Brazil and beyond. In the single captaincy of Paraíba (immediately north of Pernambuco, center of the Dutch presence) an estimated 1,100 blacks became its victims. Three years later, smallpox caused extensive losses among the Indian villages of Maranhão.[9]

Although no observer specified the source of these epidemics, they may again have been products of arid conditions then prevailing in western and central Africa. The pace of droughts in the *sahel* had quickened as rains failed from 1639 to 1643, and Portuguese traders in Cacheu, the principal Upper Guinea source of slaves for Brazil, reported famine in 1641. Two years earlier, an extended drought had afflicted Angola from the mouth of the Zaire River south beyond the Kwanza River to the Portuguese outpost of Benguela.[10]

Western and central African climates improved during the decade and a half after about 1645, and Brazil was spared further major smallpox outbreaks during those years. But a new wave of sickness hit what was then becoming Portugal's most important colony during the early and mid-1660s. A "pestilential catarrh" (influenza or tuberculosis) swept Maranhão in 1660, and two years later a lethal attack of smallpox struck Maranhão and the adjacent captaincy of Pará. João Felippe Betendorf, a Jesuit father who ministered to the sick Indians of the north, described Maranhão as "burning with a plague of smallpox. . . . Parents abandoned their children and fled into the forests to avoid such a pestilential evil." Stricken Indians were so seriously afflicted that their skins became black, and their bodies became so fever-ridden that "pieces of their flesh fell off."[11]

No casualty estimates survive for these Maranhão epidemics, and the same is true for the second Brazilian pox pandemic that

9 Gaspar Barleu(s) (trans. and ed. Claudio Brandão), *História dos feitos recentemente praticados durante oito anos no Brasil . . .* (Rio de Janeiro, 1940), 236–237; Joan Niehof (trans. Moacir N. Vasconcelos, ed. José Honório Rodrigues), *Memorável viagem marítima a terrestre ao Brasil* (São Paulo, 1942), 81; Guilherme Studart (ed.), *Documentos para a história do Brasil e especialmente a do Ceará* (Fortaleza, 1904–1921), III, 122–137.
10 Fréderic Mauro, "L'Atlantique portugais et les esclaves (1570–1670)," *Revista da Faculdade de Letras* (Universidade de Lisboa), XXII (1956), 28.
11 John Hemming, *Red Gold: The Conquest of the Brazilian Indians, 1500–1760* (Cambridge, Mass., 1978), 338–339. See also Biblioteca Pública da Evora, cód. CVX/2-4, fls. 49^v-50^r.

raced throughout Brazil between 1664 and 1666. It was particularly devastating in the sugar-producing zone from Pernambuco to Bahia, which was absorbing most of the slaves imported to the colony after its recovery from the Dutch. In Bahia some planters lost their entire labor force to the disease. Thereafter, Brazil enjoyed a reprieve of nearly fifteen years before it was again visited by mass-killing diseases.[12]

Angola may have been the African source of the pestilence of the 1660s. Sickness of an unspecified identity had broken out there among the Kongo near the Zaire River in the mid-1650s. Possibly the disease was smallpox. In 1655 authorities in Bahia ordered quarantine for arriving Angolan slaves but could not enforce such a restriction. Drought drove other central Africans to invade the Portuguese-held river valleys near Benguela in 1656, and harvest failures and a mysterious disease described as *inchação* (swelling) caused terrible mortality in even the most fertile parts of the interior east of Luanda between 1660 and 1663.[13]

The 1680s and 1690s were the most infectious decades of the seventeenth century in Brazil. A smallpox epidemic started in Bahia in 1680 and appears to have endured for the next four years as the captaincy experienced famine, no doubt a consequence of the disease as well as of a two-year drought. In 1682, the pox spread to Pernambuco, its most unusual by-product being the publication of the first medical treatise written by a Portuguese resident in Brazil who was familiar with the manifestations of smallpox and measles.[14]

During the 1690s, *Variola* afflicted all of Brazil. A ship from Bahia brought the infection to the newly established Portuguese outpost of Colônia do Sacramento on the Plata River in 1690. Three years later, Rio de Janeiro's inhabitants, especially its slaves, suffered heavily from their first reported smallpox epidemic in half a century. And in 1695 two Jesuit fathers, one serving in the

12 Sebastião da Rocha Pitta, *História da America portuguesa* (1730) (Salvador, 1950; 3rd ed.), 227–228; Domingos de Loreto Couto, "Desagravos do Brazil e glorias de Pernambuco . . . (1757)," *Annaes da Biblioteca Nacional*, XXV (1903), 180–181.

13 João Antônio Cavazzi de Montecucculo (trans. and ed. Graciano Maria de Luguzzano), *Descrição histórica dos três reinos de Congo, Matamba e Angola* (Lisbon, 1965), I, 24, 243; II, 34, 213, 256.

14 *Documentos históricos do Arquivo Municipal, Cartas do Senado 1684–1692* (Salvador, c. 1950), III, 7–8; Morão, Rosa, and Pimenta, *Noticia dos três primeiros livros*, 73–125; Eustáquio Duarte, "Introdução histórica," in *ibid.*, 37–72.

Seven Missions of the future Brazilian state of Rio Grande do Sul and the other, Betendorf, still ministering in the state of Maranhão, watched helplessly as thousands of their Indian neophytes were devastated by the disease.[15]

These intense catastrophes seem tied to severe disasters on the eastern shores of the Atlantic. The major West African drought of the entire seventeenth century desiccated lands extending far beyond the desert fringe in the 1680s, even in usually moist Lower Guinea, where Bahian slavers were then intensifying their quest for African labor. The first significant influx of the famous "Mina" slaves from the Slave Coast may well have contributed to the exceptional virulence and persistence of the epidemics in northeastern Brazil at this time. Bahian traders simultaneously abandoned Luanda in Angola, expressing alarm at yet another smallpox epidemic there, so devastating that they foresaw years of slave exports insufficient to support Brazil's requirements for African labor.[16]

EIGHTEENTH-CENTURY EPIDEMICS   Bahian concern over the African droughts and epidemics was related to the intensified Brazilian competition for slaves following discoveries of gold in the interior after 1695. The number of slaves entering Brazil climbed to over 10,000 per year after 1700 and averaged nearly 15,000 annually at mid-century, before falling back slightly during the depression that inevitably followed the end of the mining boom after 1760. They rose again to 16,000 or so during the Brazilian agricultural renaissance after 1780. About two thirds of the new arrivals came from Angola and most of the remainder from the Mina coast.[17]

---

15 Luís Ferrand de Almeida, *A Colónia do Sacramento na época da sucessão de Espanhá* (Coimbra, 1973), 323; Coaracy, *O Rio de Janeiro no séc. 17*, 229; Anton Sepp von Reinegg (trans. Reymundo Schneider), *Viagem às missões jesuitas e trabalhos apostolicos* (1698) (São Paulo, 1972), 120.

16 Pierre Verger, *Flux et réflux de la traite des nègres entre le Golfe de Bénin et Bahia de Todos os Santos du dix-septième au dix-neuvième siècle* (Paris, 1968). Marion Johnson provided a copy of her unpub. ms., "Drought on the Guinea Coast" (London, c 1974) and made helpful comments on our approach in this essay.

17 A. John R. Russell-Wood, "Colonial Brazil: The Gold Cycle, c. 1690–1750," in Leslie Bethell (ed.), *Cambridge History of Latin America* (Cambridge, 1984), II, 547–600; Alden, "Late Colonial Brazil, 1750–1808," *ibid.*, II, 601–660.

Neither the African stations nor Brazil suffered a major contagion early in the century, but that hiatus ended abruptly in 1715. Smallpox ravaged Angola between 1715 and 1720, and Lower Guinea witnessed "thousands of Men . . . swept away" by the disease, according to a surgeon of the Royal African Company on the nearby Gold Coast. Smallpox appeared in Pernambuco on schedule in 1715 and caused serious losses in the Bahian backlands the following year. An Angolan ship bearing pox-infected chattels reached Salvador also in 1716, causing devastation in the city. By 1718 the disease appeared in Rio de Janeiro and by 1730 was in São Paulo. Between 1715 and 1730 the series of epidemics that swept the entire littoral of Brazil almost certainly originated in Africa.[18]

The 1720s, 1730s, and 1740s saw continuing frequent and severe epidemics in various parts of Brazil. The first outbreak seems to have been triggered from Angola, but West Africa may also have become a source by mid-century, when the most severe drought of the 1700s overspread the region. In 1724, the pox appeared in Maranhão and Pará and was carried from Belém to plantations and mission stations up the Amazon River, creating serious shortages of Indian laborers. São Paulo and its principal seaport, Santos, were also struck by pox between 1724 and 1725. Rains failed totally along the Angolan coast between 1724 and 1726, and food scarcities in its capital, Luanda, drove grain prices to unprecedented heights. Smallpox broke out in 1725 and, by 1727, the rise in slave mortality was ruining merchants there.[19]

The years 1729 to 1732, which were marked by low rainfall and famine in West Africa along the Senegal River, also saw renewed contagion in various parts of coastal Brazil. Between 1730 and 1732, smallpox returned to the city of São Paulo, as

18 Arquivo do Municipio da Bahia, Cartas de senado a sua magestade, XXXVIII: 9, fl. 12; Luis Lisanti (ed.), *Negócios coloniaes (Uma correspondência do século XVIII)* (São Paulo, 1973), I, 91–92; II, 131; Sergio Buarque de Holanda, "Movimentos da população em São Paulo no século XVIII," *Revista do Instituto de Estudos Brasileiros*, I (1966), 77; Elena F. Scheuss de Studer, *La trata de negros en el Río de la Plata durante el siglo XVIII* (Buenos Aires, 1958), Fig. V.

19 David Graham Sweet, "A Rich Realm of Nature Destroyed: The Middle Amazon Valley, 1640–1750," unpub. Ph.D. diss. (Univ. of Wisconsin, Madison, 1974), 82–84; Affonso de Escragnolle Taunay, *História da cidade de São Paulo no século XVIII* (São Paulo, 1950), II, 101–103; Arquivo Público da Bahia (hereafter APB), Ordens régias (OR), 20, no. 102.

well as to the captaincies of Pernambuco and Pará. In Angola drought again led to famine in 1735/36, and an epidemic of an unstated nature broke out in the latter year. Another unspecified malady claimed 3,000 lives in the captaincy of Rio de Janeiro in 1737. Very possibly its source was the pox which ravaged Bahia the same year.[20]

Infectious diseases along the entire American shore of the Atlantic reached their eighteenth-century peaks during the 1740s. In Brazil, the decade produced catastrophic losses from three separate epidemics of smallpox in São Paulo, but the captaincies of Maranhão and Pará were even more grievously stricken. The first serious poxian outbreak in two decades visited Belém in August 1743, with debilitating secondary infections of catarrhs, pleurisy, and bloody flux. Then, in 1749, just as those maladies had run their course, Belém, São Luis, and the vast Amazonian interior were hit by a lethal epidemic of measles. During most of the 1750s, waves of smallpox continued to wash over Maranhão and over all of Brazil.[21]

These middle decades of the century also saw widespread drought, hunger, and diseases among both Africans and Europeans in West Africa. Supposedly half of the population of the upper Niger River valley perished at this time. Food was in short supply along the Gold Coast in 1743 and again in the early 1750s. The drought-prone Cape Verde Islands, always a sensitive pluviometer for the climate of the adjacent West African mainland, experienced serious famine in the late 1740s and again in 1754. Slaves perished from malnutrition at the French post near the mouth of the Senegal River in 1751/52. Conditions were somewhat better in Angola, although smallpox was reported aboard a slaver en route from there to Pernambuco in 1759.[22]

20 Taunay, *História da cidade*, III, 161–164; APB/OR/26, no. 38; /27, no. 68; Inácio Accioli de Cerqueira e Silva (ed. Braz do Amaral), *Memorias históricas da Bahia* (Salvador, 1935), II, 378; Couto, "Desagravos do Brazil," 184; Sor. Mariana Bernarda and Sor. Mᵃ Margarida Bittancourt to king, *ca.* 1733, Arquivo Histórico Ultramarino (Lisbon) (hereafter AHU), Papeis Avulsos (PA)/Pará cx. 7; Gomes Freire de Andrada to António Guedes Pereira, 9 June 1737, Arquivo Nacional, Rio de Janeiro (hereafter ANRJ), col. 60, 6, fl. 224ʳ; Conde das Galveas to king, 15 May 1738, APB/OR/35, no. 75.
21 Numerous accounts scattered in AHU/PA/Maranhão, cx. 29 and maço 1, and AHU/PA/Pará, cxs. 1, 3, 12. Also Leduar de Assis Rocha, *Efemérides médicas pernambucanas, séculos XVI, XVII e XVIII* (Recife, c 1954), 53.
22 Emilio F. Moran, "The Evolution of Cape Verde's Agriculture," *African Economic History*, XI (1982), 71.

Smallpox remained the principal scourge of Brazil during the second half of the eighteenth century. Northern Brazil continued to be a major theater of the infection, all the more because the state of Maranhão shifted after the mid-1750s from its traditional reliance on Indian labor to a dependency on imported African slaves. A royally chartered Maranhão Company initially purchased cargoes in Luanda at a time when prices there fell in response to drought, famine, and epidemics. The first shipments reached Belém in 1756, and that winter the city was beset by "a terrible epidemic of catarrhs" that had not abated before smallpox also broke out in the city. Company agents purchased more slaves at Luanda in the early 1760s, and the all-but-predictable smallpox epidemics followed in Maranhão in 1762/63 and 1766/67. The latter outbreak may well have followed renewed drought and a poxian upsurge in Angola between 1765 and 1767.[23]

Brazil's east coast also suffered intermittent contagion between the late 1760s and the early 1780s. Smallpox, accompanied by jaundice and leprosy, appeared in São Paulo in 1768. Eleven years later the pox caused hundreds of persons to be admitted to Salvador's two hospitals, where most of them died. In 1780, São Paulo again suffered from an eruption of smallpox, as did Pernambuco and adjacent northern captaincies on numerous occasions between 1774 and 1787.[24]

The last seven years of the eighteenth century witnessed another major *Variola* epidemic that was especially serious in northern Brazil. As the Portuguese minister of marine in Lisbon reviewed reports from the American colony, he lamented "the great damage that the pox has been causing, and continues to cause, all over Brazil."[25]

23 Alden, "Indian Versus Black Slavery in the State of Maranhão during the Seventeenth and Eighteenth Centuries," *Biblioteca Americana*, I (1983), 91–142; Colin M. Maclachlan, "African Slave Trade and Economic Development in Amazonia, 1700–1800," in Robert Brent Toplin (ed.), *Slavery and Race Relations in Latin America* (Westport, Conn., 1974), 134–139; Arthur Vianna, *As epidemias no Pará* (Belém, 1975; 2nd ed.), 36–37; Miller, *Way of Death: Merchant Capitalism and the Angolan Slave Trade, 1730–1830*, forthcoming, drawing on Carreira, "As companhias pombalinas de navegação, comércio, e tráfico de escravos entre a costa africana e o nordeste brasileiro," *Boletim cultural da Guiné portuguesa*, XXII (1967), 5–88; XXIII (1968), 301–454; XXIV (1969), 59–188, 284–474.

24 Maria Luiza Marcilio, *La ville de São Paulo: peuplement et population 1750–1850* (Rouen, 1968), 166; Accioli, *Memorias da Bahia*, V, 513–514; Osório de Andrade, "Estudo critico," in Morão, Rosa, and Pimenta, *Noticia dos três primeiros livros*, 13.

25 Francisco Inocencio de Sousa Coutinho to Luis Pinto de Sousa, 7 June 1796, 12 Feb.

Nor was the situation better on the African side of the Atlantic. From 1787 through 1794 Angola experienced intensifying drought and disease. Plagues of locusts, not reported there since the great aridity of the early seventeenth century, consumed everything growing around the colony's capital. Still, starving refugees from the interior congregated in the city, where the governor pleaded for emergency relief after declaring that "the pox . . . this year has been extremely cruel throughout the continent." Uncounted victims became involuntary passengers on Brazil-bound slavers, which experienced exceptionally high mortality rates during the crossing to Rio de Janeiro. Aridity also punished West Africa in the mid-1790s, when North American slavers along the Gold Coast reported both measles and smallpox.[26]

END OF THE LEGAL SLAVE TRADE   Dramatic changes swept across the south Atlantic in the early decades of the nineteenth century. The Portuguese royal family fled to Brazil in 1807/08 and then returned to Lisbon in 1821. Brazil declared its independence of Portugal in 1822. Both Portugal and Brazil were subjected to intense British pressure to end the slave trade, although they managed to defend legal slaving until 1831 and then continued illicitly for another two decades. Imports may have averaged 20,000 to 25,000 slaves annually over the period, the highest levels in history. The slaves came mostly from Angola but increasingly also from Mozambique and Madagascar, which became significant exporters as British naval patrols drove slavers away from Senegambia and the Mina coast.[27]

During the first three decades after 1800, Luanda and Benguela reported epidemics with alarming regularity, specifying smallpox in 1811, 1814, 1822, and 1826, and implying it in 1805, 1816, and 1825. High mortality rates on slave ships bound from

1797, Biblioteca e Arquivo Público do Pará (hereafter BAPP), cód. 682, no. 103, cód. 702, no. 14; Vianna, *As epidemias no Pará*, 39–42; Dom Rodrigo de Sousa Coutinho to Francisco Inocencio de Sousa Coutinho, 29 July 1799, BAPP, cód. 685, no. 3.
26 Miller, "Legal Portuguese Slaving from Luanda, Angola—Some Preliminary Indications of Volume and Direction, 1760–1830," *Revue française d'histoire d'outre-mer*, LXII (1975), 135–176; Darold D. Wax, "A Philadelphia Surgeon on a Slaving Voyage to Africa," *Pennsylvania Magazine of History and Biography*, LXXXXIV (1968), 482–493.
27 Leslie Bethell, *The Abolition of the Brazilian Slave Trade: Britain, Brazil and the Slave Trade Question 1807–1869* (Cambridge, 1970).

there to Rio de Janeiro seem to confirm epidemics between 1806 and 1808 and, periodically, throughout the 1810s and 1820s.[28]

Drought, famine, and disease also disturbed West Africa and Mozambique from time to time during these decades. The Cape Verde Islands, for example, suffered from a food shortage in 1803/04 and from drought between 1810 and 1814 and again in 1825. Insufficient rainfall and famine caused hardship along the lower Senegal River in 1812. Crops may have failed along the Gold Coast in 1816 and seem likely to have done so in 1824. A series of droughts parched the Zambezi valley and adjoining districts of Mozambique at various times, particularly between 1822 and 1832. Africa thus continued to dispatch slave-borne pathogens toward Brazil in the first three decades of the nineteenth century.[29]

Nonetheless, Brazil experienced only six minor outbreaks of smallpox between 1803 and 1831. Details on the severity of an 1808 eruption in São Paulo do not survive, but it followed a significant expansion in the captaincy's sugar industry and the high mortality rates on slave ships of Angolan origin. The contagion re-entered Belém in 1819 via a slave ship from Africa, and nearly a sixth of the city's inhabitants perished between April and September of that year. Six years later, in 1825, an apparently localized eruption hit the northeastern province of Paraíba. That same year and again in 1828 and 1831 epidemics upset life in Rio de Janeiro, then Brazil's capital, largest city, and chief port.[30]

BEGINNINGS OF SMALLPOX PREVENTION IN BRAZIL AND AFRICA
The decline in frequency and intensity of smallpox in Brazil, despite the persistence of drought, famine, and smallpox at all the African sources of the burgeoning slave trade, may reflect one final change—the partial success of Jennerian vaccination introduced on both sides of the southern Atlantic after 1804. Previously, public health authorities had attempted to ward off smallpox by quarantining suspected victims, just as they had attempted

28 Miller, "Legal Portuguese Slaving," 157–158.
29 For the southeastern African climate, Gerhard Liesegang, "Famines and Smallpox in South Eastern Africa, Eighteenth to Twentieth Centuries," unpub. ms. (Maputo, 1978); idem, "Famines, Epidemics, Plagues and Long Periods of Warfare: Their Effects in Mozambique 1700–1795," unpub. ms. (Harare, 1982).
30 Marcilio, La ville de São Paulo, 166, 201; Vianna, As Epidemias no Pará, 46–50; Mary Karasch, "African Mortality and Epidemic Disease in 19th Century Rio de Janeiro," unpub. ms. (1982).

to delay debarkations from disease-ridden slave ships in Brazilian ports since the early seventeenth century. These measures had largely failed, because someone was always willing to purchase even mortally ill slaves. Inoculation, also known as variolation, had offered an alternative method of prevention since the middle of the eighteenth century. Inoculation procedures transferred a small portion of virally infected matter from a lesion on the skin of a sufferer to that of a healthy partner; a mild infection would usually result, conferring lifetime immunity from smallpox. Some Africans practiced variolation by the early eighteenth century, and the technique spread from Turkish sources to England in 1721 and to some French and British slavers in the Atlantic by the 1760s and 1770s. There and in Britain's North American colonies it sharply reduced the extent and virulence of smallpox. No comparable decline had lessened Brazil's sufferings, although missionaries in Portuguese America occasionally experimented with inoculation in the late 1720s and again in the 1740s. A standard Portuguese medical text published in 1761 reported that variolation was seldom employed, and advised against its use.[31]

Both the Portuguese Crown and its colonial agents finally became interested in the therapeutic possibilities of variolation by the 1790s, perhaps sparked by the Pernambucan-born Francisco Arruda Câmara, who wrote a thesis on smallpox inoculation at the French medical school at Montpellier, from which he graduated in 1790. The alarming reports of poxian virulence in Brazil in the 1790s led to the establishment of a special hospital in Lisbon to treat victims. In 1798, Diogo de Sousa, governor of Maranhão, promoted variolation during the smallpox outbreak there and achieved some success among whites and blacks, but less among Indians. The same year the governor of neighboring and fever-ridden Pará received royal authority to offer inoculations at state

31 Herbert, "Smallpox Inoculation," 539–540, 546–547; Herbert S. Klein and Stanley L. Engerman, "A Note on Mortality in the French Slave Trade in the Eighteenth Century," in Henry A. Gemery and Jan S. Hogendorn (eds.), *The Uncommon Market: Essays in the Economic History of the Atlantic Slave Trade* (New York, 1979), 271; José Justino Teixeira Botelho, "Acerca da vacinação e das bexigas," *Boletim da Academia das Sciencias de Lisboa (Segunda Classe)*, XVII (1927), 202–203; Carlos da Silva Araujo, *The Immortalized Cow: Smallpox Vaccine and Wright's Vaccines in Brazil* (Rio de Janeiro, 1972); Duarte Rebello de Saldanha, *Illustração medica* . . . (Lisbon, 1761), I, 351; Richard B. Sheridan, *Doctors and Slaves: A Medical and Demographic History of Slavery in the British West Indies, 1680–1834* (New York, 1985), 252–256.

to the south, Francisco Mendes Ribeiro de Vasconcelos, a military surgeon in Rio de Janeiro, won public acclaim for his efforts to variolate against the "smallpox . . . [that had] alarmed sugar planters and other agriculturalists at seeing their slaves die." By a general circular of 9 July 1799, the Crown directed all colonial governors to initiate variolation programs, especially among young black and Indian children, "since experience has shown this to be the only effective defense against the scourge . . . which has caused such considerable devastation in the Portuguese colonies."[32]

That circular followed one year after Edward Jenner, an English physician, had published his confirmation of a longstanding rural belief that persons whose skins were scored with cowpox could gain immunity to smallpox at less risk than from variolation with human viral matter. A small percentage of those inoculated succumbed to the infection and could also transmit it to others at dangerously uncontrolled levels. Jenner's vaccine carried none of these disadvantages and its use spread quickly throughout Europe and abroad.[33]

It is unlikely that the Portuguese Crown meant the inoculation program it announced in 1799 to involve the novel use of cowpox. Rather, variolation was probably intended. However, vials of Jenner's cowpox lymph were sent from London to the University of Coimbra and to Lisbon in the same year, and in 1800 the Crown advised overseas authorities of the existence of the new preventive. Copies of an account of the Jenner method by de Paiva, a popularizer of current medical knowledge, were sent to Brazil in 1801. The Jenner vaccine itself first arrived in Brazil in 1804, when a wealthy Brazilian landowner, Francisco

32 Silva Araujo, *Immortalized Cow*, 18; Ernesto de Souza Campos, "Considerações sobre a ocorrencia de variola e vacina nos séculos xvii, xviii e xix sob a luz de documentação coeva," *Revista do Instituto Histórico e Geografico Brasileiro*, CCXXXI (1956), 147–149; Vianna, *As epidemias no Pará*, 45–46; "Representação de moradores do Rio de Janeiro sobre a vantagem da vacina," 15 June 1798, Biblioteca Nacional (Rio de Janeiro) (hereafter BNRJ), II-32, 16, 9; another petition, 20 Feb. 1800, BNRJ, II-34, 15, 32; Teixeira Botelho, "Acerca da vacinação," 203.

33 The older literature preceding Hopkins, *Princes and Peasants,* includes: Genevieve Miller, *The Adoption of Inoculation for Smallpox in England and France* (Philadelphia, 1957); Peter Razzell, *Edward Jenner's Cowpox Vaccine: The History of a Medical Myth* (Firle, 1977); Dexter Baxby, *Jenner's Smallpox Vaccine* (London, 1981).

Caldeira Brant, sent seven of his slaves to Lisbon to be vaccinated and to be returned to Brazil as fresh human reservoirs of the protective lymph. Their owner met them at the Salvador dockside and had his son become the first person to be vaccinated in Brazil on 31 Decemer 1804. The boy obviously survived the experience, for he died in 1906 at the remarkable age of 104.[34]

News of the Jenner method and supplies of the vaccine traveled rapidly along the Brazilian coast, reaching Rio de Janeiro and Pernambuco in 1805. Elsewhere enlightened administrators, hearing of the success of the innovative procedure, sent children to Bahia to bring the live vaccine back to their own captaincies. In Maranhão, where some of the lymph had recently arrived, a ship arrived from Angola in 1806 bearing infected slaves but failed to ignite an epidemic. That same year, the Crown distributed throughout the empire copies of a pamphlet prepared by the surgeon-general of Portuguese India to reassure remaining doubters about the safety of vaccination and asserting its superior effectiveness over other forms of prophylaxis. In 1811, three years after the exiled Portuguese court arrived in Rio de Janeiro, a municipal vaccine commission was created in Brazil's most important city, and it continued to function down to 1835. In those twenty-four years its staff administered 102,791 vaccinations, concentrating on newly arrived slaves and on those already working on plantations. By 1819, plans were announced for the establishment of a similar clinic in São Paulo.[35]

Public vaccination began that same year in Luanda, after several unsuccessful efforts to import the vaccine live from Brazil. Luanda officials had made their first attempt in 1806 during the onset of the smallpox epidemic that lasted until 1808, but the lymph expired during the crossing. The same experiment failed again the next year. A third attempt proved successful in 1819, and by early 1821, less than a year and half after the vaccine had

---

34 Silva Araujo, *Immortalized Cow,* 23–26; Manoel Joaquim Henriques de Paiva, *Preservativo das bexigas; ou a história da origem e descobrimento da vacina* . . . (Lisbon, 1806; 2nd ed.); Visconde de Anadia to Francisco da Cunha Menezes, BNRJ, I-31, 30, 49; Luiz Monteiro da Costa, "A introdução da vacina jeneriana na Bahia," *Anais do Arquivo do Estado da Bahia,* XXXIX (1970), 145–148.

35 Campos, "Considerações," 153–157, 158–159; Vianna, *As epidemias no Pará,* 17; Visconde de Anadia to governor of Bahia, 29 March 1806, BNRJ, II-33, 28, 23; "Policia— Instituição de Vaccina, 1811–1821," ANRJ, cód. 368; Joseph François Xavier Sigaud, *Du climat et des maladies du Brézil, ou statistique médicale de cet empire* (Paris, 1844), 110–111.

been introduced, authorities had conferred immunity upon 12,292 persons, presumably including most of the 2,000 to 3,000 free inhabitants of the capital and many of its about-to-be-embarked slaves. The vaccine had been successfully transported to Benguela the previous August (1820), and reports from Brazil soon confirmed a "very sensible diminution" in the mortality of slaves arriving from both ports.[36]

Looking back from the 1840s, Sigaud, a leading physician in Brazil, reviewed the achievements of the anti-smallpox campaign in the southern Atlantic. He took satisfaction in the accomplishments of the vaccine commission in the imperial capital, noting the virtual absence of *Variola* from 1829 to 1834. The final victory lay still in the distant future, but the first steps had been taken toward eradicating the major killer in both Brazil and Africa. One persistent transatlantic link between them had been significantly weakened.[37]

Early European accounts of Brazil lavished praise on its beauty, economic potential, and salubrious ambience, but it became a less healthy land after Europeans and Africans arrived in large numbers. Contagious infections imported from abroad, including measles, yellow fever, other fevers of many sorts, influenza, pleurisy, and dysentery, all in addition to the smallpox that we have tracked here, ravaged the land from the middle of the sixteenth century onward. Clearly these disorders, as well as widespread malnutrition, poor sanitation, and the brutalizing consequences of slavery for Amerindians and Africans, diminished the quality of life in colonial Brazil.

However, the state of public health was abysmal everywhere at that time, and it may have been less so in Brazil than in Europe or even in English colonial America. According to one estimate, the break between epidemics in seventeenth-century Europe averaged only four years, and that interval decreased to only two

36 Dispatch of António de Saldanha da Gama (governor, Angola), 1 Nov. 1807, AHU/PA/Angola, cx. 57; Accioli, *Memórias históricas da Bahia*, III, 196–197; João Carlos Feo Cardoso de Castello Branco e Torres, *Memórias contendo . . . a História dos governadores e capitaens generaes de Angola desde 1575 até 1825* (Paris, 1825), III, 304; dispatches of Manuel Vieira de Albuquerque e Tovar (governor, Angola), 24 March, 18 Aug., 30 Nov. 1820, 23 Jan. 1821, AHU/PA/Angola, cx. 67; cf. Manuel dos Anjos da Silva Rebelo, *Relações entre Angola e Brasil 1808–1830* (Lisbon, 1970), 30, 390, 403.
37 Sigaud, *Du climat*, 182–183.

years in the eighteenth century. Smallpox was "absent . . . for as long as five years only on two occasions" in the mainland colonies of English North America between 1675 and 1775. In greater London, where smallpox became endemic during the seventeenth century, 6.1 percent of all deaths between 1661 and 1700 were attributed to *Variola,* and the percentage increased to 8.4 between 1721 and 1760. In smaller English rural communities smallpox accounted for one out of five deaths during the eighteenth century. Losses were even higher in contemporary Geneva, where one out of four persons above age five died of the pox, and in The Hague, where 37 percent of those above age five who succumbed to infections were victims of the dreaded disease.[38]

Although the evidence from Brazil seldom approaches the famous mortality bills in England or other European sources, and although the tropical epidemiology of smallpox differs significantly from its pattern in temperate climes, the pox may have been less devastating in Brazil than in Europe during the centuries that we have surveyed. Brazil's population was more dispersed and its dense settlements smaller than those in Europe or North America, and it was certainly the urban centers that always remained primary distribution points for contagious diseases.

Major outbreaks of the contagion began in Brazilian seaports and moved rapidly via waterways and backland trails to the interior. Smallpox, along with other maladies, reached the ports via the slave trade from Africa, where droughts, famines, and epidemics frequently anticipated major *Variola* eruptions in Brazil. Africa does not appear to have acted as a source for smallpox in Brazil during the sixteenth century, when relatively few slaves came from there to Portuguese America, but the booming slave trade of the seventeenth and eighteenth centuries seems the most likely linkage for those later years, when tens of thousands of slaves each year, many of them infected, came out from African stations to Portugal's colony across the Atlantic.

38 G. Miller, *Adoption of Inoculation,* 33 (n. 22), Appendix C; John Duffy, *Epidemics in Colonial America* (Baton Rouge, 1953), 20, 104; Charles Creighton, *A History of Epidemics in Britain* (Cambridge, 1894), II, 456, 531, 623.

APPENDIX

Summary Chronology of Droughts and Epidemics in Africa and Brazil, c 1500–c 1840

Time line	West Africa	Angola	Mozambique	Brazil	Other American
1500					1507: Slavers alleged to have introduced small-pox-infected slaves in Hispaniola.
1510					1518–20: Transfer of smallpox from Caribbean to Mexican mainland.
1520					1520s: Smallpox epidemics in highland Mexico and Peru.
1530					
1540	1541–42: Famine on Upper Guinea mainland.				1546: First smallpox epidemic in New Granada, via slaves from Santo Domingo.
	1549: Drought in Cape Verde Islands.			1549: Sick slaves (disease unknown) at Bahia.	
1550		1558–60: Hunger (?) and high mortality at São Tomé.			1558–69: Smallpox at the Rio de la Plata and elsewhere in Spanish South America.

Time line	West Africa	Angola	Mozambique	Brazil	Other American
1560		1561–63: Drought and famine in interior.		1562–65: SMALL-POX PANDEMIC, PERNAMBUCO TO SÃO VICENTE.	
1570		c 1574–88: Drought, continuing intermittently. (drought)			
1580	c 1580–82: Drought in Cape Verdes.	1584: Sickness noted at Luanda.		1585: Smallpox in Ilhéus.	1581: Smallpox in Peru.
1590	1594: Drought in Cape Verdes.			1597: French vessel from Arguin (West Africa) introduced smallpox in Rio Grande do Norte.	
1600					
1610	1609 (to 1614?): Drought in Cape Verdes.	1614–19: Serious drought.		1611: Smallpox at São Paulo (?). 1613: Smallpox at Pernambuco.	

	1617: Drought along the Niger Bend.	1616: Smallpox in the northeast, attributed to slaves from both West Africa and Angola.	1621: Quarantine measures introduced at Buenos Aires.
1620	1620: Famine and sickness in Cape Verdes.	1621–23: Smallpox in the north and northeast. 1626: Ship carrying smallpox arrives in Bahia from Angola.	1627: Smallpox at Anserma.
	1625–28: FIRST RECORDED SMALLPOX EPIDEMIC, also great drought. 1625: Extraordinarily high mortality on board slavers from Luanda.	c. 1620s: Possibly a time of great drought.	
1630			1633–34, 1636, 1639–41: epidemics at Panamá.
1640	1639–45: Drought, no report of sickness. 1639–43: Major drought and famine.	1641: Excessive rains and smallpox widespread in north, northeast. 1644: Smallpox in Maranhão.	

Time line	West Africa	Angola	Mozambique	Brazil	Other American
1650		1655: Unspecified sickness in Kongo. 1656: Drought and warfare at Benguela.		1655: Angolan slaves quarantined at Bahia.	
1660	1661: Severe but short drought on Gold Coast.	1660–63: Famine and illness described as *inchação* (swelling).		1662: Smallpox in Pará and Maranhão. 1664–66: Pandemic smallpox.	1664: RAC ships reach Barbados with smallpox aboard; great mortality among slaves in St. Christopher's and Nevis.
1670	1669–70: Very dry years along Niger Bend. 1676: Drought in lower Senegal valley.				
1680	1680s: Major drought all over West Africa. 1682–83: Famine at Accra. 1687: Famine at Ardra. 1688–90: Drought and famine in Upper Guinea.	1680s: Famine, also drought (?). 1684–85: Smallpox, with great loss of life.		1680–84: Smallpox in Bahia. 1682: Smallpox in Pernambuco. (1685–c 1692: Yellow fever in Pernambuco, Bahia, etc.) 1686: Angolan slaves with small-	

1690	c. 1690: Drought in Cape Verdes. 1695: Famine along the Niger Bend. 1696: Possible famine on Gold Coast?	1691–92: (Localized?) drought near mouth of Zaire River.	1690: Smallpox at Colônia do Sacramento. 1693: Smallpox at Rio de Janeiro. 1695: Smallpox in Rio Grande do Sul and Maranhão.	1693: Smallpox in Bogotá. 1698: Quarantine measures introduced at Charleston.
1700	1704: Drought and famine along Niger Bend. 1705–21: Prolonged drought in Cape Verdes.			1700–02, 1704: Smallpox at New Granada. 1705: Smallpox aboard a ship reaching Buenos Aires. 1708: Smallpox aboard a ship arriving in Jamaica. Epidemics in Guayaquil.
1710	1710: Serious famine in lower Senegal valley. c 1712–13: Smallpox at Whydah (Slave Coast, lower Guinea) 1719: Drought at Cape Verdes.	1713–20: Drought. 1715–20: Smallpox.	1715–18: Smallpox widespread in Brazil.	1713: Smallpox aboard RAC ship at Jamaica. 1715, 1717: Smallpox in mainland north American seaports. 1718–20: Widespread reports of smallpox from southern Spanish colonies.

Time line	West Africa	Angola	Mozambique	Brazil	Other American
1770	1770–71: Drought and famine at Timbuktu. 1773–76: Serious drought in Cape Verdes. 1773: Smallpox in Sierra Leone. 1774: "Period of starvation" on Gold Coast.			1774: Smallpox in Pernambuco and Rio Grande do Norte. 1776: Smallpox at Belém. 1779: Smallpox at Bahia. 1779: Smallpox at São Paulo.	
1780	1786: Smallpox at Upper Guinea. 1787: Smallpox at Porto Novo (Slave Coast).	1781: Food shortages and high mortality at Benguela. 1786: Famine, smallpox. 1787: Extraordinary food shortages, smallpox.		1787: Smallpox at Pernambuco and Maranhão.	1782–83: Smallpox epidemics in New Granada. 1788–89: Epidemics in New Granada (?). 1789: Smallpox in Buenos Aires.

	West Africa	Slave ships	South / Natal	Brazil	New Granada
1790	1789–91: Drought in Cape Verdes. 1790s: Generally dry in West Africa.	1789–94: Extreme famine and disorder, repeated epidemics.	1791–96: Drought in the south.	1791: "Febres miasmaticas" in Ceará. 1793–99: Pandemic smallpox throughout Brazil.	
	c 1790: Smallpox on River Sherbro (upper Guinea).	1793(?)–94: High mortality aboard slave ships.			
	1795: Measles and smallpox on the Gold Coast.	1796–97: Second mortality peak on slavers.	1796: Smallpox aboard slave ship, suppressed by inoculation.		
1800	1803–04: Drought in Cape Verdes 1804–05: Drought in Sahara	Recurrent epidemics. Smallpox implied in 1805 1806–08: Mortality rises on slavers at sea.	1799–1803: Dry period in Nguniland (Natal).	1808: Smallpox in São Paulo	1801–02: Smallpox epidemics in New Granada, "less severe."
1810	1810: Drought in Cape Verdes.	Smallpox further specified in 1811, 1814.			
	1812: Drought and famine in lower Senegal. 1813–14: Drought in Cape Verdes.	Continuing episodes of drought.			

Time line	West Africa	Angola	Mozambique	Brazil	Other American
1820	1816: Possible dearth on Gold Coast. 1822–23: Serious epidemics in Sahara. 1824: Crop failure on Gold Coast. 1825: Drought in Cape Verdes.	Continuing epidemics. Smallpox specified in 1822 and 1826, implied in 1825.	1817: Drought in Madagascar. 1822–32: Widespread drought. 1824: Famine and wars at Delagoa Bay.	1819: Smallpox at Belém from a ship from Africa. 1825: Smallpox in Paraíba, Rio de Janeiro. 1828: Smallpox (minor?) at Rio de Janeiro.	
1830–1840	c. 1828–39: Severe drought climaxing lengthy period of climate deterioration.	1830: Drought	Drought continues. 1832–36: Smallpox epidemics.	1831: Smallpox (minor?) at Rio de Janeiro. 1834–36: Smallpox reappears at Rio de Janeiro.	

Kenneth F. Kiple and Virginia H. Kiple

Deficiency Diseases in the Caribbean

The historiography of slavery in the Americas has recently taken on a new biological dimension as historians have begun to appreciate the importance of pathogenic agents in any holistic understanding of their subject. Of special interest is the impact of these agents on slave mortality and, more specifically, the extent of the role that they played in preventing most Caribbean slave populations from sustaining a natural rate of growth.

Historians are also looking beyond pathogens to the nutritional factor, which may have figured prominently in the etiologies of slave diseases. Seldom does a new work appear which does not allege that malnutrition was a serious problem of Caribbean slave health. However, no attempt has been made to single out specific nutritional deficiencies in the Caribbean slave diet and in the process prove that Caribbean bondsmen were malnourished. Nor for that matter has any effort been made to link suspected nutritional deficiencies with some of the more important West Indian slave diseases.

This study makes such an attempt by investigating the West African nutritional heritage of Caribbean slaves, by analyzing the Caribbean slave diet, and by matching nutritional deficiencies revealed by this analysis with the symptoms of the diseases which plagued slaves exclusively.

Kenneth F. Kiple is Associate Professor of History at Bowling Green State University. He is the co-author with Virginia H. Kiple of a book-length study on the biological history of blacks in the United States.

This study is an elaboration of the Caribbean portion of the paper "Slave Nutrition and Disease during the Nineteenth Century: The United States and the Caribbean," which was delivered at the annual meeting of the Organization of American Historians (1979). The authors wish to thank the Joint Committee on Latin American Studies of the Social Science Research Council and the American Council of Learned Societies for an award to support the project out of which this research was generated. They are grateful also to the Bowling Green Faculty Research Committee for assistance with supplementary travel funds.

0022-1953/80/020197-19 $02.50/0

THE AFRICAN NUTRITIONAL HERITAGE   Although there were some exceptions, West African diets were poor. Prior to the sixteenth century, they consisted of bananas, taro, the small African yam, millet, and rice crops, which researchers believe did little more than sustain life. In the sixteenth century, American cassava and maize were imported, and are credited with stimulating the growth of West Africa's population—a growth that kept pace, or even exceeded, the drain of the slave trade.[1]

Although the introduction of these two starchy plants may have resolved problems of quantity, the quality of West African diets remained deficient. Animal protein has never played a major role in West African nutrition, with much of the blame belonging to the tsetse fly—a bloodsucking insect which imparts African sleeping sickness to animals as well as to man. In much of West Africa the tsetse fly was so prevalent that it made the raising of cattle and other large animals, if not in all cases impossible, at least unprofitable. Thus many West Africans were limited to keeping a few goats, chickens, and dogs and sometimes a pig— animals so scarce and highly prized that they were slaughtered only on special occasions.[2]

Bovine milk was thus excluded from West African diets, which may be a reason for the high frequency of lactose intolerance today among blacks of West African origin. Such intolerance occurs among people with a history of low milk consumption. Also excluded in many places were eggs, for some because of taboos against their consumption, and for others because it seemed wasteful to eat the egg rather than wait for the chicken. Finally, because of cultural beliefs, fruit consumption was frequently frowned upon as was the use of most vegetables, except the yam, taro, cassava, and maize.[3]

---

1 Oliver Davis, *West Africa Before the Europeans: Archaeology and Prehistory* (New York, 1967), 8, 149; Alfred W. Crosby, *The Columbian Exchange: Biological and Cultural Consequences of 1492* (Westport, Ct., 1972), 186–188; Bruce F. Johnston, *The Staple Food Economics of Western Tropical Africa* (Stanford, 1958), 174–181.
2 J. P. Glasgow, *The Distribution and Abundance of Tsetse* (London, 1963), 1–3; John Ford, *The Role of the Trypanosomiases in African Ecology: A Study of the Tsetse Fly Problem* (Oxford, 1971), 88–89; Frederick J. Simoons, *Eat Not This Flesh: Food Avoidances in the Old World* (Madison, 1961), 56.
3 Although West Indian figures are not available, about three-quarters of the Afro-Americans living in the United States are lactose intolerant, meaning that, because they have low levels of the lactase enzyme which breaks down milk sugars, they cannot drink

One consequence of this background was that many West Africans must have reached the New World with a history of malnutrition. Empirical data suggest that this was the case. Research conducted by Fogel, Engerman, and Higman concerning the height of some 25,000 Trinidadian slaves indicates that newly imported Africans were significantly shorter on average than Creole-born slaves. Fraginals has found the same to be true for Cuba. First-generation Creole slaves were significantly taller than freshly imported Africans.[4]

Research has demonstrated that a radical change in dietary habits produces a dramatic increase in height. The rapid growth of New World slaves over the course of a generation or so implies that West Indian diets were at least more protein laden than those of West Africa and were probably also of better overall quality. We discuss West Africa in order to emphasize the poor nutritional status of a sizable portion of slaves in the Caribbean.[5]

West Indian slave populations were seldom self-sustaining so long as the slave trade endured. Rather, they received massive injections of fresh imports from that traffic until the beginning of the nineteenth century and, in the case of Cuba, through the middle of that century. Hence Caribbean slave populations always had many badly nourished newcomers crowding their ranks—a condition which the circumstances of the Middle Passage could only have aggravated. The standard menu for slaves making the passage was a boiled cereal (usually rice) with a "sauce" made by boiling salted fish—a diet lacking in many important nutrients.

milk. For a discussion, see K. and V. Kiple, "Slave Child Mortality: Some Nutritional Answers to a Perennial Puzzle," *Journal of Social History*, X (1977), 284–309. For West African dietary habits, consult Simoons, *Eat Not This Flesh*, 73–78; Tadeuz Lewicki, *West African Food in the Middle Ages* (London, 1974), 79, 116–127; Michael Gelfand, *Diet and Tradition in African Culture* (Edinburgh, 1971), 206.

4 Robert W. Fogel and Stanley L. Engerman, "Recent Findings in the Study of Slave Demography and Family Structure," *Sociology and Social Research*, LXIII (1979), 566–589; Barry W. Higman, "Growth in Afro-Caribbean Slave Populations," *American Journal of Physical Anthropology*, L (1979), 373–385; Manuel Moreno Fraginals, "Africa in Cuba: A Quantitative Analysis of the African Populations in the Island of Cuba," in Vera Rubin and Arthur Tuden (eds.), "Comparative Perspectives on Slavery in New World Plantation Societies," *Journal of the New York Academy of Science*, CCXCII (1977), 197–198.

5 J. M. Tanner, "Earlier Maturation in Man," *Scientific American*, CCXVIII (1968), 26–27; Albert Damon, "Secular Trend in Height and Weight within Old American Families at Harvard, 1870–1965: Within Twelve Four-generation Families," *American Journal of Physical Anthropology*, XXIX (1968), 45–50; Phyllis Eveleth and Tanner, *Worldwide Variation in Human Growth* (Oxford, 1976), 274.

Moreover, the dysentery and diarrhea, always rife aboard a slaver, would have leached away many of those nutrients which such a diet could have provided.[6]

Thus many West Africans, badly nourished to begin with and then subjected to the disastrous nutritional circumstances of the Middle Passage, reached the New World in a malnourished condition. Doubtless some never recovered, which must count as an important reason for the high incidence of "seasoning" mortality.

Malnutrition, in addition to its own inherent destructiveness, also renders the body more susceptible to pathogenic invasion and, in the case of slaves moving into a new disease environment, to pathogens and strains of pathogens against which they had inefficient defenses. Assuming, however, that the newly imported slaves did survive, they did so on a diet which, although in many ways superior to their accustomed diets in West Africa, may nonetheless have been seriously deficient in some nutrients.

DIET   Our technique for constructing the Caribbean slave diet reflected in Table 1 has been to assign to slaves the amount of meat and cereal that planters claimed that they issued—the kind of standardized *ideal* allotment which is mentioned over and over again in everything from instructions to overseers, to travel accounts, to tracts on slave care—and then "build up" that basic allotment with the most commonly mentioned and readily available or easy to store supplements to reach a caloric intake of about 3,000 calories daily. Three thousand calories would be too low for a young male laboring during a sugar harvest; 3,200 to 4,000 calories would be closer to his requirement for this fraction of the year. However, not all islands employed a majority of their slaves in sugar cultivation, and female requirements run on the average about 1,200 calories fewer than males. Thus 3,000 calories seems a reasonable intake for the average adult slave for at least most of the year.[7]

6 Philip D. Curtin, *The Atlantic Slave Trade: A Census* (Madison, 1969), remains the authority for measuring the magnitude of the various slave trades to the Americas. See also Herbert S. Klein, *The Middle Passage: Comparative Studies in the Atlantic Slave Trade* (Princeton, 1978). For the diets of blacks in the middle passage consult *ibid.*, 200–201; John Riland, *Memoirs of a West-India Planter* (London, 1827), 56.
7 Food and Agriculture Organization, *Calorie Requirements* (Washington, D.C., 1950), 23–24.

By employing this technique, we may assume that, ideally, Caribbean slaves received an allotment of a little less than a half pound of animal protein daily, either as dried beef or salted fish, and about a pint of cereal in the form of either cornmeal or rice. This core allotment would have provided in the neighborhood of a third of the daily calorie requirements but about twice as much protein as today's recommendations suggest.[8]

Because of a lack of calories provided by the core, Caribbean slaves were dependent upon supplements to that core, which explains the importance of their provision grounds and vegetable gardens often mentioned in the literature on Caribbean plantations. Although West Indian plants and dietary preferences varied from place to place, yams, taro, plantains, and bananas are the most frequently cited supplements. The usual practice was to boil all of these foods (save the bananas) with the ration of animal protein and cereal; and, assuming that out of the cooking pot the average slave plucked a half pound of yam, another of taro root, and perhaps a pound of plantains, he would have satisfied his caloric needs for the day.[9]

Surprisingly, despite the usual description of these basic diets as "starchy" and "protein poor," they seem to have supplied most of the basic nutrients. The diets were poor in calcium, and with milk—the one food which might have remedied the problem—in

8 The fish or meat ration in particular varied erratically from the ideal. For example, slave laws in the Leeward Islands required planters to issue a slave 1¼ lbs. of salt fish weekly. Elsa V. Goveia, *Slave Society in the British Leeward Islands at the End of the Eighteenth Century* (New Haven, 1965), 193. Barbadan planters, however, claimed that they issued a pound of fish daily. A Report on a Committee of the Council of Barbados, Appointed to Inquire into the Actual Condition of the Slaves (London, 1824), 106, 113. Yet Jerome S. Handler and Frederick W. Lange in *Plantation Slavery in Barbados* (Cambridge, 1977), 87, an investigation on the Newton plantation, found that its slaves received only one-half pound of salt fish every two weeks, although for the island as a whole the norm was about one pound weekly. Richard N. Bean, "Food Imports into the British West Indies: 1680–1845," *Journal of the New York Academy of Sciences*, CCXCII (1977), 581–590, also found the average to be "just a bit over one pound of preserved fish per slave per week" (587). For Cuba, Fraginals, "Africa in Cuba," 198, states that "the daily norm was some 200 grams [about one-half pound] of jerked beef." The point is that by accepting planters' claims of about one-half pound of fish or meat daily, we are doubtless erring on the high side.

9 For two contemporaries who stressed the importance of slave provision grounds see Robert Collins, *Practical Rules for the Management and Medical Treatment of Negro Slaves in the Sugar Colonies* (London, 1811; reprint ed. 1971), 87, 99; Bryan Edwards, *The History, Civil and Commercial, of the British Colonies in the West Indies* (London, 1807; 4th ed.), II, 160–163.

short supply and most slaves lactose intolerant, a widespread calcium deficiency must have been a nutritional fact of life. Caribbean slaves seem also to have been slightly deficient in vitamin A, but, superficially at least, the slave diets of the Caribbean might be characterized as not that poor by eighteenth and nineteenth-century standards.[10]

A closer look, however, reveals some serious problems, in part because of the chemical composition of some of the foods in question and in part because of the peculiar relationships among some of the nutrients. For example, an enormously complicating factor is the absence of sufficient fats. In both the beef and fish slave diets the animal protein and cereal were the only items to supply any amount of fat. However, because of the low fat content of dried fish and jerked beed, this meant only 20 grams of fat daily for West Indian slaves on a beef-corn core, and a measly 3 grams for those on a fish-rice core. Yet the established world standard for fat intake suggests 80–125 grams as a safe minimum.[11]

Although the low fat intake of slaves may have been good for cholesterol levels, such a diet means that the amount of vitamin A that Table 1 shows West Indian bondsmen as receiving is considerably overstated. Vitamin A is fat-soluble; hence a low fat diet impairs the ability of the body to absorb that vitamin. Moreover, the fish or meat allotment to slaves was usually reported as rancid; indeed, slaves allegedly preferred it that way. Unfortunately rancidity has a destructive effect on fat-soluble vitamins. Thus, instead of being only mildly vitamin A deficient, many West Indian slaves, because of an absence of dietary fat and the rancidity of much of the fat that they did ingest, must have been severely vitamin A deficient.[12]

10 Ignio Abbad y Lasierra, *Historia Geográfica de Puerto Rico* (San Juan, 1886; reprint ed. 1970), 183; Humphrey E. Lamur, "Demography of Surinam Plantation Slaves in the Last Decade before Emancipation: The Case of Catharina Sophia," *Journal of the New York Academy of Sciences*, CCXCII (1977), 161–173; Michael Craton, "Hobbesian or Panglossian? The Two Extremes of Slave Conditions in the British Caribbean, 1783–1834," *William and Mary Quarterly*, XXXV (1978), 345.

11 League of Nations Technical Commission on Nutrition, *The Problems of Nutrition* (New York, 1936).

12 Edward Long, *The History of Jamaica* (London, 1774), II, 413; Craton and James Walvin, *A Jamaican Plantation, The History of Worthy Park* (Toronto, 1970), 135. Leonard W. Aurand and A. E. Woods, *Food Chemistry* (Westport, Ct., 1973), 122.

Less well known is the relationship between fat and thiamine or vitamin B_1. Because thiamine is part of the water soluble vitamin B complex, fat has little to do with its absorption. But in the case of low fat diets, such as those of Caribbean slaves, carbohydrates replace fat as the major energy source, and carbohydrates require thiamine for metabolism. Thus the low fat/high carbohydrate content of the Caribbean slave diets would have greatly accelerated thiamine requirements. For West Indian slaves thiamine requirements would have been higher than for the whites on the islands whose diets were heavily fat-laden. But even more to the point, it is highly doubtful that Caribbean bondsmen actually received as much thiamine as is suggested by Table 1.[13]

The process of pickling, salting, and drying beef or fish treats thiamine poorly. Both alkaline solutions and prolonged dehydration have a destructive effect on thiamine, the least stable of the B complex vitamins. This lack of stability also means that heat is more destructive to thiamine than to riboflavin or niacin. Thus data on the thiamine content of foods are usually given, as they are in Table 1, before cooking because of the losses which occur in the process. The loss from cornmeal, for example, runs between 15 and 25 percent. In the case of meat, however, that loss can be as high as 85 percent.[14]

Moreover, because thiamine is so highly soluble in water, it is readily leached out of the food during boiling, the standard method of cooking on most West Indian plantations. Fish or beef was tossed into the family or communal pot where it simmered all day along with yams, plantains, taro root, and, quite possibly, the cereal ration as well. Because of such factors as dehydration

13 L. E. Lloyd, B. E. McDonald, and E. W. Crampton, *Fundamentals of Nutrition* (San Francisco, 1978; 2nd ed.), 166. Roger J. Williams et al., *The Biochemistry of B Vitamins* (Austin, Tx., 1950), 276, 282; Aurand and Woods, *Food Chemistry*, 210. The relationship between fat and thiamine requirements may help to explain a puzzle that nutritionists recently encountered in Puerto Rico. The diet of their subjects clearly supplied a sufficiency of thiamine, yet measurements revealed them to be slightly deficient. Throughout the article, frequent mention is made of the extremely *low fat* yield of the diet. Nelson A. Fernandez et al., "Nutrition Survey of Two Rural Puerto Rican Areas Before and After a Community Improvement Program," *American Journal of Clinical Nutrition*, XXII (1969), 1639–1651.
14 Aurand and Woods, *Food Chemistry*, 211; E. E. Rice, "The Nutritional Content and Value of Meat and Meat Products," in J. F. Price and B. S. Schweigert (eds.), *The Science of Meat and Meat Products* (San Francisco, 1971; 2nd ed.), 307; Lloyd, McDonald, and Crampton, *Fundamentals of Nutrition*, 163.

and cooking losses, the thiamine delivered by the West Indian slave diet is probably overstated by at least 50 percent. Those slaves especially whose cereal allotment was rice were bound to be seriously B_1 deficient because, when rice is subjected to a polishing process to retard spoilage, the process also strips away the thiamine-rich husk of the grain.[15]

Finally, it bears repeating that the low fat diet of Caribbean slaves would have severely exacerbated a condition of thiamine deficiency by elevating thiamine requirements. To this factor should be added two more exacerbating difficulties: a diet high in carbohydrates also accelerates thiamine requirements; and thiamine is the most poorly stored of all of the B vitamins.[16]

Not all Caribbean bondsmen suffered from deficiencies of calcium, vitamin A and thiamine. Red peppers provided much in the way of vitamin A, as did mangoes and ackee, both of which came into widespread West Indian use at about the turn of the nineteenth century. Milk was not totally unavailable to Caribbean slaves and, although most blacks were lactose intolerant, a few ounces in cornbread or coffee would have made a nutritional contribution—especially in the areas of sorely needed tryptophan and calcium—without necessarily producing symptoms of lactose intolerance.[17]

DISEASE   Not all slaves had access to a variety of supplementary comestibles, and many had access to very few. Even assuming that slave diets were marginally, rather than severely, deficient in one or another vitamin, economic, political, and climatic circumstances could quickly have changed those diets for the worse. The English-French global struggle frequently deprived West Indian slaves of their meat and cereal core diet, as did the end of North American imports to the British West Indies after the American Revolution. Hurricanes were always destructive to slave provision

---

15 A. Barclay, *A Practical View of the Present State of Slavery in the West Indies* (London, 1827; 2nd ed.), 307. Analysis of Caribbean diets today consisting principally of rice, beans, bananas, and codfish indicates that they would be seriously thiamine deficient were it not for "enriched" rice. See for example Diva Sanjur, *Puerto Rican Food Habits: A Socio-Cultural Approach* (Ithaca, 1970), 23.

16 Lloyd, McDonald, and Crampton, *Fundamentals of Nutrition*, 163.

17 John H. Parry, "Plantation and Provision Ground: An Historical Sketch of the Introduction of Food Crops into Jamaica," *Revista de Historia de America*, XXXIX (1955), 16–17.

grounds, particularly to the fragile plantain and banana trees, and high prices for meat and cereal or low prices for sugar reduced supplies for slave rations.[18]

Even during good times Caribbean slave diets were badly out of balance, and times were often far from good. Yet all that a nutritional analysis of the basic foodstuffs in the slave regimen has done is to create the suspicion of widespread deficiencies of vitamins A and B_1. That suspicion can only be transformed into something more concrete if the diseases triggered by these deficiencies can be found to have afflicted slaves in large numbers. A correlation could then be established between a nutritional deficiency and a deficiency disease.

In any search for a deficiency disease one is quickly confronted with the phenomenon of so-called "Negro diseases," given much prominence by West Indian physicians of the period. These were diseases from which blacks were far more likely to suffer than whites. Yaws, for example, was reportedly an affliction with an enormous color prejudice. The prejudice, however, is easily explicable in terms of a slave trade which constantly introduced persons infected in West Africa. Because of skin-to-skin transmission, the disease flourished among a people who lived in close contact and wore few clothes. Another such disease—a major killer of infants—was the "jawfull," or neonatal tetanus. The affliction singled out black infants for special grim attention because of the frequency of umbilical stump infections. The unsanitary condition of many slave quarters, on the one hand, and West African practices such as packing the stump with mud, on the other, guaranteed a high black as opposed to white death rate from the disease. There are, however, other Negro diseases the etiologies of which are not so easily understood in terms of pathogenic discrimination, but the symptoms of which do suggest problems of nutrition.[19]

18 David Lowenthal, "The Population of Barbados," *Social Economic Studies,* VI (1957), 445–501; Richard B. Sheridan, "The Crisis of Slave Subsistence in the British West Indies during and after the American Revolution," *William and Mary Quarterly,* XXXIII (1976), 615–641; Berta Cabanillas, *Origenes de los Habitos Alimenticios del Pueblo de Puerto Rico* (Madrid, 1955), 274–275, 290.
19 For works that deal exclusively with West Indian black-related diseases see Jean Barthelemy, *Observations sur les Maladies des Negres, leurs causes, leurs traitemens, et les moyens de les prevenir* (Paris, 1892; 2nd ed.), 2 v.; James Thompson, *A Treatise on the Diseases of Negroes as They Occur in the Island of Jamaica* (Kingston, Jamaica, 1820).

Nutritional analysis has suggested that many Caribbean slaves would have been vitamin A and thiamine deficient, both because the diet itself was low in these vitamins and because a low fat diet meant that much vitamin A was not absorbed and that thiamine requirements were elevated. Considering vitamin A first, one discovers among those peculiarly "Negro afflictions" which occupied the attention of Caribbean slave physicians the malady "sore eyes." Eye afflictions were so widespread among the slaves that whole chapters in books on slave medicine were devoted to the problem, which is characteristic of several nutrient deficiencies. Night blindness, described as a "disease which is so frequently seen among Negroes," is prominently mentioned in those chapters, and is a classic sign of vitamin A deficiency. Its prevalence among the slaves, along with the high incidence of sore eyes, does much to strengthen the suspicion born of nutritional analysis that many Caribbean bondsmen were vitamin A deficient.[20]

Another sizable body of literature amassed by Caribbean physicians concerns one of the worst curses to befall a West Indian slave—the *mal d'estomach*. Also called *mal de estomágo, hati-weri, cachexia africana,* and just plain dirt-eating, the disease afflicted the black population of the West Indies exclusively. In Puerto Rico it was reportedly one of the two worst diseases of the slaves. In Jamaica it was portrayed as "common upon almost every plantation" and on some estates the cause of about half of the deaths. At first, doctors were powerless against it, and iron masks were used to break the pica habit. However, by the last decades of the eighteenth century, physicians were nearly unanimous in their prescribed cure—a better, more balanced diet.[21]

This mysterious malady, as described by eighteenth-century

20 See William Hillary, *Observations on the Changes of the Air and the Concomitant Epidemical Diseases, in the Island of Barbados* (London, 1811; 2nd ed.), 297–304, for a discussion of nyctalopia. See also Collins, *Practical Rules,* 287; James Grainger, *Essay on the More Common West Indian Diseases* (London, 1807; 2nd ed.), 60.

21 Bengt Anell and Sture Lagercrantz, *Geophagical Customs* (Uppsala, 1958), 60; John Stewart, *An Account of Jamaica* (London, 1808), 273; Abbad y Lasierra, *Historia de Puerto Rico,* 207; John Imray, "Observations on the Mal d'estomach or Cachexia Africana, as it Takes place among the Negroes of Dominica," *Edinburgh Medical and Surgical Journal,* CIX (1843), 314; John Williamson, *Medical and Miscellaneous Observations Relative to the West India Islands* (Edinburgh, 1817), I, 177–182; II, 267; Edwards, *History of British in West Indies,* II, 167; Collins, *Practical Rules,* 274.

physicians, made its victims "languid and listless," "short breathed," and "giddy," and afflicted them with "palpitations of the heart" and "loss of appetite." With the progression of the sickness, legs swelled, the countenance became bloated and "dropsy ensue[d]." These symptoms are a classic portrayal of beriberi advancing from the dry to wet stage—and beriberi is caused by thiamine deficiency.[22]

In addition to these outstanding symptoms of thiamine deficiency, many other reasons exist for suspecting that *mal d'estomach* was in fact beriberi. Pregnant and lactating females were reported as the most susceptible to the disease, and pregnant and lactating females have historically proven the most vulnerable to beriberi because of accelerated requirements for most nutrients, including the B complex. Also vulnerable were young girls who suffered a disproportionately heavy incidence of the disease "at a certain time in their life . . . [just] before their periodical evacuations appear." The females in question, who probably consumed less food than their brothers of the same age, would have been experiencing the period of growth when requirements for all the B vitamins accelerate. The children susceptible to *mal d'estomach* were depicted as nutritionally deprived and often rickety in appearance. Whether the disease struck at the young or old, male or female, the remedy that physicians prescribed was "wholesome food"; that the cure worked does nothing to weaken the hypothesis that the disease was indeed beriberi.[23]

There are other explanations for the symptoms. Slaves who manifested dirt-eating symptoms were sometimes thought to be attempting suicide, and slaves who developed *mal d'estomach* often personally diagnosed their problem as the result of having been poisoned or cursed by an "obeah man." More recently *mal d'estomach* has been pronounced to be the result of ankylostomiasis or hookworm infection, and indeed dirt-eating among slaves in the United States has also been attributed to hookworm. Yet this

22 *Ibid.*, 293, 295; Williamson, *Medical and Miscellaneous Observations*, I, 110; Abbad y Lasierra, *Historia de Puerto Rico*, 207; John Hunter, *Observations on the Diseases of the Army in Jamaica* (London, 1808; 3rd ed.), 249.

23 David Mason, "On Atrophia a Ventriculo (Mal d'Estomac) or Dirt-Eating," *Edinburgh Medical and Surgical Journal*, XXXIX (1833), 292; Orlando Patterson, *The Sociology of Slavery* (London, 1967), 102; Williamson, *Medical and Miscellaneous Observations*, I, 182; II, 267; Collins, *Practical Rules*, 294; Imray, "Mal d'Estomac or Cachexia Africana," 314; Edwards, *History of British in West Indies*, II, 167.

explanation ignores the relative immunity that blacks have to hookworm "expressed as a resistance both to invasion by the parasite and to the injurious effects after invasion." Another problem with hookworm infection as the culprit is that the disease was not unknown to colonial physicians; rather it was commonly diagnosed in British troops and thus presumably would have been recognized in blacks had they manifested similar symptoms.[24]

Others have confused the *mal d'estomach* with the dry belly ache, which was also frequently fatal. This affliction, however, was accompanied by enormous intestinal pains that often had individuals begging to be shot or otherwise put out of their misery and which terminated in convulsions or epileptic seizures. Benjamin Franklin became interested in the problem and speculated in a letter to a West Indian physician that the dry belly ache was the result of drinking rum distilled in apparatuses using lead fastenings and pipes. Franklin's speculation may have been correct, for other physicians observed that the dry belly ache often caused lead poisoning. *Mal d'estomach* and dry belly ache were clearly two separate afflictions, with only the former, according to contemporary doctors, having a nutritional etiology.[25]

Evidence of a general B vitamin deficiency in the West Indies is contained in a seasonal phenomenon which occurred at crop time on sugar plantations; despite the long hours of extraordinarily hard labor, blacks paradoxically enjoyed better health throughout the harvest. Physicians commented on the "peculiar glossiness of the skin, so indicative of health [which] is never seen to the same extent at any other season." Moreover, it was accepted wisdom that slaves purchased during crop time would do better in terms of health than slaves purchased at any other time of the year. Physicians and planters attributed this condition to the drinking of sugar cane juice. Custom allowed slaves to drink as much as they wished of the "hot liquor" from the "last copper," which contained a mixture of brown sugar and molasses. Thus

24 This "very pronounced" black resistance to hookworm infection was discovered by investigators in the American South during the early decades of this century. See for example, A. E. Keller, W. S. Leathers, and H. C. Ricks, "An Investigation of the Incidence and Intensity of Infestation of Hookworm in Mississippi," *American Journal of Hygiene,* XIX (1934), 629–656.
25 Hillary, *Diseases in Barbados,* 182; Hunter, *Diseases of the Army in Jamaica,* 195, 211–216; Grainger, *West Indian Diseases,* 32.

slaves who drank from the "last copper" were imbibing a liquid rich in iron and the B vitamins. If island physicians were not certain why, they nonetheless knew that this annual infusion of minerals and vitamins was beneficial for slaves.[26]

Physicians also (significantly in terms of thiamine deficiency) periodically suspected rice of producing bad health. A Jamaican physician reported early in the nineteenth century that rice had lately "fallen into disuse" because it caused "dropsical swellings." Edema can be symptomatic of many disorders but, because they were linked to rice consumption, the "dropsical swellings" do suggest beriberi, and dropsy had the reputation of being a major killer of adult Caribbean slaves.[27]

Mortality records bear out dropsy's deadliness; in those consulted for Barbados, dropsy dominated as a cause of plantation deaths. In Jamaica, on the Worthy Park estate between 1811 and 1834, dropsy accounted for fully 10 percent of the 222 deaths, ranking only behind deaths from old age (53) and fever (23); of 357 slave deaths in St. James Parish, Jamaica, between 1817 and 1820, dropsy accounted for 11 percent of the deaths, second only to old age. If dirt-eating and *mal d'estomach* deaths are added to those from dropsy, the three accounted for 16 percent of the deaths. Dropsy alone claimed 11 percent of the 288 deaths on three other Jamaican estates from 1817 to 1829. If other diseases with symptoms suggestive of beriberi, such as "fits," "convulsions," and "bloated," are included with dropsy, the diseases in question accounted for 22 percent of the deaths registered.[28]

On the Newton plantation in Barbados from 1796 to 1801 and from 1811 to 1825, dropsy accounted for 9 percent of the 153 deaths (14), tying with consumption for third place behind old

26 Claude Levy, "Slavery and the Emancipation Movement in Barbados, 1650–1833," *Journal of Negro History,* LV (1970), 6; Williamson, *Medical and Miscellaneous Observations,* I, 73; Long, *History of Jamaica,* II, 548, 551; Frank Wesley Pitman, "Slavery on the British West Indian Plantations in the Eighteenth Century," *Journal of Negro History,* II (1926), 632; Richard Henry Dana, *To Cuba and Back: a Vacation Voyage* (Carbondale, Ill., 1966; reprint ed.).

27 Collins, *Practical Rules,* 85; Patterson, *Sociology of Slavery,* 99; J. Harry Bennett, *Bondsmen and Bishops: Slavery and Apprenticeship on the Codrington Plantations of Barbados, 1710–1838* (Berkeley, 1958), 56–58; George W. Roberts, *The Population of Jamaica* (Cambridge, 1957), 175; Richard S. Dunn, *Sugar and Slaves: The Rise of the Planter Class in the English West Indies, 1624–1713* (Chapel Hill, 1972), 302, 305–306; Higman, *Slave Population and Economy in Jamaica* (Oxford, 1976), 112–113.

28 Craton and Walvin, *A Jamaica Plantation,* 113, 197–198; Higman, *Slave Population,* 112. Deaths were substantially understated because of a failure to report infant deaths.

age (22) and "no cause given" (19). By race the death records for the dioceses of Havana for 1843 recorded a black death rate from *anasarea* (general dropsy) of about three times that for whites. Finally, slave death statistics compiled by a West Indian physician during the 1820s for a Jamaican parish credits dropsy, plus other beriberi-like afflictions, with fully 20 percent of the victims aged over one year of age in the district in question.[29]

As with *mal d'estomach* and "cachexias," there was a cure for dropsy. In the words of Long, "Sometimes they [the slaves] fall into dropsies, which generally prove mortal; for this disorder requires a very nutritious diet." In the minds of white planters good nutrition was equated with fresh meat, and fresh meat contains that thiamine which could have cured the "dropsies."[30]

FERTILITY AND INFANT MORTALITY   Beriberi is one of those nutritional diseases, like pellagra, which escaped identification as a disease *sui generis* for many years, largely because its protean symptoms misled physicians into thinking that they were confronting a number of diseases. Because it was in the Far East that beriberi was finally identified, it subsequently was associated with rice-eating cultures; hence, beriberi is not usually thought of in a Caribbean context. Yet in 1865, early in the effort to conquer beriberi, Hava reported that the disease was epidemic among blacks on Cuban plantations and described all of the symptoms of wet beriberi. In 1871 a French physician observed the disease on Cuban *ingenios* (plantations) and attempted, not very successfully, to treat it with arsenic. Finally in 1873 the disease was reported as raging with virulence on some Cuban plantations, causing a mortality rate between 60 and 75 percent. Because the slave diet in Cuba could and did produce beriberi, there are grounds for the suspicion that the disease was fairly widespread among West Indian slaves and that many of those who died from *mal d'estomach*, dropsy, or convulsions were actually dying of beriberi.[31]

29 Handler and Lange, *Plantation Slavery in Barbados*, 99; D. Angel Jose Crowley (ed.), *Un Ensayo Estadistico-Medico de la Mortalitad de la Diocesis de la Habana durante el Ano de 1843* (Havana, 1845); William Sells, *Remarks on the Condition of the Slaves in the Island of Jamaica* (London, 1823; reprint ed. 1972), 19–20.

30 Long, *History of Jamaica*, II, 433; Pitman, *The Development of the British West Indies, 1760–1763* (New Haven, 1917), 13, 386.

31 Juan G. Hava, "Communicacion Dirigida a la Academia sobre una Epidemia de Beriberi," *Academia de Ciencias Medical de la Habana. Anales*, II (1865), 160–161; J. Min-

If these deaths were caused by beriberi, then the dietary deficiency which produced this disease may have significantly altered the demographic history of West Indian slave populations—not so much because of the adult deaths, but because of infant mortality. For all the major nutritional diseases, only beriberi is a killer of otherwise normal infants receiving an adequate supply of breast milk. Adult slaves in the United States, for example, suffered from pellagra caused by niacin deficiency. Yet it is almost impossible for infants to be niacin deficient, because human milk supplies an adequate amount of both niacin and tryptophan (niacin's precursor), even if the mother is niacin deficient. However, a mother deficient in thiamine will invariably have milk deficient in that vitamin. To complicate matters for medical personnel, she may show few or even no signs of thiamine deficiency herself; in other words, a mother whose child develops infantile beriberi may not display overt signs of the malady.[32]

Infantile beriberi symptoms are very different from adult symptoms, and edema is only occasionally seen. The disease begins with vomiting, pallor, restlessness, loss of appetite, and insomnia and terminates life with convulsions and/or cardiac failure. Clearly the variety of symptoms makes it difficult to pin down the disease on West Indian plantations of yesterday. But if beriberi were fairly widespread, then infantile beriberi had unquestionably to be a major destroyer of West Indian slave infants. How major a destroyer may be gauged by looking at the Philippines, where beriberi has been and still is a chronic problem; in the late 1950s between 75 and 85 percent of the 25,000 beriberi deaths reported there annually were infants. By the turn-of-the-century, nearly half of all infants born alive in Manila failed to reach one year of age; infantile beriberi bears much of the blame for this mortality.[33]

How major a killer beriberi was in the West Indies can only

---

teguiaga, "Lettre sur le Beriberi," *Gazette Medicale de Paris*, XLV (1874), 35; August Hirsch, *Handbook of Geographical and Historical Pathology* (London, 1883), II, 576.

32 C. C. de Silva and N. G. Baptist, *Tropical Nutritional Disorders of Infants and Children* (London, 1969), 114–115; Robert R. Williams, *Toward the Conquest of Beriberi* (Cambridge, 1961), 153, 156–157.

33 Michael Latham et al., *Scopes Manual on Nutrition* (New York, 1972), 39; Stanley Davidson et al., *Human Nutrition and Dietetics* (Edinburgh, 1975; 6th ed.), 415; Williams, *Toward the Conquest of Beriberi*, 81.

be speculated upon. The disease usually strikes infants between the first and sixth months of life, before supplements have been added to their diets. If the attack is acute, the infant has difficulty in breathing, becomes cyanosed, and dies of cardiac failure with "unnerving rapidity." If it is chronic, the infant grows thin and wasted, edema occasionally occurs, and convulsions are frequently seen in the terminal stages.[34]

To be sure, the infant slave had to live long enough to contract infantile beriberi by first escaping that primary destroyer of the newborn in the Caribbean—neonatal tetanus. The fearsome reputation of this affliction was well deserved; indeed, the ailment has been credited with carrying off about one quarter of all slave infants within their first two weeks of life. However, as pointed out by students of Caribbean slave mortality, "it is evident that the majority of fatalities among slave children born at Worthy Park occurred not at birth but in the children's early years."[35]

A consultation of the literature produced by West Indian physicians and of the mortality data suggests that the latter statement applies not only to Worthy Park but to the Caribbean slave population as a whole. Rivaling neonatal tetanus as major causes of infant deaths were marasmus, convulsions, and tetanic convulsions. Researchers today looking for evidence of beriberi's presence in a region scrutinize any death that is classified under the rubric of convulsions or marasmus. Convulsions were also associated with teething difficulties, yet infants do not convulse simply because of teething. However, the months of teething are also those months during which infants would be most likely to succumb to beriberi.[36]

Another signal to researchers is the phenomenon of mothers with a history of losing one baby after another within the first few months of life. The West Indian literature offers many ex-

34 Davidson et al., *Human Nutrition*, 415; Latham et al., *Scope on Nutrition*, 39.
35 Craton and Walvin, *A Jamaican Plantation*, 134. See also the parochial records for Barbados: the parish of St. Thomas, for example, buried 168 slave children aged ten and under for the period 1816–1834. Only 36 of the deaths were one year of age or less. In St. Phillips parish, 33 of their 106 burials were infants. The records for other parishes are incomplete, yet what data are available continue to suggest that only about one third of those aged ten and under of those slave children who died were infants aged one or less.
36 Collins, *Practical Rules*, 393–394; Roberts, *Population of Jamaica*, 175; Williams, *Toward the Conquest of Beriberi*, 85.

amples of mothers who had produced fifteen children and lost all but two, or who "had borne ten children, and yet has now but one alive," or "the instances of those who have had four, five, six children, without succeeding in bringing up one in spite of the utmost attention and indulgence . . ."[37]

Further analysis of mortality data and plantation records is needed. But this study does show that there is a correlation between a thiamine deficiency in the West Indian slave diet and diseases with beriberi-like symptoms, which ranked among the most important causes of slave mortality. If beriberi were as widespread as the evidence gathered thus far suggests, then thiamine deficiency must join with other factors produced by the slave trade and sugar monoculture to explain why Caribbean slave populations did not sustain themselves by natural means as did the slave population of the United States. It has often been urged that low fertility was at fault. Yet none of the islands have adequate birth records either to confirm or refute this suggestion. A possible measure of fertility relates the number of children under one year to the number of women able to bear those children. But if something is killing those infants at a brisk rate, then this kind of fertility ratio is a very misleading statistic.

Finally, it has been suggested that low fertility may have been partially the result of the practice of West African mothers to nurse their children for periods as long as three years. West Indian planters tried to discourage prolonged nursing but were not so successful in combating West African cultural practices as were United States' planters, who were dealing with a people much further removed in time from their homeland. United States' slaves tended to nurse their babies for a year or less. Although the ability of lactation to prevent pregnancy after a few months of nursing is in doubt, there seems no question that prolonged lactation substantially increased the risk of death by thiamine deficiency for many West Indian slave infants.[38]

---

37 M. G. Lewis, *Journal of a West Indian Proprietor, 1815–1817* (London, 1929), 97, 111.
38 Engerman, "Some Economic and Demographic Comparisons of Slavery in the United States and the British Indies," *Economic History Review*, XXIX (1976), 264–266; Anrudh K. Jain, "Demographic Aspects of Lactation and Postpartum Amenorrhea," *Demography*, VII (1970), 250–271; Lamur, "Demography of Surinam Plantation Slaves in the Last Decade before Emancipation," 168; Klein and Engerman, "Fertility Differentials between Slaves in the United States and the British West Indies: A Note on Lactation Practices and their Possible Implications," *William and Mary Quarterly*, XXXV (1978), 357–374; Collins, *Practical Rules*, 146.

Although the slave diets of both the United States and the West Indies contained the potential for precipitating a B vitamin deficiency disease, pellagra, the deficiency disease of United States slaves would not have killed the very young. But beriberi, the disease of Caribbean slaves, most certainly would have. The result may well help to account for the "astounding fact, that while the blacks in the United States have increased *tenfold,* those of the British West Indies [and the West Indies] generally have decreased in the proporation of five to two." [39]

39 Josiah Clark Nott, and George R. Gliddon (eds.), *Indigenous Places of the Earth; or New Chapters of Ethnological Inquiry* (Philadelphia, 1857), 387.

Daniel Blake Smith

Mortality and Family in the
Colonial Chesapeake
Colonial Chesapeake society is currently receiving a vigorous reexamination. After a decade of important demographic studies written about New England communities in the seventeenth and eighteenth centuries,[1] social historians have begun to explore the largely neglected areas of population growth, life expectancy, and family structure in early Virginia and Maryland. Some of the research is unpublished, but the intensity and quality of recent work on early Chesapeake society suggest that the findings of these social historians will be of major importance to students of colonial America. When completed, this reassessment of the Chesapeake should underscore the differences between the social history of early New England and the colonial South.[2]

Daniel Blake Smith is Visiting Assistant Professor of History at Northern Illinois University.

The author would like to thank Kevin Kelly, Darrett B. and Anita H. Rutman, Daniel Scott Smith, Russell R. Menard, and Allan Kulikoff for their useful comments on an earlier version of this essay.

1 Demographic work on colonial New England was first published in the mid-1960s. See John Demos, "Notes on Life in Plymouth Colony," *William and Mary Quarterly*, XXII (1965), 264–286; *idem*, "Family in Colonial Bristol, R.I.: An Exercise in Historical Demography," *William and Mary Quarterly*, XXV (1968), 40–59; *idem*, *A Little Commonwealth: Family Life in Plymouth Colony*; Philip J. Greven, Jr.: "Family Structure in Seventeenth-Century Andover, Massachusetts," *William and Mary Quarterly*, XXIII (1966), 234–256; *idem*, "Historical Demography and Colonial America," *ibid.*, XXIV (1967), 438–454; *idem*, *Four Generations: Population, Land, and Family in Colonial Andover, Massachusetts* (Ithaca, N.Y., 1970); Kenneth Lockridge, "The Population of Dedham, Massachusetts, 1636–1736," *Economic History Review*, XIX (1966), 318–344; *idem*, "Land, Population and the Evolution of New England Society, 1630–1790," *Past & Present*, 38 (1968), 62–80; *idem*, *A New England Town: The First 100 Years, Dedham, Massachusetts, 1636–1736* (New York, 1970). Other important articles are Susan Norton, "Population Growth in Colonial America: A Study of Ipswich, Massachusetts," *Population Studies*, XXV (1971), 433–452; Daniel Scott Smith, "The Demographic History of Colonial New England," *Journal of Economic History*, XXXII (1972), 165–183; Maris Vinovskis, "Mortality Rates and Trends in Massachusetts Before 1860," *ibid.*, 184–213; Robert V. Wells, "Quaker Marriage Patterns in Colonial Perspective," *William and Mary Quarterly*, XXIX (1972), 415–442.

2 Craven sketched the basic outline of population growth in seventeenth-century Virginia through a study of land patents. See Wesley Frank Craven, *White, Red and Black: The Seventeenth-Century Virginian* (Charlottesville, 1971). Two critiques of his work have recently appeared: Edmund S. Morgan, "Headrights and Headcounts: A Review Article," *Virginia Magazine of History and Biography*, LXXX (1972), 361–371; Russell R. Menard, "Immigration to the Chesapeake Colonies in the Seventeenth Century: A Review Essay,"

The scarcity of adequate population sources for colonial Virginia and Maryland, such as parish registers, censuses, and tithable lists, has confined research to only a very few counties along the tobacco coast.[3] Nevertheless, studies completed thus far have already come to some significant conclusions about the key demographic trends in the early Chesapeake. These may be briefly summarized as follows: the combination of a high mortality rate among immigrants and natives—especially the former—and a persistent shortage of females stifled natural population increase in the Chesapeake colonies during the seventeenth century. As a result, population growth in early Virginia and Maryland depended almost entirely on the influx of immigrants whose numbers peaked near the third quarter of the century. It was not until around 1700 that improved life expectancies, an earlier mean age at marriage for native women—thereby increasing the number of childbearing years—and more balanced sex ratios—due in part to a decline in the largely male stream of white immigrants—permitted most regions

Maryland Historical Magazine, LXVIII (1973), 323–329. For family life in the seventeenth-century Chesapeake, see Irene W. D. Hecht, "The Virginia Muster of 1624/5 as a Source for Demographic History," *William and Mary Quarterly*, XXX (1973), 65–92; Lorena S. Walsh, "Till Death Us Do Part: Marriage and Family in Maryland in the Seventeenth Century," in Aubrey C. Land, Lois Green Carr, and Edward C. Papenfuse (eds.), *Law, Society, and Politics in Early Maryland: Essays in Honor of Morris Leon Radoff* (Baltimore, 1977).

Mortality studies are only now beginning to appear for the early Chesapeake. See Lorena S. Walsh and Russell R. Menard, "Death in the Chesapeake: Two Life Tables for Men in Early Colonial Maryland," *Maryland Historical Magazine*, LXIX (1974), 211–227; Darrett B. and Anita H. Rutman, "'Now-Wives and Sons-in-Law': Parental Death in a Seventeenth-Century Virginia County," in Thad. W. Tate and David Ammerman (eds.), *Chesapeake in the Seventeenth Century: Essays on its Euramerican Society and Politics* (Chapel Hill, forthcoming). Two recently-completed dissertations analyze colonial Chesapeake population history: Kevin P. Kelly, "Economic and Social Development of Seventeenth-Century Surry County, Virginia," unpub. Ph.D. diss. (University of Washington, 1972); Allan Kulikoff, "Tobacco and Slaves: Population, Economy, and Society in Eighteenth-Century Prince George's County, Maryland," unpub. Ph.D. diss. (Brandeis University, 1975).

3 For a discussion of available census and tithable records, see Edmund S. Morgan, *American Slavery, American Freedom: The Ordeal of Colonial Virginia* (New York, 1975), 395–432. Fourteen parish registers have survived for Virginia during the colonial period, but most of these contain only short runs of data and thus are of limited value for family reconstitution or long-range aggregative analysis. For information on early Virginia parish records, see W. Edwin Hemphill, "Parish Records of the Diocese of Southern Virginia and Southwest Virginia, 1648-1900," *Fifth Annual Report of the Archivist, University of Virginia Library, 1934-35*, (Charlottesville, 1935), 9–24; "Parish Records of the Diocese of Virginia, 1653-1900," *Fourth Annual Report of the Archivist, University of Virginia Library, 1933-34*, (Charlottesville, 1934), 9–24; "Public Officers in Virginia, 1702, 1712," *Virginia Magazine of History and Biography*, I (1894), 361–377.

in the Chesapeake to achieve significant natural increase for the first time. More important for population growth, slave importations rose precipitously beginning in the late seventeenth century and continued strong in the early eighteenth century. Thus both components of population growth—sustained natural increase and rapid immigration (in the form of black slaves)—emerged at roughly the same time, providing the Chesapeake colonies with steadily expanding populations by 1700.

Clearly the central demographic phenomenon in the early Chesapeake was low life expectancy produced in large part by an endemic malarial environment. In this disease environment men and women struggled with chronic sickness and the prospect of early death.[4] As difficult and short as existence seems to have been in the colonial Chesapeake, there is evidence for at least one area of early Virginia that even higher levels of mortality prevailed.

The demographic history of Charles Parish in York County, Virginia, suggests that the expectation of life for men was considerably lower than in other areas of the Chesapeake and far below what has been discovered for colonial New England communities. And in contrast to the basic demographic trend in the Chesapeake of gradually improving mortality schedules by the eighteenth century, Charles Parish's persistently high death rate created a population that barely managed to reproduce itself throughout the colonial era. In short, the mortality experience of Charles Parish indicates that this part of tidewater Virginia must have been one of the unhealthiest areas in the colonial Chesapeake.

Charles Parish was established around 1645 between the Poquoson River and Back Creek in the eastern end of York County. It was but one of four parishes in the county during the latter half of the seventeenth century and one of three after 1706 when two other parishes in the county were merged.[5] Unfortunately, the absence of tax lists or tithable lists makes it impossible to

4 Darrett B. and Anita H. Rutman, "Of Agues and Fevers: Malaria in the Early Chesapeake," *William and Mary Quarterly,* XXXIII (1976), 31–60.
5 Charles Parish was called New Poquoson and New Towson until 1692 when it was re-named Charles Parish after the renaming of the New Poquoson River as Charles River in the same year. York County Deeds, Orders, Wills, etc., no. 9, (1691–1694), 227, Virginia State Library, Richmond.

measure the size of the parish population during the colonial era.[6] The survival of Charles Parish's birth and death registers, however, which run without significant interruption from the mid-seventeenth to the mid-eighteenth centuries, permits a unique glimpse of the effect of mortality on the pattern of natural increase in this Virginia parish community.[7]

Although neither the birth nor the death register for Charles Parish (especially the latter) is free from the problem of underrecording of vital events, there is sufficient evidence to assume that, except for the recording of infant deaths (which will be dealt with later in the essay), underregistration was not so great as to seriously distort an analysis of natural growth in the parish. For example, demographers have suggested that an important test of the accuracy of a set of birth records is the calculation of sex ratios at birth in a given population (the number of male births for every 100 female births recorded). A normal range for the sex ratio at birth runs between 102 and 108, with a typical figure of 105.[8] In fact, the sex ratio for children listed in the Charles Parish birth register was calculated at 107.0 for the entire period 1660 to 1760, suggesting at the very least that no distortions occurred in the registration by sex. That births were conscientiously recorded in the parish register receives further support from the fact that only 6

---

6 A study of the 1702 tithable list and the 1704 quit rent roll for York County indicates that Charles Parish contained between 300 and 350 tithes in 1702. Using a multiplier of 2.57 suggested by Edmund Morgan for York County in 1699 ("Headrights and Headcounts," 367–368), one can estimate that Charles Parish may have had a population of between 770 and 900. If so, Charles Parish was a relatively small parish in early eighteenth-century Virginia. The mean size of parishes reporting their tithes in 1702 (28 of 49) was 468 tithes, or about 1258 souls (using the 2.57 multiplier). The tithable figures were drawn from "Public Officers in Virginia," 373–377.

7 The Charles Parish registers which span the year 1648 to 1789 have records beginning before any other parish in Virginia. Seven clerks and nine ministers served the parish without absence during this century and a half. And except for a two-year gap in the death register in 1715 and 1716 (due to a lost register), there do not appear to be any defects in the records. Before 1660 and after 1760, however, the number of annual vital events in the registers is too small for demographic analysis. The original registers do not exist for births recorded during the period 1648 to 1714 and for deaths recorded from 1665 to 1725. But copies of these earlier registers were made by a Charles Parish clerk in 1716 and 1725, respectively, and are available in photostatic copy at the Virginia State Library, Richmond. For further information on the history of Charles Parish and its registers, see Landon C. Bell's introduction to the published version of the registers, *Charles Parish, York County, Virginia, History and Registers* (Richmond, 1932), 1–42.

8 George W. Barclay, *Techniques of Population Analysis* (New York, 1958), 83.

percent of the children named in York County wills as Charles Parish residents are not listed in the birth register.[9]

As a later discussion of mortality will indicate more precisely, the Charles Parish death register is less reliable. Emigration and the common failure to register the deaths of infants contributed to the incompleteness of parish death records. The underregistration of deaths may have been offset, however, by the influx of immigrants into the parish whose deaths were added to the death register but whose births were not recorded in the birth register.[10] Moreover, a close examination of the Charles Parish death register suggests that it was kept with considerable care—relatively few deaths (6.2 percent) are listed out of chronological order and no serious gaps in recording are discernible.[11] The uncertain extent of underregistration in the parish records prevents any precise measurement of natural growth but the likelihood that deaths were less diligently recorded than births only underscores the pattern of slow natural population increase described below.

It is clear from the registers that reproductive population increase was rare in colonial Charles Parish. As displayed in Fig. 1, Charles Parish grew almost imperceptibly until the early 1680s. Indeed, from 1665 to 1680 births exceeded deaths (256 to 217) for a net natural increase of only 39 in these 15 years, a gain of less than 3 per year. Heavy mortality impeded natural growth as the deaths recorded in this period comprised a high 84.8 percent of the number of births recorded during the same years.

Charles Parish failed to achieve any significant natural growth in the first half of the eighteenth century as well. In fact, during the three decades from 1695 to 1724, the ratio of deaths to births grew to 79 percent, up over 9 percent from the previous thirty-year period (Table 1). And as Fig. 1 shows, mortality reached its high-

---

9 York County Deeds, Orders, Wills, etc., nos. 3–18, photostat, Virginia State Library, Richmond. This 6% figure may be too high, since some of these children named in wills but missing from the birth register may have been born elsewhere before their families entered Charles Parish.

10 On the underregistration of parish deaths, see D. E. C. Eversley, "Exploitation of Anglican Parish Registers by Aggregative Analysis," in E. A. Wrigley (ed.), *An Introduction to English Historical Demography From the Sixteenth to the Nineteenth Century* (New York, 1966), 81–85.

11 Two years are missing from the death register, 1715 and 1716. The number of deaths for these years has been estimated based upon the mean number of annual deaths during five-year periods surrounding the missing records: 1710–1714 and 1717–1721.

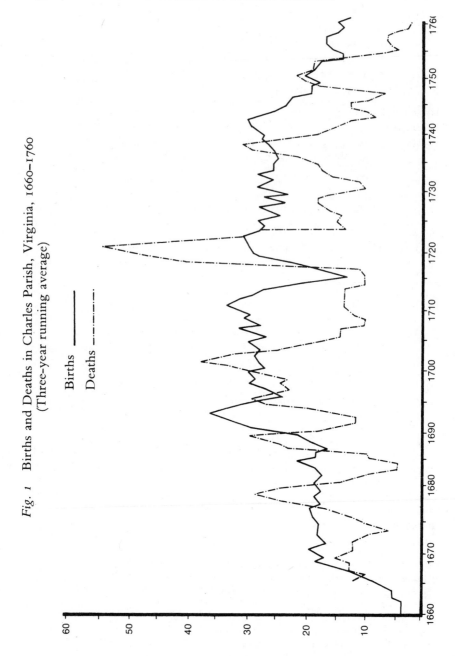

Fig. 1 Births and Deaths in Charles Parish, Virginia, 1660–1760
(Three-year running average)

Births ——————
Deaths —·—·—·—

est level in the parish's history during 1717 and 1718. In these two years 117 deaths were recorded compared to only 58 births. Most of the deaths (62.4 percent) occurred between November and the end of March, indicating that a particularly deadly winter epidemic swept through the parish in these years. In the final thirty-year period, 1725–1754, parish mortality remained high with deaths comprising 72.4 percent of the recorded births, about the same proportion of deaths to births as in the latter third of the seventeenth century (Table 1).

Table 1   Natural Increase in Charles Parish, Virginia, 1665–1754

PERIOD	TOTAL BIRTHS RECORDED	TOTAL DEATHS RECORDED	RATIO OF DEATHS TO BIRTHS IN PERCENT
1665–1674	165	100	60.6
1675–1684	195	148	75.9
1685–1694	272	210	77.2
Total 1665–1694	632	458	70.2
1695–1704	284	239	84.2
1705–1714	300	126	42.0
1715–1724	254	302[a]	118.9
Total 1695–1724	838	667	79.5
1725–1734	267	168	62.9
1735–1744	280	213	76.1
1745–1754	185	149	80.5
Total 1725–1754	732	530	72.4
Totals	2202	1655	75.2

a   Because of a two-year gap in the Charles Parish death register for the years 1715 and 1716, the number of deaths in this period is an estimate. See note 11.
SOURCE: Charles Parish Registers, Virginia State Library, Richmond.

All of which stands in contrast to what is known thus far about natural increase elsewhere in the early Chesapeake. Most counties in Virginia and Maryland managed to achieve rapid natural growth by the 1690s.[12] And there is some indication that at least in the early eighteenth century other Virginia parishes did not experience the withering mortality that prevailed in Charles Parish. Two extant lists of births and deaths in Virginia parishes

12   Walsh and Menard, "Death in the Chesapeake," 220.

for 1714 and 1725 reveal that recorded deaths made up 38.3 percent of the births in all parishes in these two years, while Charles Parish showed a much higher mortality with 69.9 percent of its births cancelled by deaths.[13] Because of the unknown quality of death registration in other parishes, these figures are only rough estimates of the varying mortality levels in early eighteenth-century Virginia. But they do suggest that rapid natural increase may have come more slowly to Charles Parish than to most regions of the early Chesapeake.

Although the pattern of natural increase in Charles Parish does not quite fit that of the colonial Chesapeake, its mortality experience diverges significantly from the demographic trends reported for early New England towns. The number of deaths in Andover, Massachusetts, for example, never exceeded 24 percent of the births recorded for any period until the eighteenth century—about one third of the ratio of deaths to births in Charles Parish.[14] Actually, the sluggish growth of colonial Charles Parish more closely resembled the pattern of mortality of the English villages Clayworth and Colyton in the seventeenth century and Barbados and Jamaica in the seventeenth and eighteenth centuries, where burials nearly always outnumbered baptisms.[15]

What explains the near failure of natural increase in Charles Parish during most years of the colonial period? The shortage of women in early Virginia was partly responsible for limiting growth. Estimates of sex ratios during the seventeenth century indicate that men outnumbered women by as much as three or four to one, resulting in a large pool of unmarried men whose potential fertility could not be used for the colony's growth.[16] Indeed, an examination of the headright entries for seventeenth-

---

13   The lists are in C.O.5/1317/127–129; C.O.5/1320/74, Colonial Virginia Records Project, University of Virginia. The figure 75.9% for Charles Parish represents the mean proportion of deaths to births between 1705 and 1725.

14   Greven, Four Generations, 89.

15   Peter Laslett and John Harrison, "Clayworth and Cogenhoe," in H. E. Bell and R. L. Ollard (eds.), Historical Essays, 1600–1750, Presented to David Ogg (London, 1963), 182; E. A. Wrigley, "Mortality in Pre-Industrial England: The Example of Colyton, Devon Over Three Centuries," Daedalus, XCVII (1968), 556; Richard S. Dunn, Sugar and Slaves: The Rise of the English Planter Class in The English West Indies, 1624–1713 (Chapel Hill, 1972), 328–329. See also his article, "The Barbados Census of 1680: Profile of the Richest Colony in America," William and Mary Quarterly, XXVI (1969), 3–30.

16   Morgan, American Slavery, 407.

century York County shows that from 1620 to 1660 male immigrants settling in Charles Parish outnumbered female settlers by four to one and in the county as a whole the sex ratio (the number of males for every 100 females) was 460. In the subsequent forty years, from 1660 to 1700, the sexes became more balanced among the immigrant population, as the sex ratio for Charles Parish dropped to 268.9, while that of the county fell to 273.7.[17] Despite this drop in the surplus of men (due mainly to an abrupt decline by the late seventeenth century in the predominantly white male immigration to Virginia), men continued significantly to outnumber women in the early eighteenth century.[18]

The chief hindrance to growth in Charles Parish, however, was the unusually low life expectancy in the area. The high death rates also had an important impact on the life of the family. Data on life expectancy in Charles Parish was obtained from a variety of sources. The reconstitution of all families listed in the birth and death registers was an essential beginning. But because of name confusion in the records (children often being given the same first name as their parents or other relatives), information was gathered from a number of local and provincial records—such as wills, deeds, inventories, land patents, rent rolls, court order books, and genealogies—to insure the proper identification of individuals in the parish. Unfortunately, no marriage register has survived for Charles Parish (thereby preventing one from tracing the careers of women in the records after marriage); consequently, the analysis of adult life expectancy was confined to the men of the parish.

Children were probably the most susceptible to the parish disease environment. Although the persistent problem of under-registration of infant deaths (children dying before age one) masks the full extent of infant and childhood mortality (ages 0 to 14) in the parish, the existing evidence suggests that a large proportion of children did not survive to adulthood.

The central difficulty in estimating infant mortality is that most children who did not survive their first year died within the

17 Headright records for York County are in Nell M. Nugent, *Cavaliers and Pioneers: Abstracts of Virginia Land Patents and Grants* (Richmond, 1934), I; Virginia State Land Office, Land Patents, Books 5–9, *passim*.
18 Robert V. Wells, *The Population of the British Colonies in America before 1776* (Princeton, 1975), 154. Both the headrights and county servant importation records for York County suggest that by the early 1680s white immigration to the county had come almost to a standstill.

first few weeks of life and received private burials which were usually not recorded in the parish death register.[19] To develop a good estimate of infant mortality, then, one must try to establish the proportion of early infant deaths omitted from the death register. Louis Henry has created a useful technique for estimating unrecorded infant deaths through an analysis of birth intervals. His method assumes that if a child dies in his first year, the interval between this and the next birth will be smaller than if the child had lived beyond the first year. Using his formula, I calculated that 50 percent of all infant deaths were not recorded in the Charles Parish death register. Thus, two sets of infant and childhood death rates are presented in Table 2—one computed from the raw data and one computed after the mortality figures for the first year were increased by 50 percent.

The unadjusted infant death rates in Charles Parish of 66 per 1000 for males and 92 per 1000 for females during the last third of the seventeenth century are extremely low compared to New England and England during the same period. Despite the apparently healthier climate of seventeenth-century New England communities, Andover and Ipswich, Massachusetts, had higher infant death rates of 115 and 112 respectively.[20] In the English village of Colyton infant mortality was between 118 and 147 in the second half of the seventeenth century.[21] Clearly the adjusted infant death rates in Charles Parish of 132.2 for males and 184.6 for females, although probably still too low, more accurately reflect the parish's high mortality during the seventeenth century.

The death rates for children in the age group 1 to 4 are of particular importance for understanding mortality in Charles Parish. In most populations infants die in much larger proportions than the children who survive their first year. But as the Rutmans have recently discovered, inhabitants of the early Chesapeake endured a severe malarial environment which created important age-specific mortality rates. In this disease environment, infants frequently received from diseased mothers a short-term immunity to malaria which allowed many to survive infancy only later to succumb to

19 Wrigley, "Mortality in Pre-Industrial England," 564–566.
20 Susan L. Norton, "Population Growth in Colonial America," 442; Greven, *Four Generations*, 189.
21 Wrigley, "Mortality in Pre-Industrial England," 571.

the disease as small children when their immunity had worn off.[22] Thus, we find Charles Parish boys aged 1 to 4 dying at almost the rate of male infants during the last third of the seventeenth century, while girls in this age group experienced a higher death rate than female infants (Table 2).

Table 2   Life Table Death Rates of Infants and Children in Charles Parish, 1665–1734[a] (per 1000)

MALES BORN 1665–1699			FEMALES BORN 1665–1699		
	Raw Data	Adjusted		Raw Data	Adjusted
0–1	66.1	132.2	0–1	92.8	184.6
1–4	107.0	117.9	1–4	149.0	191.2
5–9	28.3	32.1	5–9	67.5	84.6
10–14	38.4	57.1	10–14	57.1	60.3
1–14	133.3	145.4	1–14	174.9	198.0

MALES BORN 1700–1734			FEMALES BORN 1700–1734		
	Raw Data	Adjusted		Raw Data	Adjusted
0–1	91.9	183.8	0–1	90.4	180.8
1–4	85.5	100.9	1–4	100.0	157.5
5–9	58.5	74.4	5–9	59.9	80.2
10–14	75.2[b]	107.7	10–14	130.0[b]	229.7
1–14	128.1	145.2	1–14	133.8	151.1

a   The correction made for the underregistration of infant deaths follows a method suggested by Louis Henry in his *Manuel de démographie historique,* (Paris, 1970), 22–25.
b   Because an unusually large number of persons dropped from observation during these years, the death rate is highly inflated for this age group.
SOURCE: Charles Parish Registers, Virginia State Library, Richmond.

Of course, those children who survived their early contacts with malaria and other childhood diseases could expect increasingly improved chances to live to maturity. This is reflected in the declining death rates for children 5 to 9 and 10 to 14 in the seventeenth century. (The eighteenth-century figures for children 10 to 14 are much too high due to emigration from the parish). Overall childhood mortality (1 to 14) in Charles Parish reached about

22   Rutman and Rutman, "Malaria in the Early Chesapeake," 38; Peter H. Wood, *Black Majority: Negroes in Colonial South Carolina from 1670 through the Stono Rebellion* (New York, 1974), 90.

145.4 per 1000 for males and 198 for females in the seventeenth century. In contrast, childhood mortality rates for colonial New England communities did not exceed 95 per 1000.[23]

Movement out of the parish was likely to be greatest among children aged 15 to 19, so it is difficult to determine mortality rates for this age group or for all the childhood years, 0 to 19. But if one assumes that the mortality rate was the same between 15 to 19 as between 10 to 14, then of all the children born between 1665 and 1699, 315 per 1000 died before reaching the age of 20. Thus mortality before adulthood remained about as high in the early decades of the eighteenth century: of those children born between 1700 and 1734, 311 per 1000 did not survive to their twentieth birthday. That these figures represent a relatively high level of mortality is evident from a comparison with rates calculated for a New England community. In Andover, Massachusetts, the chances of surviving to maturity were substantially greater than in Charles Parish—and until well into the eighteenth century. Of children born in Andover between 1670 and 1699, 170 per 1000 died before reaching age twenty. Indeed only during the years 1730–1759 when the throat distemper was raging in Andover did mortality rates begin to equal those that had prevailed in Charles Parish since the latter third of the seventeenth century.[24]

Even those who reached maturity in Charles Parish could not expect to live long lives. Evidence on the age at death exists for

---

23   Norton, "Population Growth in Colonial America," 443; Greven, *Four Generations,* 197. In Colyton childhood mortality for both sexes was 200 per 1000: Wrigley, "Mortality in Pre-Industrial England," 571.

24   Greven, *Four Generations,* 189–190. Little is known as yet about infant and childhood mortality elsewhere in the Chesapeake. In a recent study of mortality in seventeenth-century Charles County, Maryland, however, Walsh and Menard have used model life table estimates to suggest that a large proportion of children (46.6%) failed to reach maturity. They developed their "preferred estimate" on the assumption that 80% of infant deaths were unrecorded because of late birth registration—estimated as an average delay of six months from birth. The Charles Parish materials allow us to modify these estimates. Beginning around 1715 both the date of birth and baptism are often given in the registers, permitting the calculation of an estimated mean interval between birth and registration. What one finds for Charles Parish is an average time lag of four weeks between birth and registration (64.1% of the births were recorded within four weeks and 97.0% within eight weeks). If the pattern of birth registration in Charles Parish were common for most of the early Chesapeake, then it appears that Walsh and Menard may have exaggerated the extent of underregistration of infant deaths (by overestimating the delay in registration); consequently, their estimates of infant and childhood mortality are probably too high. See Walsh and Menard, "Death in the Chesapeake," 221–222.

only 118 out of 240 males who were born between 1665 and 1699 and who are known to have survived to at least age twenty. These incomplete data suggest that men were struck down by death long before they had reached an advanced age.

Table 3, Column A shows the life expectancy for those men whose age at death is known. The average lifespan for the 118 men who survived to at least age 20 was only 39.9 years. But since these men comprise only about one half of all males known to have reached adulthood in Charles Parish, it is possible that their mean life expectancy is unrepresentative of most men in the parish. Thus, for a more comprehensive view of adult male mortality, it is necessary to account for the experience of the remaining 122 men for whom the age at death is not known.

Using a method developed by Walsh and Menard, I have followed the careers of these 122 men in all the available county rec-

Table 3 Life Expectancy for Males Born in Charles Parish, Virginia, 1665–1699

ACHIEVED AGE	EMPIRICAL TABLE[a]	HIGH MORTALITY[b]	LOW MORTALITY[c]	PREFERRED ESTIMATE[d]
20	19.9	16.7	23.2	20.8
25	17.9	14.5	20.7	18.2
30	16.3	13.3	17.6	16.4
35	14.3	11.6	15.8	14.4
40	11.7	10.9	13.7	11.8
45	10.9	10.5	12.2	11.3
50	9.5	9.2	11.5	9.5
55	8.3	8.0	10.6	8.5
60	6.8	6.6	7.3	6.9
65	5.1	4.7	6.0	5.2
70	4.0	3.8	4.9	4.0

a   includes only those whose age at death is known.
b   assumes that unknowns died the day after their last appearance in the records. Unknowns participate only through the age at which they last appear.
c   assumes that unknowns lived for ten years after their last appearance and then followed the rate of knowns. Unknowns participate only through the age at which they last appear.
d   assumes that unknowns lived until the last day of appearance and then followed the rate of knowns.

   This life table was constructed according to a method suggested by Lorena S. Walsh and Russell R. Menard, "Death in the Chesapeake: Two Life Tables for Men in Early Colonial Maryland," *Maryland Historical Magazine* LXIX (1974), 212–213.
SOURCE: The prosopography described in the text.

ords and have determined the date at which they could last be proven to have been alive in York County.[25] Since the mean age at which men first appeared in the records was 20.4, age 20 was designated the age when the unknowns were first placed at risk. A high mortality estimate was then constructed on the assumption that these men died the day after their last appearance in the records (Table 3, Column B). A low mortality estimate was also established which assumes that all unknowns lived an additional ten years beyond their last appearance in the records and then followed the mortality experience of those whose age at death is known (Column C). These two extremes in mortality experience are sufficiently broad so that the actual life expectancy of the unknowns fell within this range. Finally, a preferred estimate that assumes that the unknowns lived until the last day of their appearance in the records and then shared the mortality rate of the knowns represents the closest estimate of life expectancy between the high and low assumptions (Column D).

The high mortality assumption is too extreme because it indicates that men upon reaching age 20 could expect to live only another 16.7 years, well below the short life expectancy already established for the men whose age at death is known. Undoubtedly the unusually low figures produced in the high mortality estimate is a reflection of the difficulty in tracing the careers of Charles Parish men in a county that contained several parishes. The low mortality estimate is somewhat more reliable for it corrects for the problem of overrepresentation of youthful deaths in the records.[26] But because few of the unknowns could be followed beyond age forty-five, the life expectancies shown in this estimate are probably more reliable in the earlier years. The preferred estimate that a man could expect to live an additional 20.8 years beyond age 20 is in all likelihood the most accurate estimate of life expectancy in the parish.

Life expectancies were low in other parts of the early Chesapeake, but clearly not as low as in Charles Parish. Life tables constructed by the Rutmans for Middlesex County, Virginia, and

25 *Ibid.*, 212–213. For a general guide to the construction of life tables, see Barclay, *Techniques of Population Analysis,* 93–122.
26 Unless it can be shown that mortality was higher among migrators than "stable" members of a community, it seems likely that fewer young deaths than old ones were omitted from parish registers. See Wrigley, "Mortality in Pre-Industrial England," 562.

by Walsh and Menard for Charles County, Maryland, show that in these areas the expectation of life for men was several years beyond that for Charles Parish men. The Rutmans have determined that men who achieved age 20 in Middlesex could expect to live another 28.8 years, while Walsh and Menard have found that native men of Charles County who survived to maturity lived an additional 26 years[27] (Table 4). Apparently, living in Charles Parish meant that most men would die from five to eight years earlier than their contemporaries elsewhere in the Chesapeake.

However uncertain existence was for men in the early Chesapeake, it was not as harsh as that endured by Englishmen in the West Indies. Planters who came to these tropical islands, according to Dunn, "died young, married irregularly, and had too few children to maintain the population." Most men remained single and those who did marry normally died before they could produce large families. The 1715 Barbados census depicts a strikingly youthful society, not unlike Charles Parish, in which only 16 percent of the inhabitants had passed age forty and only 3 percent were over sixty.[28]

The similar experience of colonists in Virginia, Maryland, and the West Indies demonstrates that Englishmen suffered in the hot climate of these islands and the Chesapeake. Contributing to the unhealthy living conditions in Charles Parish were the low, marshy soil, mosquitoes, hot temperatures, and poor drinking water. All of these together could have produced dangerous outbreaks of malaria which seem to have been responsible for much of the heavy mortality in the colonial Chesapeake.[29] However susceptible to disease men were upon their arrival in the parish, conditions such as these increased the likelihood that they would not survive long.

27 Rutman and Rutman, "Malaria in the Early Chesapeake," 48; Walsh and Menard, "Death in the Chesapeake," 213. Due to the severities of the "seasoning" process, immigrants fell victim to disease more easily than natives and consequently had a shorter life expectancy of 22.7 years beyond age 20. Walsh and Menard, *ibid.*, 218, 224.

28 Dunn, *Sugar and Slaves*, 325, 332.

29 L. G. Tyler, *Narratives of Early Virginia* (New York, 1907), 21–22, 36–37, 127, 210–211, 220, 423–424; John Duffy, *Epidemics in Colonial America* (Baton Rouge, 1953), 214–222; Rutman and Rutman, "Malaria in the Early Chesapeake," 36, 38. See also the following letters from Virginia governors in the 1680s complaining about their debilitating health in the harsh Virginia summers and winters: Lord Effingham to King, 1687, McDonald Papers, VII, 262–263; Lord Jenkins to Lord Howard, 1683, McDonald Papers, VI, 272. Virginia State Library, Richmond.

Demographic research into colonial New England communities suggests a rather different mortality experience. In seventeenth-century Plymouth and Andover, Massachusetts, survival to maturity gave men the prospect of living an additional forty-four to forty-eight years—more than twice the average life expectancy of adult males in Charles Parish [30] (see Table 4). Although too little is known about life expectancy throughout early America, it does appear that mortality may have decreased as one travelled northward along the Anglo-American coast from the West Indies to New England in the seventeenth century.

Table 4 Life Expectancy for Men in the Seventeenth-Century Chesapeake and New England

ACHIEVED AGE	CHARLES PARISH	MARYLAND IMMIGRANTS	MARYLAND NATIVES	MIDDLESEX COUNTY	PLYMOUTH COLONY	ANDOVER, MASS.	SALEM, MASS.
20	20.8	22.7[a]	26.0	28.8	48.2[b]	44.6	36.1
30	16.4	17.4	20.4	19.4	40.0	39.3	29.2
40	11.8	13.2	15.6	13.0	31.2	31.8	24.1
50	9.5	10.3	12.0	7.7	23.7	23.5	19.1
60	6.9	10.0	9.3	5.8	16.3	15.6	14.5
70	4.0	5.5	7.0	3.6	9.9	10.3	10.0

a   age 22
b   age 21

SOURCES: Charles Parish: Table 3, Column D; Maryland: Lorena S. Walsh and Russell R. Menard, "Death in the Chesapeake: Two Life Tables for Men in Early Colonial Maryland," *Maryland Historical Magazine* LXIX (1974), 224; Middlesex County: Darrett B. and Anita H. Rutman, "Of Agues and Fevers: Malaria in the Early Chesapeake," *William and Mary Quarterly* XXXIII (1976), 48; Plymouth: John Demos, *A Little Commonwealth: Family Life in Plymouth Colony* (New York, 1970), 192; Andover: Philip J. Greven, Jr., *Four Generations: Population, Land, and Family in Colonial Andover, Massachusetts* (Ithaca, 1970), 27, 108; Salem: Rutman and Rutman, "Malaria in the Early Chesapeake," 48.

An important consequence of the shortened lifespans of men born in Charles Parish was the distinct shape it gave to their families. With the death of many fathers long before they reached the end of their normal procreative years, the size of most families remained small. The reconstitution of 386 families of men born between 1660 and 1689 discloses that the mean number of children known to have been born to all of the wives of these Charles

30   Demos, *A Little Commonwealth*, 192; Greven, *Four Generations*, 27, 108. Salem is an exception to the New England communities studied thus far. Still, Salem's estimated life expectancy for men of thirty-six years from age twenty suggests that it was considerably healthier than Charles Parish. For the Salem figures, see Vinovskis, "Mortality Rates and Trends in Massachusetts," 198–199.

Parish men was 2.99. Almost two-thirds of these families (63.9 percent) contained fewer than four children and nine out of ten (90.3 percent) had under seven children. A large family of ten or more children was clearly a rare occurrence for only four families of that size (about 1 percent) could be found during this period (Table 5). Families remained small among fathers born between

Table 5 Size of Families of Fathers Born Before 1689

NUMBER OF CHILDREN		NUMBER OF FAMILIES	PERCENTAGE OF FAMILIES
1–3		247	64.0
4–6		102	26.4
7–9		33	8.8
10 or more		4	1.0
mean	2.99		
median	3.00		
total		386	100.2

1690 and 1719. The mean number of children per family rose to 3.65, but the proportion of large families—those with seven or more children—stayed at about 10 percent. Again, families of one to three children predominated as 59.5 percent were of this size (Table 6).

Table 6 Size of Families of Fathers Born Between 1690 and 1719

NUMBER OF CHILDREN		NUMBER OF FAMILIES	PERCENTAGE OF FAMILIES
1–3		147	59.5
4–6		75	30.3
7–9		20	8.1
10 or more		5	2.0
mean	3.65		
median	3.00		
total		247	99.9

SOURCE: Charles Parish Registers, Virginia State Library, Richmond.

Reconstituting families from the parish register can create difficulties, however. A married couple may have begun raising a family elsewhere before entering Charles Parish or may have had additional children after leaving the parish. In either case the size of the family as reflected in the parish register would be underestimated. Thus, a separate study was made of only those families headed by men who were known to have spent their entire lives in the parish. Limited in this way, only seventy-seven families can be analyzed in Charles Parish from 1660 to 1719. Even this restricted sample confirms our initial observation that families grew to only modest proportions. Indeed, the mean number of children born to all the wives of these 77 men was 3.6, roughly the same as that determined for all families reconstituted from the register from 1690 to 1719. Although about a third of these families contained from four to six children, only four could have been considered large, with seven or more children[31] (Table 7).

Table 7   Size of Families of Fathers Born Between 1660 and 1719 and Who Remained in Charles Parish Until Death

NUMBER OF CHILDREN		NUMBER OF FAMILIES	PERCENTAGE OF FAMILIES
1–3		42	54.5
4–6		29	37.6
7–9		6	7.7
10 or more		0	0.0
mean	3.60		
median	3.00		
total		77	99.8

SOURCE: The prosopography described in the text.

31 This analysis of family size was based on the procreative years of the husband rather than the wife because of the lack of marriage records, which prevents tracing the lives of women after marriage. Since the reproductive years of men are not usually limited as are those of women, the average family size indicated here may be somewhat larger than what would be found if the wife's period of fertility were used. Moreover, if men outlived women in Charles Parish to the same extent as they did in Middlesex County, the period of female fertility would have been considerably shortened. Rutman and Rutman, "Malaria in the Early Chesapeake." Child-bearing came somewhat less frequently to Charles Parish women than to women in other parts of early America, with a mean birth interval of thirty-two months. Other studies indicate that children were usually spaced from twenty-four to thirty months apart in seventeenth- and eighteenth-century America and Europe. See Wells, "Quaker Marriage Patterns," 440–441.

Parental death frequently led to remarriage and the merging of two families could sometimes produce rather large households. Unfortunately, the absence of marriage records for Charles Parish precludes a study of remarriage. An illustration from the parish register, however, suggests how the development of large households from remarriage may have been a limited phenomenon. Buford Pleasants had one son, John, by his first wife, Mary. After her death in 1725, he quickly remarried and within two years he and his new wife Elizabeth, had the first of seven children. Infant and childhood deaths, however, reduced what might have developed into a large family of eight children. Indeed, by 1743 when Buford and Elizabeth's last child, George, was born, only four children were still alive. Thus, while second and third marriages on occasion forged large and complex households for a few years, the constant presence of death made swift and frequent changes in these families and limited most of them to three or four children.

Clearly, the controlling demographic fact in colonial Charles Parish families was the early death of parents rather than of children. With a rather high proportion of persons dying in childhood and adolescence, even those few parents who survived to an advanced age could expect to nourish only one or two children to maturity. Grandparentage was an even rarer phenomenon. From 1660 to 1760 only a dozen men in Charles Parish are known to have lived to see their grandchildren. In light of this, Murrin's recent suggestion that grandparents were a New England "invention" takes on added plausibility.[32]

For children early parental loss had an important and immediate consequence: orphanhood. According to the Rutmans, orphanhood was part of the fabric of life in seventeenth-century Middlesex County, where about three-fourths (73.2 percent) of all children had lost at least one parent before reaching twenty-one or the age of marriage. Over a third (36.0 percent) were fully orphaned at maturity. The same phenomenon can be followed in the Charles Parish materials throughout the colonial era.[33] During the

---

32 See John Murrin's review essay of several of the demographic and community studies of colonial New England in *History and Theory*, XI (1972), 238.

33 Orphanhood appears slightly more prevalent in the Middlesex figures probably because the data analyzed by the Rutmans focus mainly on the seventeenth century, when mortality and early parental loss were particularly high.

years 1660 to 1740, fully two-thirds (66.8 percent) of the parish children for whom evidence exists on the death of their parents were at least half-orphaned, while one of seven (13.9 percent) became full orphans[34] (Table 8).

Table 8   Orphanhood in Early Virginia

	CHILDREN KNOWN TO SURVIVE TO MATURITY[a]	CHILDREN WITH BOTH PARENTS AT MATURITY	CHILDREN WITH ONLY ONE PARENT AT MATURITY	CHILDREN ORPHANED AT MATURITY
Middlesex Co.[b]	164 (100%)	44 (26.8%)	61 (37.2%)	59 (36.0%)
Charles Parish	459 (100%)	152 (33.1%)	243 (52.9%)	64 (13.9%)

a   For the Middlesex data, maturity means age twenty-one or the age of marriage, whichever came first; for Charles Parish maturity is defined as twenty-one for men and eighteen for women.
b   The Middlesex data are based on children born between c. 1660 and 1710. See Darrett B. and Anita H. Rutman, "'Now-Wives and Sons-in-Law': Parental Death in a Seventeenth-Century Virginia County," in Thad. W. Tate, (ed), *The Chesapeake in the Seventeenth Century: Essays on its Euramerican Society and Politics* (Chapel Hill, forthcoming). The Charles Parish data cover children born between 1660 and 1740.
SOURCE: The prosopography described in the text.

Early parental death not only created an abundance of orphans in colonial Virginia, but also permitted young men to gain their autonomy rather early in life. This is reflected in the relatively young age at which sons married. Although marriage records are not available for Charles Parish, a crude estimate of the average age at marriage for men can be made by establishing a man's age at the birth of his first child. Given this figure, calculated from the birth register, one can subtract the average interval between marriage and first birth. In a recent paper Menard has suggested that despite a fairly high incidence of bridal pregancy, most Chesapeake couples experienced an interval of fifteen months between marriage and first birth. Using this fifteen-month interval as a guide for Charles Parish families, one can arrive at an estimated maximum age at marriage for men.[35]

34   Data concerning the date of death for at least one parent were available for 164 families. Of these 164 known deaths, 109, or 66.4%, were fathers, 16, or 9.9% were mothers, and in 39 cases, or 23.7%, the deaths of both parents were known. That so few deaths of mothers are known is simply a reflection of the difficulty in following the lives of women in the records without the benefit of a marriage register.
35   Russell R. Menard, "The Demography of Somerset County, Maryland: A Preliminary Report," paper presented to the Stony Brook Conference on Social History (1975). Since the first marriage for a man might have ended in the death of his wife before having a child,

Evidence for sixty-one men born between 1660 and 1699 reveals that they had reached an average age of 25.9 years at the birth of their first child. Although this would suggest that the mean age at marriage was around 24.7, a significant number of men married and started families much earlier than this. In fact, about one half (50.8 percent) had their first child before they were twenty-five, and about one third (34.4 percent) between the ages twenty-one and twenty-four (Table 9).

Table 9 Age at Birth of First Child of Fathers Born Between 1660 and 1699

AGE		N	PERCENTAGE
under 21		10	16.4
21–24		21	34.4
25–28		18	29.6
29 or more		12	19.6
mean	25.9		
median	24.0		
total		61	100.0

During the subsequent forty years, 1700–1739, young men in the parish had even earlier opportunities for marriage and independence. Fewer data are available for these years, but the experience of thirty-seven men discloses that they began raising families at a mean age of 24.8 years, indicating 23.6 as a maximum age at marriage. Twenty-two of the men, or 59.5 percent, had become parents by age 24, or about 22.8 when married, which was almost a 10 percent increase over the previous four decades (Table 10).

Despite the awkward nature of these calculations, it is apparent that from 1660 to 1740 the mean age at marriage was not higher than 24.8 years.[36] For the first four decades of the

---

this estimated mean age at marriage may still be too high. On the other hand, without marriage records, it is impossible to control for the effect of premarital pregnancies, which in most cases would place the estimated interval between marriage and first birth around six to nine months, rather than fifteen.

36 A demographic study of 100 gentry families in eighteenth-century Virginia corroborates this pattern of relatively early age at marriage, at least among the elite. From 1695 to 1750 the mean age at marriage for men was 24.4, while for women it was 20.3 years. Karen Dawley, "Childhood in Eighteenth-Century Virginia," unpub. master's thesis (University of Virginia, 1973).

Table 10 Age at Birth of First Child of Fathers Born Between 1700 and 1739

AGE		N	PERCENTAGE
under 21		5	13.8
21–24		17	45.8
25–28		8	21.6
29 or more		7	18.9
mean	24.8		
median	24.0		
total		37	100.1

SOURCE: Charles Parish Registers, Virginia State Library, Richmond.

eighteenth century, in fact, it declined to a maximum of 23.6 years. Particularly persuasive of the early age at marriage in Charles Parish is the fact that over half (54.1 percent) married before age 24. Similar marriage patterns have been discovered in portions of early Maryland. By comparison, men in colonial Andover waited until they were 26 or 27 before marriage, as did Quaker men in the early eighteenth century. Indeed, no region studied thus far in colonial America exhibited such early marital patterns for men as the Chesapeake.[37]

In a farming community such as Charles Parish, the ability to marry and to establish an independent household depended largely on gaining an inheritance of land or slaves. The age, then, at which a man could marry and become self-sufficient was often closely linked to the timing of his father's death. Young men in Charles Parish found conditions favorable for their early independence. Since most fathers died in their early forties, sons usually received their inheritance before they had come of age at twenty-one. Moreover, with the normally small number of surviving sons in each family, parents could bequeath rather generous portions of their land and personal property. Consequently, many young men

---

37 Menard, "Demography of Somerset County"; Greven, *Four Generations,* 33, 35, 118, 120, 206, 208; Wells, "Quaker Marriage Patterns," 417. The one region outside the Chesapeake where men may have married as early as they did in Charles Parish was Bristol, R.I., where the mean age at marriage for men before 1750 was 23.9. See Demos, "Families in Colonial Bristol," 55.

had the wherewithal quite early in life to consider marriage and assert their economic independence.[38]

The link suggested here between early parental loss and early marriage can be tested by comparing the marital patterns of children who were orphaned before reaching the mean age at marriage with those whose fathers were still alive. As Table 11 shows, the

Table 11   Impact of Early Parental Loss on Age at First Marriage for Males in Charles Parish

	MEAN AGE OF MEN AT BIRTH OF 1ST CHILD	ESTIMATED MEAN AGE AT MARRIAGE (15 MO. INTERVAL— MARRIAGE TO 1ST CHILD)
Father living when child reached estimated mean age at marriage	27.2 (N = 27)	26.0
Father dead when child reached estimated mean age at marriage	23.5 (N = 33)	22.3

SOURCE: Charles Parish Registers, Virginia State Library, Richmond.

timing of a father's death appears to have made an important difference in marriage opportunities, for orphaned children married almost four years earlier than children whose fathers were still alive. Admittedly, the evidence on this question is too small to be conclusive, but the data presented do suggest the strong impact of early parental loss on the marital autonomy of children.

The incomplete and often intractable vital records for Charles Parish have of necessity made this a tentative study of family structure and mortality. More work remains to be done on family life and demographic patterns in other areas of the early Chesapeake before solid conclusions can be drawn. Nevertheless, it may be

38 Williams has emphasized the important connections between inheritance and the independence of sons in an English village. See William M. Williams, *The Sociology of an English Village: Gosforth* (London, 1956), 49–51. See also William G. Hoskins, *The Midland Peasant: The Economic and Social History of a Leicestershire Village* (London, 1957); William J. Goode, "Family Systems and Social Mobility," in Reuben Hill and René König (eds.), *Families in East and West: Socialization Process and Kinship Ties* (The Hague, 1970), 315–336.

worthwhile to consider some possible implications from what is known about this parish.

If the demographic experience of Charles Parish were at all common, then the population of colonial Virginia had a distinctive age structure. Indeed, the oppressive mortality that prevailed in the seventeenth century virtually eliminated the development of an elderly generation, which may have had important consequences for the character of family life and authority in the parish. In the absence of grandparents, uncles, aunts, and family friends became especially important in caring for a rather large population of orphans. Many children, then, encountered more than one set of parents while growing up in Charles Parish. As a result, any tendency toward strong patriarchal authority was probably diverted amid these often abrupt changes in the life of the family.

Moreover, without a watchful, paternalistic group of elders in the parish, the forces for authority and tradition may have been considerably weaker than in New England towns where the influence of old Puritan patriarchs was keenly felt. That Virginia experienced more social and political unrest in the seventeenth century than the New England colonies may in part have been a reflection of the extremely youthful composition of the adult population.[39] "Conversation across the generations," as Laslett has put it, was rare in early Virginia, allowing men of roughly the same age to scramble for power and wealth relatively unimpeded by a sense of tradition or a concern for the opinion of an elderly generation.[40]

Above all, the demographic experience of Charles Parish indicates that little had changed in terms of family structure and longevity for Englishmen arriving in Virginia after the middle of the seventeenth century. Conditions in the colony could be rather harsh, but most English villages also suffered the effects of high mortality. Men in both England and Virginia lived relatively short lives (to about age fifty in England to age forty-five in Virginia) and very few survived to boast about grandchildren. English and

39 Timothy Breen, "Labor Force and Race Relations in Virginia, 1660–1710," *Journal of Social History*, VII (1973), 1–20; Edmund S. Morgan, "Slavery and Freedom: The American Paradox," *Journal of American History*, LIX (1972), 5–30.
40 Peter Laslett, *The World We Have Lost* (New York, 1965), 98–99; Bernard Bailyn, "Politics and Social Structure in Virginia," in James Morton Smith (ed.), *Seventeenth-Century America* (Chapel Hill, 1959), 90–118.

Virginia families were small, usually no more than a husband and wife and two or three children. In seventeenth-century Virginia, however, land was more abundant and the early deaths of fathers reduced paternal authority in the family and cleared the way for their sons' early autonomy, several years before young men in England could expect an independent life.[41]

41 Laslett, *ibid.*, 81–106.

David Northrup

African Mortality in the Suppression of the Slave Trade: The Case of the Bight of Biafra

Studies of the magnitude and causes of African mortality in the Atlantic slave trade have been hampered by the absence of reliable records at both ends of slaving voyages, a problem which worsened in the early nineteenth century as trade from portions of Africa and by a growing number of European nations became illegal and forced the adoption of more clandestine measures. This study partially solves the problem by using the very complete records of that portion of the slave trade which was intercepted by the British navy's West African Squadron. These captured ships were escorted along the coast for adjudication before the binational Courts of Mixed Commission at Freetown in the British colony of Sierra Leone, where the slaves on them were registered, liberated, and resettled. These sources not only provide a record (differentiated by the age and sex of the captives) of the astonishingly high losses between capture and adjudication, but also permit calculation of the factors responsible for these losses. Although the conditions on captured ships were not precisely the same as those on the much larger number of ships that eluded the patrol, these records do provide some indication of mortality in the overall slave trade in this period.[1]

In order to limit the number of variables, this study is confined to the slave trade from the most important slaving coast in West Africa during the first third of the nineteenth century, the Bight of Biafra, which extends east and south from the mouth of the Niger River to the equator. This coast included the main slaving ports of Bonny, New Calabar, and Brass in the eastern Niger

David Northrup is Professor of History at Boston College.

Special thanks are due to David Eltis, who most generously shared the bounty of his own research, offered much useful advice and encouragement, and made helpful comments on an earlier draft of this study. Thanks are also due to Stanley L. Engerman and Stephen Baier for valuable suggestions and comments on earlier drafts. Some of the research was made possible by a grant from the Fulbright-Hays Commission of the United States Office of Education.

1 For accounts of the operation of the patrol see William Law Mathieson, *Great Britain and the Slave Tade 1839–1865* (London, 1928); Christopher Lloyd, *The Navy and the Slave Trade* (London, 1949); W. E. F. Ward, *The Royal Navy and the Slavers* (New York, 1969).

trading areas further east and south known as the Cameroon and Gabon rivers. The study is based on the records of 100 ships from the Bight of Biafra apprehended by the West African Squadron between 1821 and 1839, the slaves from which were emancipated and registered in Sierra Leone.[2] These 100 ships include all but a few of the ships apprehended with slaves on board from this coast, and these records account for most of the Africans originally loaded on these vessels. Excluded are the small number of captured ships lost at sea en route to Freetown and a few others that were judged to have been stopped illegally and were restored to their owners along with the captive Africans on board. Also excluded are those slave cargoes or portions of cargoes that were deposited on the island of Fernando Po and were not subsequently registered in Sierra Leone. Although these omissions are significant (since their inclusion would raise the total losses connected with the captured ships to over 19 percent) the calculations in this essay are possible only when such anomalies have been removed. Except for indicating a slightly lower number of captures and deaths than in fact occurred, the cases included here accurately mirror the actual circumstances of the trade.[3]

The losses in transit to Sierra Leone are not calculated on exactly the same basis as is customary for those ships completing the middle passage to the Americas. In the first place, the losses and durations of the voyages are counted not from the point of embarkation at a port in the Bight of Biafra, but from the point

2 The accounts of the capture of these ships and the tallies of the Africans on board are found in the British Foreign Office Slave Trade Series (F.O. 84). The records of the emancipation and registration of liberated Africans are also scattered throughout this series, but are more conveniently consulted in the "Registers of Slaves Emancipated," originally kept in Sierra Leone and now in the Public Record Office (F.O. 315/31-36). Most of the correspondence on this subject can also be found in the British *Parliamentary Papers* along with useful (but sometimes imperfect) summaries of African liberation figures. The registers of emancipation have not been printed. Most of the information for the sample used here was compiled from the original files. The transit times used here are entirely from the following summaries: *Parl. Papers* 1830, x (661), appendix 8, "Return of the Number of Vessels which have been adjudicated in the Courts of Mixed Commission" (1819–29); *ibid.* 1832, xlvii (Correspondence, Class A), enclosure in no. 2, "Cases adjudicated in the year 1830"; *ibid.* 1842, xliv (385), "Return of Vessels brought before the Courts of Mixed Commission 1830–41."

3 A list of the 109 ships from the Bight of Biafra captured by the British navy while carrying slaves will appear in David Northrup, *Trade Without Rulers: Pre-Colonial Economic Development in South-Eastern Nigeria* (Oxford, 1978).

of their capture by the British patrol. The latter point seems preferable because the number of slaves alive at capture is normally based on an actual count, whereas the total at embarkation must be selected from the often conflicting testimony of the captured ship's officers and crew. In any event, since nearly all of these captures took place in port or within a short time after sailing and before many deaths could occur, this decision introduces only a very slight downward bias in the overall mortality rate, a bias that is more than offset by the fact that the losses in transit and the duration of the voyages are not calculated on the basis of identical time periods. A captured ship's voyage ended upon its arrival at Freetown, but the emancipation and registration of liberated Africans did not take place until the ship had been officially judged and condemned by the appropriate binational Mixed Commission there, a process which generally took only a few days, but when backlogs or disputes occurred could drag on for weeks. Until this process was completed captive Africans generally remained on board the slave ship, where they were given medical care, food, and water. Because these circumstances delayed the registration of Africans, the mortality figures used here represent deaths over a somewhat longer period of time than the actual duration of the voyage to Freetown, and because deaths were more likely to occur at the end of a voyage than at the beginning, this fact produces a small upward bias in the mortality figures when compared to transatlantic losses. At the same time, this manner of accounting does provide a more complete picture of the mortality in the slave trade since deaths occurring after the arrival in Freetown were directly attributable to the rigors of the trade.[4]

One of the most obvious factors governing the rate of mortality on ships from the Bight of Biafra, as from elsewhere in Africa, was the length of the time at sea. Slave ships were crowded and insanitary to begin with, so the longer the voyage the more likely were shortages and spoilage in food and water supplies and

4 Using records of the Africans alive upon arrival in Sierra Leone generously supplied by David Eltis, it has been possible to compute the difference between losses at arrival and those at registration for a significant portion of my 100 ships. For the period from 1821 to 1825 there was no significant difference from the losses reported in Table 2, but the losses at registration were higher by 1.1 percentage points for 1826 to 1830, by 2.1 points for 1831 to 1835, and by 3.0 points for 1836 to 1839.

Table 1 Mortality between the Bight of Biafra and Sierra Leone related to Length of Voyage and compared with Transatlantic Mortality

DAYS	TO SIERRA LEONE, 1821–39		TO AMERICAS, 1817–43[a]		TO RIO DE JANEIRO, 1825–30[b]	
	% OF SHIPS	AVERAGE LOSS (%)	% OF SHIPS	AVERAGE LOSS (%)	% OF SHIPS	AVERAGE LOSS (%)
10–19	11	9.6	>1	7.9	—	—
20–29	32	15.5	23	4.8	22	4.0
30–39	31	18.1	40	5.9	45	5.2
40–49	13	23.8	12	8.5	12	5.3
50–59	3	22.6	10	13.1	9	9.1
60–69	7	28.0			6	10.9
70–79	1	} 31.4	} 14	} 22.0	4	20.1
80–89	1				2	23.1
90+	1				>1	34.9
Total	100	17.9	100	9.0	100	7.0

a From Philip D. Curtin, *The Atlantic Slave Trade: A Census* (Madison, 1969), Table 81, based on a sample of 206 ships known to the British Foreign Office listed in *Parl. Papers* 1845, xlix (73).
b From Herbert S. Klein and Stanley L. Engerman, "Shipping Patterns and Mortality in the African Slave Trade to Rio de Janeiro, 1825–30," *Cahiers d'Etudes Africaines*, XV (1975), Table 9, based on the newspaper records of 386 ships.

the more common the spread of infectious diseases. The relationship between the losses suffered and the length of the voyage from the Bight of Biafra is shown in Table 1 along with two transatlantic series which are drawn primarily from other parts of the continent. Although all three series show that mortality increased with the time at sea, deaths on captured ships mounted less rapidly on the longest voyages since shortages of food and water were less likely to occur. More significant is the higher magnitude of loss on short and average length voyages in the series of captured ships. In part this is because neither transatlantic series includes ships from the Bight of Biafra, which other records suggest had an especially high mortality rate in crossing the Atlantic. This and other possible causes of these differences will be considered below.

The distribution of ships over time in Table 1 might be taken to suggest that voyages to Sierra Leone were generally faster than those to the Americas were it not for the fact that both transatlantic tabulations include ships from Mozambique, which had enormously long crossings (and notoriously high mortality rates).

Table 2 Mortality between Capture and Registration by Quinquennia and Decades, 1821–1839

	NUMBER OF SHIPS	AVERAGE DAYS IN TRANSIT	ALIVE AT CAPTURE	REGISTERED IN SIERRA LEONE	AVERAGE LOSS (%)
1821–25	12	49	2,630	2,103	20.0
1826–30	26	39	6,311	4,850	23.1
1821–30	38	43	8,941	6,953	22.2
1831–35	31	30	10,668	9,020	15.4
1836–39	31	28	9,037	7,536	16.6
1831–39	62	29	19,705	16,556	16.0
1821–39	100	34	28,646	23,509	17.9

SOURCE: The sources for Tables 2–6 are indicated in footnote 2.

In fact it appears that the transit time to Sierra Leone was actually about the same as the average transatlantic time. The transit time to Sierra Leone of the sample from the Bight of Biafra captured by the British navy from 1821 to 1839 averaged thirty-four days (Table 2), while twenty-seven ships arriving in Bahia during the first half of 1830 "chiefly from the Ports of Onim [Lagos], Bonny, New Calabar, &c." took an average of thirty-two days.[5]

The main reason for this long transit time was that Sierra Leone, from a navigational point of view, was a poor choice as the seat of the Mixed Commissions. Situated far from the Bights of Benin and Biafra, the principal slaving centers in West Africa during the nineteenth century, Sierra Leone could be reached only by sailing against the prevailing winds and currents along the coast. The shortcomings of the Colony as the seat of the Commissions were accurately stated by an investigating committee of Parliament in 1830:

> . . . it is the opinion of this Committee, That the situation of the Mixed Commission Court at Sierra Leone, for the adjudication of

5 Consul John Parkinson to Earl of Aberdeen, Bahia, Oct. 13, 1830, in *Parl. Papers* 1831, xix (Correspondence, Class A), no. 62. This is the source, imperfectly copied, for entries 1138–1171 in the summary list entitled "Return of the Number of Slave Vessels arrived in the Transatlantic States since 1814," *Parl. Papers* 1845 xlix (73). The extensive work by Eltis on the whole range of British records of the slave trade in this era strongly suggests that, despite the Consul's statement, nearly all of these twenty-seven ships to Bahia were from Lagos. Nevertheless, on the basis of presently available evidence this is as close as one can come to calculating sailing times from the Bight of Biafra to the New World in this era.

captured Slaves, is highly inconvenient for that purpose, considering that the Slaves are captured chiefly at the distance of 800 or 1,200 miles to the Eastward; and that as a current constantly sets from West to East, the captured ships are sometimes eight or nine weeks, and on the average, upwards of five weeks, on their passage from the place of capture to Sierra Leone; occasioning a loss of the captured Slaves, amounting to from one-sixth to one-half of the whole number, whilst the survivors are generally landed in a miserable state of weakness and disease.[6]

The solution to this regrettable situation, in the Committee's view, was to relocate the Mixed Commissions on Fernando Po, an island in the Bight of Biafra within easy sailing distance from the major slaving ports of West Africa. Some slaves were landed on the island about this time and it was later used as a residence for the Consul to the Bights of Benin and Biafra, but this sensible recommendation was never carried out because Spain, which claimed Fernando Po but had never occupied it, refused to sell the island to Britain. Without sovereignty Britain could not legally guarantee the freedom of liberated Africans and so the project was abandoned.[7]

Despite this major setback some reduction in losses en route to Sierra Leone did take place after 1830 as the result of other efforts begun in the previous decade. Changes made in the British patrol in the late 1820s had increased the number of captures and reduced the transit time to the Colony by an average of ten days between the period 1821 to 1825 and 1826 to 1830, although there was no corresponding reduction in mortality, which in fact increased (Table 2). One of the major problems with the patrol had been the poor quality of its ships. Most patrol vessels were either large, slow frigates, the tall masts of which rounding the horizon gave slave ships enough advance warning to escape, or "smaller ships, . . . mostly Seppings brigs, which everyone agreed sailed like haystacks, compared with the clean lines of the slaving schooners." However, encouraged by the practice of granting "prize-money" to the captors, enterprising naval officers had be-

6 *Parl. Papers* 1830, x (661), "Report from the Select Committee on the Settlements of Sierra Leone and Fernando Po," 4.
7 K. Onwuka Dike, *Trade and Politics in the Niger Delta 1830–1885* (Oxford, 1956), 55–60, based on the British Colonial Office file C.O. 82.

Table 3   Mortality between Capture and Registration related to Length of Voyage, by Decades

	1821–30			1831–39		
DAYS	NUMBER OF SHIPS	ALIVE AT CAPTURE %	AVERAGE LOSS %	NUMBER OF SHIPS	ALIVE AT CAPTURE %	AVERAGE LOSS %
10–19	3	7.6	8.4	8	13.8	9.9
20–29	4	10.6	23.6	28	42.8	14.6
30–39	13	39.0	21.9	18	28.2	15.8
40–49	5	11.9	18.4	8	15.2	25.7
50+	13	30.9	27.1	—	—	—
Total	38	100.0	22.2	62	100.0	16.0

gun buying condemned slave vessels to serve as tenders to their official ships. The incorporation of the *Henriqueta* (renamed *Black Joke*) into the patrol in this manner in 1828 had greatly increased captures and reduced sailing times. Other measures aimed specifically at saving African lives, when combined with better sailing times, had cut losses so that by the 1830s the transit time to Sierra Leone had been reduced from an average of six weeks in the previous decade to an average of four weeks.[8]

As Table 3 shows, this faster sailing time was accompanied by a reduction in losses from 22.2 percent to 16.0 percent. Not all of this reduction can be attributed to the shorter sailing time since changes in the condition of slaves at the point of supply, in carrying techniques, and in the care provided by the British patrol also would have affected this figure. It is possible to isolate the reduction in losses attributable to the shorter sailing time from these other factors by redistributing the slaves captured from 1821 to 1830 according to the faster sailing times of the 1831 to 1839 ships.[9] Such a projection gives a mortality rate of 20.2 percent, indicating that the faster sailings of the 1831 to 1839 period would have reduced the 1821 to 1830 losses by 2 percentage points. Since

8 Lloyd, *Navy*, 71; Ward, *Royal Navy*, 128. From 1830 patrol ships were required to place a medical officer on captured vessels to treat those who were ill; see *Parl. Papers* 1831–32, xlvii (Correspondence, Class A), no. 4.

9 This is accomplished by multiplying the percentage of slaves in each sailing category from 1831 to 1839 by the average mortality rate for the same category from 1821 to 1830. Thus for 10–19 day voyages: .138 × .084 = .0116. Similarly for 20–29 days we get .1010, for 30–39 days, .0618, for 40–49 days .0280, giving a total loss of 20.2% in this projection versus actual losses of 22.2%.

Table 4 Mortality between Capture and Registration by Month of Capture and by Principal Month en route to Sierra Leone, 1821–39

	BY MONTH OF CAPTURE			BY MONTH EN ROUTE		
	NUMBER OF SHIPS	AVERAGE DAYS IN TRANSIT	AVERAGE LOSS (%)	NUMBER OF SHIPS	AVERAGE DAYS IN TRANSIT	AVERAGE LOSS (%)
January	7	45	18	10	38	23
February	9	42	16	8	41	19
March	8	39	21	8	40	21
April	13	31	17	8	41	19
May	5	29	28	12	33	18
June	3	25	16	4	22	30
July	4	28	11	4	20	12
August	10	39	25	9	32	22
September	10	31	16	7	38	14
October	13	30	14	11	29	14
November	8	30	10	14	33	14
December	10	34	24	5	26	11
Total	100	34	18	100	34	18

the actual reduction in mortality from the earlier period to the later one was 6.2 percentage points, it may be concluded that the various other factors influencing mortality rates were twice as important for this reduction as was the shortened sailing time.

Another factor linked with the mortality rate was the time of year in which the sailing took place. In order to explore possible links between weather and mortality two series were constructed, both shown in Table 4. The first distributes ships and mortality by the month of capture; the second by the month during which they spent the greatest number of days en route to Sierra Leone after capture. Neither arrangement shows any consistent linkage between the time of year and the rate of mortality. What does show up is a remarkably consistent reverse congruence between the average rainfall per month in the Bight of Benin and the average number of days required to reach Sierra Leone. This trend exists in both series but is stronger in the arrangement by month of capture, indicating a strong influence of the weather during the early part of the voyage on the length of its overall duration. It was not the rain itself which sped the ships on their way but the accompanying winds, the amount of rainfall being a convenient quantifiable measure of the seasons along the West African coast. During the long dry season in November-February and the short dry season in August winds were lighter and consequently the voyages took much longer.[10]

The health of the slaves might be expected to have varied more directly with the amount of rain since many travelled exposed on the main deck and the others had to endure the stifling heat and foul air below decks when rain and rough seas necessitated closing the ventilators. However, the ill effects of the storms were partly offset by the shorter duration of the voyage in the rainy season except when either factor was acute. Then the mortality rate swung upward. This is illustrated most clearly by using the distribution of ships by the principal month of voyaging (rather than by the month of capture), indicating the cumulative nature of these effects. Thus the three peaks in mortality (the dotted line in Fig. 1) in January, June, and August correspond to the extremes either in the amount of rainfall or in the duration of the voyages. The January and August extremes correspond with the peaks of the dry seasons (and longest sailing times), while the apex of mortality occurred in June at the peak of the rains (despite the shortest average sailing times). At other times of the year the mortality rate was pulled in opposite directions by these two factors and occupied an intermediate position.

A cause of mortality on slave ships that has not been measured here is overcrowding. Although it was once common to attribute large numbers of deaths to cruel and greedy captains who maltreated their slaves, especially by packing excessive numbers of them into their ships, several recent studies have dis-

10   In studying the Congo-Angola slave trade, Herbert S. Klein and Stanley L. Engerman found a strong correlation between high mortality and sailing times made during the stormy season: "Shipping Patterns and Mortality in the African Slave Trade to Rio de Janeiro, 1825–30," *Cahiers d'Etudes Africaines*, XV (1975), 394. Whether the slave traders were aware of these seasonal variations and were influenced by them is a question that cannot be answered on the basis of the present sample, which may reflect the sailing preferences of the British patrol as likely as those of the slavers. A study by W. E. Minchinton suggests that reaching the Americas during the summer months was the prime concern for slavers to South Carolina and Virginia. See his "The Slave Trade of Bristol with the British Mainland Colonies in North America 1699–1770" in Roger Anstey and P. E. H. Hair (eds.), *Liverpool, the African Slave Trade, and Abolition* (Liverpool, 1976), 47–49.

Fig. 1 Monthly Variations in Rainfall, Mortality, and Transit Time to Sierra Leone, 1821–1839.

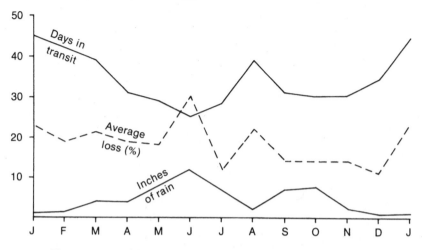

SOURCE: The average rainfall in the Bight of Benin measured in inches at Lagos–Ikeja is from William A. Hance, *The Geography of Modern Africa* (New York, 1975; 2nd ed.), 48. The average number of days in transit (by month of capture) from the Bight of Biafra to Sierra Leone and the average loss of life among slaves (by principal month en route) are from Table 4.

counted the importance of overcrowding as a factor directly linked to high transatlantic mortality.[11] In the case of the ships captured in the Bight of Biafra the possibility of more than ordinary mistreatment was reduced through supervision by the British captors, although overcrowding was sometimes relieved by transferring some Africans to other captured ships or by disembarking some on the island of Fernando Po. Because of these and other anomalies in the sample used here, which made conditions on captured ships significantly different from those which existed during the middle passage to the Americas, and because of the difficulties of accurately converting different measures of capacity to a single system, no attempt has been made to produce slave/capacity ratios.[12] However, the records of individual ships

11 Klein and Engerman, "Shipping Patterns," 394; *idem,* "Slave Mortality on British Ships 1791–1797," in Anstey and Hair, *Liverpool,* 118; Johannes Postma, "Mortality in the Dutch Slave Trade 1675–1795," in Henry A. Gemery and Jan S. Hogendorn (eds.), *The Uncommon Market: Essays in the History of the Atlantic Slave Trade,* forthcoming.
12 Some ships were taken before they had completed their cargoes; others after partly unloading their slaves as the patrol ship approached, since until "equipment" treaties were signed in the 1830s and 1840s only ships actually carrying slaves could be captured.

do support the subjective impression that little correlation existed between mortality rates and the conditions on the captured ships.

In the case of the ship *Invincival*, which was captured in the Cameroon estuary just before Christmas in 1826, only 250 of 440 slaves on board at capture survived the journey to Sierra Leone, a loss of 43 percent. The British captors reported that the ship carried food and water "in abundance and of the best quality," but that it was "terribly overcrowded" with 200 African boys being kept on deck and in the lifeboats sheltered only by spare sails. Despite these crowded conditions, the ship was actually carrying sixty slaves *less* than the 500 a ship of its size was permitted under Brazilian law. In part, the captors attributed this high mortality to the fact that the captain and crew had fallen sick while trading in Cameroon and had also become embroiled in a dispute with the African slave traders there. As a consequence the slaves had been loaded with unusual haste into an ill-prepared and dirty ship, a fact which promoted the rapid spread of disease among the slaves. As was usual on Brazilian ships there was no doctor to minister to the sick. Moreover, during the voyage to Sierra Leone the ship had the extreme ill-luck to the struck by lightning twice and to encounter twenty-seven consecutive days of heavy rains. Temporary repairs to the damaged masts and these storms delayed the ship's progress so that it took two months to reach Freetown. Another two weeks elapsed before the adjudication was completed.[13]

Although the lives of 190 African captives were lost on this voyage, there seems little in the circumstances of it to warrant placing unusual blame on the Brazilian captain and crew, who could not have anticipated their own illness, the dispute, the capture, or the necessity of navigating against foul weather en route to Sierra Leone. This does not mean that they were blameless, but in carrying no medical officer and in filling the decks with slaves they were doing no differently than other slave traders who did not suffer such enormous losses.

13 *Parl. Papers* 1828, xxvi (Correspondence, Class A) no. 53: Commissioners to Canning, Sierra Leone, Mar. 31, 1827; *Parl. Papers* 1830, x (661). "Report from the Select Committee," evidence of Captain William Jardin Purchase, 24–25. Brazilian law limited the number of slaves to 5 per 2 tons of registered burden, while British law from 1788 to 1799 limited its slavers to 5 slaves for every 3 tons up to 200 registered tons and 1 slave per ton thereafter. See Klein and Engerman, "Slave Mortality," 119–121.

Two other Brazilian cases will underline the vagaries of the trade. The *Silveirinha* was captured at Old Calabar in March 1827 with 266 slaves on board, sixty-one more than its small size (eighty-two tons) permitted even by the lax Brazilian law, making it grossly overcrowded. Since the small ship sailed poorly against the wind and currents, it took over eleven weeks to reach Freetown, but its losses, although substantial enough, were still not far from average for this period: 21.4 percent.[14] A month later the *Creola* was taken with 308 slaves from Old Calabar, and the record of the captor is vehement with denunciations of her captain:

> Although she was limited to carry only 214 slaves, the rapacity of her inhuman master induced him to cram nearly 100 more into her, making upwards of seven for every two tons, aggravating in a most cruel degree the horrid misery of his victims by such studied barbarity; putting the law of his own government at defiance, as well as the treaty and the convention [with Britain]. On her arrival here she presented the shocking spectacle of a living mass, etc.[15]

Yet, taken in tow by her captor, she arrived in Sierra Leone after a remarkably short voyage of only two weeks having lost twenty of her slaves for a mortality rate of only 6.5 percent. Compared to the captain of the *Invincival*, the masters of these other two ships were surely less mindful of the safety of their slaves, yet their cruelty is not reflected in the actual rates of mortality aboard their ships, leading one to doubt that overcrowding was directly linked to loss of life in a significant way.

The causes of mortality considered so far refer primarily to the conditions on captured ships; the remainder of this essay examines factors that should apply equally to captured ships and to those successfully reaching the Americas. Because of poor records for the transatlantic slave trade in this period calculations of mortality have varied. James Bandinel, long time chief clerk and superintendent of the British Foreign Office's Slave Trade Department, advised Parliament in 1848 that the transatlantic mortality during the previous two decades had been about 24

14 *Parl. Papers* 1828, xxvi (Correspondence, Class A), no. 69: Commissioners to Canning, Sierra Leone, June 20, 1827.
15 *Ibid.*, no. 68: Commissioners to Canning, Sierra Leone, June 18, 1827.

percent, a figure he arrived at by calculating losses on captured ships taken to Freetown at 18 percent and adding another 6 percentage points to account for the longer distance to the Americas. This figure can no longer be accepted, not least because, as was suggested above, sailing times to the Americas from key slaving points such as the Bight of Biafra were generally not longer than those to Sierra Leone. In contrast, a study by Curtin of British records from 1817 to 1843 has arrived at a mortality rate of only 9 percent, and a more limited study by Klein and Engerman of the slave trade to Rio de Janeiro based on Brazilian records for the period from 1825 to 1830 has arrived at a mortality rate of 7 percent (See Table 1). However, new work by Eltis making more critical use of a broader range of sources, strongly suggests that these figures are much too low, both because the samples used include few ships from high loss areas such as the Bight of Biafra and because the records themselves probably underreport losses for the regions that they do consider. Eltis estimates that transatlantic mortality from 1821 to 1843 ranged from 7 to 25 percent depending on the African region of origin and the American region of importation.[16]

Significantly, Eltis postulates a mortality rate of 17.2 percent for ships from the Bights of Benin and Biafra to the Spanish and French Caribbean, the primary destination of slaves from these coasts in this era. He also maintains that ships from the Bight of Biafra had the highest losses on the Atlantic side of Africa. This reinforces the conclusion of another study by Klein and Engerman of British ships trading in slaves to the West Indies in the 1790s which reports that ships from the Bight of Biafra suffered losses double the average for this group. There are several reasons why losses from the Bight of Biafra ought to have been higher than those from elsewhere on the Atlantic side of Africa, but the full explanation may still be obscure. Sailing times and sailing conditions on this coast were certainly one factor. Because the winds and currents ran strongly from the west, ships leaving the Bight commonly sailed south and east before swinging round near the

---

16 James Bandinel, "Memoranda on the Mortality of Slaves in their Passage in Slave Ships from *Africa* to the West Indies," in Reports from Committees, Slave Trade, Second Report, Appendix, *Parl. Papers* 1847–48, xxii, 175–179. David Eltis, "The Volume and Direction of the Transatlantic Slave Trade 1821–43: A Revision of the 1845 Parliamentary Paper," in Gemery and Hogendorn (eds.), *Uncommon Market*.

equator to head for the Americas, a detour that added one or more weeks to their voyages. Klein and Engerman's figures show, for example, that ships from the Bight of Biafra took longer to reach their destinations than those from any other African coast (except the Bight of Benin, which is represented in their study by only three ships). Moreover, as was shown above, the weather conditions encountered in the Gulf of Guinea during the early days of the voyage markedly affected the losses on captured ships and presumably (though the routes were different) on those that escaped detection as well. However, Klein and Engerman found too little correlation in their sample from the 1790s to warrant attributing the losses to these conditions of shipment, arguing instead that the high losses from the Bight of Biafra "must relate to the nature of the African supply source," that is, to the conditions under which the Africans were enslaved, taken to the coast, and readied for shipment.[17]

Since the identification of African supply conditions as most responsible for these high losses was arrived at by eliminating other possibilities rather than by an analysis of the actual African supply conditions, this conclusion must remain open to some doubt. Many conditions could have been significant and most are known imperfectly if at all. Certainly what is known of the general conditions of supply to this coast suggests no obvious circumstance that can be used to explain the high mortality rates encountered. The hinterland of the Bight of Biafra was densely populated and may have been experiencing some shortages of food at that time, but there is no reason to think that this produced conditions notably worse than elsewhere on the continent. Rather the density of the population meant that the slaves exported were drawn principally from among the Igbo (Ibo) and Ibibio peoples just behind the coast and thus were not subjected to the long marches that have been suggested as causes of high mortality elsewhere.[18] Moreover, the absence of large-scale states among

17 · Eltis, "The Export of Slaves from Africa, 1820–1843," *Journal of Economic History*, XXXVII (1977), Table 3, 5, and personal communication; Klein and Engerman, "Slave Mortality," 117.
18 The operation of the slave trade in this region is discussed in considerable detail in Northrup, *Trade Without Rulers*, esp. chs. 3–6. The main lines of this region's economy in the period under consideration are described in Northrup, "The Compatibility of the Slave and Palm Oil Trades in the Bight of Biafra," *Journal of African History*, XVII (1976), 353–364.
Faced with a discrepancy between the losses in transit on slave ships from West Africa

Table 5 Proportion of Children in Cargo related to Mortality between Capture and Registration

CHILDREN %	NUMBER OF SHIPS	ALIVE AT CAPTURE	REGISTERED IN SIERRA LEONE	AVERAGE LOSS (%)
0–24	9	1,889	1,651	12.6
25–49	70	21,169	17,674	16.5
50–74	19	5,298	4,006	24.4
75–99	2	290	178	38.6
Total	100	28,646	23,509	17.9

these peoples meant an absence of the major conflicts and disruptions which sent so many prisoners of war and refugees into the overseas slave trade elsewhere. Instead, most of those enslaved seem to have been the victims of kidnapping or of sales for various reasons by fellow villagers. Perhaps because of these circumstances the Bight of Biafra supplied a greater proportion of female slaves than was usual elsewhere in Africa as is attested by a small sample of cargoes near the end of the seventeenth century and by a larger sample near the end of the eighteenth century. However, there is no known connection between sex ratios in the slave trade and mortality. In any event, by the 1820s and 1830s the proportion of males (62 percent) was more typical of the Atlantic trade overall.[19]

Although the proportion of females had fallen, the proportion of children had increased from one-eighth in the late seventeenth century to two-fifths of the total in the first half of the nineteenth century. Table 5 suggests a strong link between the proportion of children in a cargo and the mortality rate incurred. Because the age ratios at capture are unknown, it is impossible to

compared with those from the Congo area, Philip D. Curtin, *The Atlantic Slave Trade: A Census* (Madison, 1969), 280–282, adopted a line of reasoning parallel to that developed here, suggesting that slaves from the Congo area were likely to have been drawn from further inland and that they were thus loaded onto ships in an already weakened condition. Using different data, Klein and Engerman, "Shipping Patterns," 394, also suggested that the much lower rate of loss for slaves north of the Congo River, compared to losses from Angola, might be accounted for in a similar manner.

19 The earlier sample (5 ships) contained 56% males and 13% children; see Northrup, *Trade Without Rulers*, Table 1. The latter sample (over 100 ships) contained 56.6% males and about 13% children; see Klein and Engerman, "Slave Mortality," 119 and Table 3.

calculate the actual mortality ratios of adults to children on these voyages and thus the precise nature of this link is unknown. Children may simply have died more readily or there may have been some more complex contagion effect which also raised adult mortality.[20]

Another approach to the African supply situation is to consider the variations in mortality among the ports of call in the Bight of Biafra. Table 6 shows that mortality and transit times rose with the distance of the trading sites from Freetown, being lowest at the Nun branch of the Niger and progressively higher at points to the east. The direction of this trend is not surprising, but the rate at which mortality rose appears out of proportion to the additional time and distance involved. The losses are particularly out of line in the eastern part of the Bight at Old Calabar and even more in the Cameroon estuary.

Part of the explanation of the higher losses in the eastern Bight seems to be the higher proportion of children shipped from these ports than from the Rio Real (Table 6, column 6).[21] It is possible that a higher mortality on the arduous voyage to Freetown also resulted from slaves from Old Calabar and the Cameroon estuary being in a weaker physical condition than those shipped from elsewhere in the Bight. Although the information on this point is short on details, oral traditions and other sources suggest the strong possibility that in the 1820s and early 1830s a large proportion of the slaves shipped from the Cameroon estuary were in a weakened condition. During this period the highlands of central Cameroon were rocked by a succession of raids and wars separately initiated by the Chamba-led Bali (Ba'ni), the Fulani of the Adamawa Emirate, the Bamum, and others. These conflicts created widespread disruption and dislocation that resulted in many persons being sold into the overseas slave trade.[22]

20 Whether children formed a significantly larger share of the slaves from the Bight of Biafra than from elsewhere in Africa in this period is not known.
21 Children appear to have been particularly vulnerable to long sailing times. Table 6 shows that ships from Brass, which carried slightly more than the average proportion of children but had much shorter than average sailing times, suffered losses averaging only 9%, although ships from the Cameroon estuary, which had much longer sailing times as well as a much higher proportion of children than was average, had losses over three times as severe. The Gabon figures do not agree with this pattern, a fact that is probably to be explained by the statistically inadequate number of ships from that port.
22 There is no single reliable account of this area in that era, but aspects of its history are treated in Merran McCulloch, Margaret Littlewood, and I. Dugast, *Peoples of the*

Table 6 Mortality and Proportion of Children in Cargo by Area of Origin, 1821–39

	NUMBER OF SHIPS	AVERAGE DAYS IN TRANSIT	ALIVE AT CAPTURE	REGISTERED IN SIERRA LEONE	AVERAGE LOSS %	CHILDREN %
Nun River (Brass)	9	26	2,611	2,376	9.0	41.0
Rio Real (Bonny and New Calabar)	51	32	15,180	12,847	15.4	34.6
Cross River (Old Calabar)	26	37	7,377	5,803	21.3	43.8
Cameroon River (Bimbia, etc.)	12	35	2,943	2,039	30.7	53.0
Gabon River	2	40	535	444	17.0	51.4
Total	100	34	28,646	23,509	17.9	39.4

Koelle's biographies of liberated Africans in Sierra Leone from central Cameroon show that many victims of these disruptions were sold from the Cameroon estuary and Old Calabar, a fact that may have raised losses from these ports. However, the effects would have been less pronounced in Old Calabar, which drew many more slaves from other areas, than in the Cameroon estuary, which was more dependent on central Cameroon supplies.[23]

In conclusion, it may be said that the factors governing the mortality on slave ships from the Bight of Biafra captured and condemned in Sierra Leone in the period from 1821 to 1839 fall into two broad categories. First are those general circumstances which determined that the overall mortality would be high. These include the normally high proportion of children supplied along this coast, the distance to be covered to Sierra Leone, and the difficulties of navigating along that route, particularly in the Gulf of Guinea. The second category includes those factors which governed the sizeable variations in mortality from ship to ship. The most significant of these were the time of the year in which the sailing took place (because of variations in winds and rains) and the port at which the slaves were purchased (because of

Central Cameroons (London, 1954), 20–21, 53; Edwin Ardener, *Coastal Bantu of the Cameroons* (London, 1956), 48; E. M. Chilver, "Nineteenth Century Trade in the Bamenda Grassfields, Southern Cameroons," *Afrika und Übersee*, VL (1962), 237–238; E. M. Chilver and P. M. Kaberry, "Sources of the Nineteenth-Century Slave Trade: Two Comments. I. The Cameroons Highlands," *Journal of African History*, VI (1965), 119. For distance as a factor producing weakened slaves see note 18 above.
23 S. W. Koelle, *Polyglotta Africana* (London, 1854), 11–13, 20–21.

of children offered for sale, and the distance to be covered to Sierra Leone).

Some of these factors would also have affected mortality rates on transatlantic voyages, notably the condition of the slaves at loading and the proportion of children. Problems of navigation were common to all ships, but the actual circumstances were different enough that the normal transatlantic crossing might well have been less costly of life than the hard passage to Sierra Leone. However, any lessening of the relative mortality thus achieved would probably have been offset by the measures that the patrol took to relieve congestion and shortages of supplies on captured ships. Finally, it is possible that ships captured by the patrol were not a random sample of the total trade, since faster ships and more alert crews may have been more successful in eluding capture. Measurement of some of these variations may come from future research, but it seems reasonable to conclude that the mortality in the transatlantic slave trade from the Bight of Biafra to the Americas in this era (when measured to include passage-related deaths occurring within a reasonable period after the actual end of the voyage) was of a comparable order of magnitude to that reported here for captured ships.

Myron P. Gutmann and Kenneth H. Fliess

The Social Context of Child Mortality in the American Southwest

The health of children was an important subject of debate among doctors, reformers, and government officials at the beginning of the twentieth century, as evidenced by a grand tide of proposals for reform and research studies. The United States Department of Labor established the Children's Bureau to marshal information and set up procedures for improving child health and reducing infant and childhood sickness and mortality. Individual states also acted for improved child welfare and health, spurred on by a women's reform movement that saw children's health and welfare as fundamental. The emphasis on children's health reform was inspired, in part, by the poor health and sanitation conditions of the poorest and least well-educated families, relative to the healthier families within the privileged class of the reformers. The early studies of rural health conditions, such as Bradley and Williamson's study of North Carolina, focus on how the differences between families effect their health. Studies of rural health in the Midwest, when compared with those of conditions in the South, further highlighted the wide variations between the childhood health and mortality

Myron P. Gutmann is Professor of History, The University of Texas, Austin. He is the author of *Towards the Modern Economy: Early Industry in Europe, 1500–1800* (New York, 1988); *War and Rural Life in the Early Modern Low Countries* (Princeton, 1980).

Kenneth H. Fliess is Associate Professor of Anthropology, The University of Nevada, Reno. He is the author of "Mortality Transition among the Wends of Serbin, Texas, 1854–1884: Investigation of Changes in the Pattern of Death Using Parochial Records," *Social Biology*, XXXVI (1991), 266–276; "Fertility, Nuptiality, and Family Limitation among the Wends of Serbin, Texas, 1854–1920," *Journal of Family History*, XIII (1988), 251–263.

This research was supported by Grant # R01 HD23693 from the National Institute of Child Health and Human Development, and by grants from the University of Texas Project Quest and the University Research Institute of the University of Texas, Austin. We are grateful to the other members of the Texas Historical Demography project staff, and especially to John Vetter, Jane Zachritz, Judy McArthur, and Christie Sample for their assistance and advice. This article was originally presented to a seminar organized by the International Union for the Scientific Study of Population on the subject of "Infant and Child Mortality in the Past." We are grateful to the organizers for giving us the opportunity to present our work, and to the other participants for their helpful suggestions. We also wish to thank the Economic History Seminar at the University of Arizona for useful comments.

situations of different family, ethnic, and social groups in the rural United States.[1]

Mortality conditions were improving in the United States in the late nineteenth and the early twentieth centuries, largely because of the continuing growth of cities and the continuing improvements in urban public health and sanitation. In rural areas, sanitation was not improving as rapidly, yet levels of mortality declined. Many reformers and public health officials saw their task as speeding the development of sanitation in the countryside, and eliminating, so far as possible, the differences between groups. Much of the historical literature about rural mortality in the United States has concentrated on the causes of the decline in mortality, debating the extent to which it was due to improvements in sanitation and health, or to improvements in standards of living and nutrition. Although the evidence is not unequivocal, there is reason to believe that both factors were important, even in the countryside.[2]

Scholars still measure the rates of infant and childhood mortality within the United States and debate the cause of the differences between groups. In the Southwest, where the research of this article is focused, a number of important differentials have appeared. Racial and ethnic differences are the most commonly cited in American child health, made more complex in Texas and the rest of the Southwest by the large number of Mexican-origin Hispanics and African-Americans. As Powell-Griner has shown, racial and ethnic differences interact with other forces—most prominently social and economic conditions and the quality and quantity of prenatal medical care available to the mother. What is remarkable in the recent research is the favorable experience of

1 Judith N. McArthur, "Motherhood and Reform in the New South: Texas Women's Political Culture in the Progressive Era," unpub. Ph.D. diss. (Univ. of Texas, Austin, 1992); Emma L. M. Jackson, "Petticoat Politics: Political Activism among Texas Women in the 1920s," unpub. Ph.D. diss. (Univ. of Texas, Austin, 1980); Molly Ladd-Taylor, *Raising a Baby the Government Way: Mothers' Letters to the Children's Bureau, 1915–1932,* (New Brunswick, 1986), 19; Frances Sage Bradley and Margaretta A. Williamson, *Rural Children in Selected Counties of North Carolina* (Washington, D.C., 1918); Elizabeth Moore, *Maternity and Infant Care in a Rural County of Kansas* (Washington, D.C., 1917); Florence Brown Sherbon and E. Moore, *Maternity and Infant Care in Two Rural Counties in Wisconsin* (Washington, D.C., 1919).

2 Samuel H. Preston and Michael R. Haines, *Fatal Years: Child Mortality in Nineteenth-Century America* (Princeton, 1991); Robert Higgs, "Mortality in Rural America, 1870–1920: Estimates and Conjectures," *Explorations in Economic History,* X (1973), 177–195.

Mexican Americans in terms of infant and childhood mortality, relative to the rest of the population, especially considering their relatively low socioeconomic position.[3]

This article is a report about the social context of infant and childhood mortality levels in six rural counties in Texas. Because Texas did not require public birth and death registrations until 1903, and because registration was incomplete for a long time thereafter, our evidence derives from the set of questions asked of married women in the 1900 and 1910 census about the number of children born, the number of children surviving, and the number of years married. To these facts we have added other evidence about wealth, as reported in County tax assessments.[4]

Our goal is to show the nature of social differences in childhood mortality in Texas, as well as to emphasize a number of issues. The idea of social difference goes beyond the common descriptors, social status and occupational socioeconomic condition. In Texas, as in much of the South (and eventually all of the United States), racial and ethnic differences were major determinants of the demographic experiences of population groups. Blacks and whites differed, of course, but so did important groups within the white population. In Texas, there were important differentials between whites of Mexican origin and ancestry, whites of central European origin and ancestry, and all other whites. The early sections are concerned with the explication of childhood mortality differences by racial and ethnic group and by occupational group. Our research indicates that differences in childhood mortality evade the readily identifiable social characteristics of families. We refer to these extended differences in our population as local mortality attributes, which, in our analysis, initially take the form of county differences in mortality, when

3 Eve Powell-Griner, "Differences in Infant Mortality among Texas Anglos, Hispanics, and Blacks." *Social Science Quarterly*, LXIX (1988), 452–467; Richard G. Rogers, "Ethnic Differences in Infant Mortality: Fact or Artifact?", *Social Science Quarterly*, LXIX (1989), 722–736; Powell-Griner, "Differences."

4 Texas' immigrant communities of European and Mexican origin had a strong tradition of infant baptism with registration, and a weak tradition of church burial registration (especially for children). White immigrants and their children from other states were not likely to be active church participants, and the churches were not likely to register vital events. The immigrant communities accepted public vital registration quickly, but the communities of native whites of native parentage had inadequate registration for some time after it was mandated in 1903. Gutmann and Fliess, *How to Study Southern Demography in the Nineteenth Century: The Early Lessons of the Texas Demography Project* (Austin, 1989)

ethnicity, social status, and other variables are held constant. Further pursuit of the matter suggests that contact with disease, through general conditions of poverty and density, was a significant factor. These findings help to shape a fuller description of the social conditions in rural Texas at the turn of the century.

SIX COUNTIES IN RURAL TEXAS   The six counties of rural Texas under investigation, in 1900 and 1910, are Red River, Angelina, and DeWitt Counties, in the eastern portion of the state, and Jack, Gillespie, and Webb Counties, in the central and western portion of the state (see Figure 1). These counties were chosen for their spatial and environmental arrangement, the presence of ethnic populations of interest, and the available manuscript sources. This study does not include any large urban locations, although Webb County has much of its population in Laredo, a city of 15,000 in 1910.[5]

The basic source is a sample drawn from the United States Census manuscript population schedules, supplemented by wealth information from each county's *ad valorem* tax assessments. Not every household paid taxes, but we have linked as many tax assessment records as possible to census records. In the absence of tax assessment data for a household, we assigned a wealth value to that household that was consistent with other households having similar characteristics for the age, sex, occupation, and ethnic group of the household head. We oversampled for Germans and Mexicans, and we compensated for this oversampling by weighting the data so that our total population reflects the ethnic distribution of the state in each census year as well as possible. All the categorical analyses herein make use of weighted data. The regression analyses, which take ethnicity into account, do not use the weighted data. The discussion employs a subset of married women as the basic unit of analysis, as reported in Tables 1 and 2. It is important to realize that the weight applied to each

5 We describe these counties in Gutmann and Fliess, *How to Study Southern Demography;* Gutmann, "Older Lives on the Frontier: The Residential Patterns of the Older Population of Texas, 1850–1910," in David I. Kertzer and Peter Laslett (eds.) *Aging in the Past: Demography, Society, and Old Age* (Berkeley, 1995), 175–202. We include no counties in the far western part of Texas because this phase of the research involved longitudinal coverage from 1860 to 1910, and rural west Texas had little population before 1880. Even Jack County had a tiny, largely transient population in 1870.

Fig. 1 Six Counties in Rural Texas

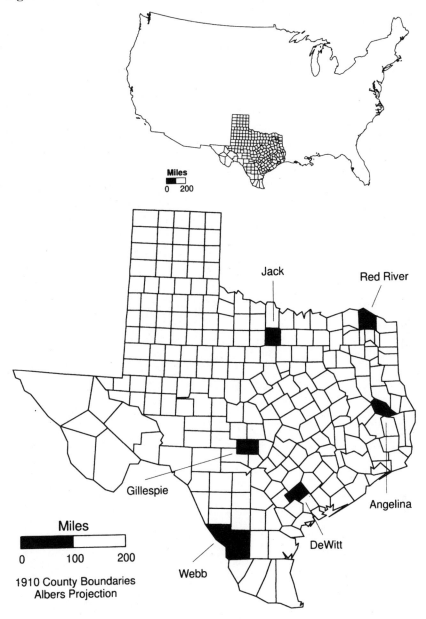

Table 1 Characteristics of Women in the Texas Project Sample Counties, 1900

		ANGELINA	DEWITT	GILLESPIE	JACK	RED RIVER	WEBB	TOTAL
TOTAL NUMBER OF WOMEN		468	371	584	394	1,395	239	3,451
			ETHNIC ORIGIN GROUPS					
African	N	66	113	18	5	454		656
	%	14.0	30.5	3.1	1.2	32.6	0.0	19.0
German (all generations)	N	10	72	369	19	21	7	498
	%	2.2	19.4	63.2	4.9	1.5	2.8	14.4
1st generation	N	1	29	38			1	70
	%	0.1	7.9	6.6	0.0	0.0	0.5	2.0
2d generation	N	0	28	230	3	1	2	264
	%	0.1	7.5	39.3	0.8	0.1	0.8	7.6
3rd generation	N	9	15	101	16	20	3	164
	%	2.0	4.0	17.3	4.1	1.4	1.4	4.8
Mexican (all generations)	N	0	31	12	0	2	202	247
	%	0.0	8.3	2.0	0.1	0.1	84.8	7.2
1st generation	N	0	8	5	0		108	121
	%	0.0	2.0	0.8	0.1	0.0	45.3	3.5
2d generation	N	0	12	3		0	38	53
	%	0.0	3.2	0.5	0.0	0.0	15.9	1.5
3d generation	N	0	11	5		1	56	74
	%	0.0	3.1	0.8	0.0	0.1	23.6	2.1
Other whites	N	393	155	185	370	919	30	2,050
	%	83.8	41.7	31.7	93.8	65.8	12.4	59.4
			OCCUPATIONAL STATUS OF HUSBAND					
Farm owner	N	133	67	353	147	364	11	1,075
	%	28.4	18.2	60.4	37.3	26.1	4.7	31.2
Farm tenant	N	101	124	98	127	721	9	1,179
	%	21.5	33.4	16.8	32.2	51.7	3.9	34.2
Farm laborer	N	73	83	36	36	95	84	406
	%	15.5	22.3	6.2	9.1	6.8	35.0	11.8
High white collar	N	13	16	28	25	47	11	139
	%	2.7	4.2	4.8	6.3	3.4	4.6	4.0
Low white collar	N	31	20	25	33	49	17	174
	%	6.5	5.3	4.3	8.3	3.5	7.3	5.1
Skilled work	N	38	29	32	15	43	48	204
	%	8.1	7.8	5.5	3.9	3.0	20.0	5.9
Non-farm laborer	N	74	11	5	5	47	48	190
	%	15.8	2.9	0.9	1.2	3.4	20.2	5.5
No occupation	N	7	22	6	7	30	10	83
	%	1.5	6.0	1.1	1.8	2.2	4.2	2.4
			HOUSEHOLD WEALTH (DOLLARS)					
Mean		359	740	1,171	673	372	627	
Median		100	105	740	355	107	295	

Table 2 Characteristics of Women in the Texas Project Sample Counties, 1910

		ANGELINA	DEWITT	GILLESPIE	JACK	RED RIVER	WEBB	TOTAL
TOTAL NUMBER OF WOMEN		711	421	855	480	1,216	316	3,451
ETHNIC ORIGIN GROUPS								
African	N	69	107	8	3	366	2	555
	%	9.7	25.5	0.9	0.7	30.1	0.5	16.1
German (all gens)	N	15	67	565	16	23	6	692
	%	2.1	15.9	66.1	3.4	1.9	1.9	20.1
1st generation	N	2	29	27	2		0	59
	%	0.3	6.8	3.1	0.4	0.0	0.0	1.7
2d generation	N	2	5	223	2	2	2	236
	%	0.3	1.1	26.1	0.3	0.2	0.8	6.8
3d generation	N	10	34	315	13	21	3	397
	%	1.5	8.0	36.9	2.7	1.7	1.1	11.5
Mexican (all gens)	N	3	51	38	0	3	243	338
	%	0.4	12.1	4.4	0.1	0.3	76.8	9.8
1st generation	N	0	12	19	0	1	141	173
	%	0.0	2.9	2.2	0.1	0.1	44.6	5.0
2d generation	N	0	17	11		0	35	64
	%	0.1	4.0	1.3	0.0	0.0	11.2	1.9
3d generation	N	2	22	8		2	66	101
	%	0.3	5.2	0.9	0.0	0.2	20.9	2.9
Other white	N	624	152	244	460	824	66	2,371
	%	87.8	36.2	28.6	95.9	67.7	20.8	68.7
OCCUPATIONAL STATUS OF HUSBAND								
Farm owner	N	177	78	412	135	266	26	1,095
	%	24.9	18.7	48.2	28.2	21.9	8.3	31.7
Farm tenant	N	85	148	164	213	667	17	1,294
	%	11.9	35.3	19.2	44.4	54.8	5.4	37.5
Farm laborer	N	20	47	58	17	73	65	281
	%	2.8	11.1	6.8	3.6	6.0	20.7	8.1
High white collar	N	34	24	54	23	53	19	207
	%	4.8	5.7	6.3	4.8	4.4	6.1	6.0
Low white collar	N	72	27	46	22	58	40	264
	%	10.1	6.5	5.3	4.6	4.7	12.6	7.7
Skilled work	N	133	43	70	25	32	62	365
	%	18.7	10.2	8.2	5.2	2.6	19.5	10.6
Non-farm laborer	N	181	44	44	41	56	86	451
	%	25.4	10.4	5.1	8.5	4.6	27.1	13.1
No occupation	N	10	9	4	3	11	1	39
	%	1.4	2.2	0.5	0.7	0.9	0.3	1.1
HOUSEHOLD WEALTH (DOLLARS)								
Mean		761	1,720	1,931	1,199	830	1,099	
Median		265	260	1,320	300	250	300	.

woman is drawn from the overall characteristics of the population, and not from the female population. Hence, the distribution of women's characteristics shown in the tables may not be the same as that in the overall census population, and especially not the same as that in the published census volumes.

The racial and ethnic makeup of the population is crucial to the analysis. A large majority of the Texas population was white, and most of them were either English-speaking immigrants from other states, or the children and grandchildren of those immigrants. The rest of the Texas population was comprised of three other relatively sizable groups, plus a small group of immigrants from Western Europe, Canada, Asia, and the Americas that we have merged with the white immigrants from other states, to form the large and heterogeneous group "other whites." This large group is called "Anglos" in other studies, but we give it a more general name in light of the diverse origin of the English-speaking white population of Texas that was not of Mexican or German origin.[6]

The second largest group in Texas was of African origin—slightly more than one-sixth of the population in 1910. At the turn of the century, it consisted mainly of former slaves and their children, and an ever-increasing number of their grandchildren and other descendants. Texas did not have a large slave population distributed throughout the state at the time of the Civil War (c. 30 percent of the state's population was black in 1860), but some of the plantation areas in the eastern section had a large amount. Over time, the arrival of other immigrants gradually diminished the proportion of African-Americans in Texas. The African-Americans in our sample lived in Red River, Angelina, and DeWitt counties, where they were farm tenants and farm laborers in various kinds of agriculture.

The third important group in Texas in the early twentieth century were the immigrants from central Europe, and their descendants. These immigrants came to Texas in two important shifts, one that began in the 1840s and ended before the Civil

6 For the size of ethnic groups in Texas, see Jane Zachritz and Gutmann, "Residence and Family Support Systems for Widows in Nineteenth and Early Twentieth Century Texas," in Tamara Hareven (ed.), *Aging and Generational Relations in Historical and Cross-Cultural Perspective,* (Berlin, forthcoming), Table 1.

War began in 1861, and another that took place in the 1880s and 1890s. In 1910, more than 6 percent of the population of Texas comprised individuals born in central and eastern Europe, or who had at least one parent born in those regions. An equally large group were the third-generation descendants of immigrants. We call this population "German" in the rest of this chapter, both for convenience and in recognition of the strong role of the German speakers in the evolution of the state's culture.

Many Germans landed at Texas ports and settled large communities in Galveston and San Antonio, as well as in a broad stretch of land from the Gulf Coast to the Texas hill country west of Austin and northwest of San Antonio. These settlements quickly established a reputation as prosperous, conservative, and stable—a reputation justified by our research into the German and mixed European communities in Gillespie and DeWitt counties. The first-generation Germans are easy to identify because they were born in Germany or some other German- or Slavic-speaking place. The members of the second generation are also readily identifiable because they have at least one parent born in a German- or Slavic-speaking territory. The third generation is more difficult to identify. Consequently, we have constructed a dictionary of "German" surnames based on our first- and second-generation populations, and we treat the wives of third-generation men as third-generation, based on their names, unless their places of birth or parentage suggests another categorization.[7]

The fourth group in the Texas population—immigrants from Mexico and their descendants—was almost as large as the Germans in 1910, and has grown rapidly since 1880, when rail transportation between Mexico and the United States became available. Mexicans brought a strong culture, and like the other minority groups in the state, a tradition of hard work that has contributed to the region's development and prosperity. Mexicans first settled in the counties that bordered Mexico, and in San Antonio. Later, they moved throughout the state, taking up agricultural work in areas deserted by the laboring population of English-speaking whites and African-Americans who were attracted to the cities.

---

7 Gutmann, John E. Vetter, Gregory Joslyn, and Fliess, *Staying Put or Moving On? Ethnicity, Migration and Persistence in Nineteenth-Century Texas* (Austin, 1990). We have not categorized ambiguous names, such as Miller, as "German."

We use the same general scheme for identifying Mexican-Americans as German-Americans. The first and second generation categories are defined by place of birth and parents' place of birth. The third generation is defined by a dictionary of surnames. We began with the Hispanic surname dictionary from the 1980 United States census, which we supplemented with information from the Mexican-born and Mexican-parentage populations in our sample.[8]

MORTALITY IN TEXAS AT THE TURN OF THE CENTURY   The census asked women who had been married various lengths of time how many children they had borne, and how many of them still survived. An empirical investigation showed that it is possible to estimate the average ages of the children, according to the number of years their mothers were married. For all women who had been married fewer than twenty-five years (the group we used), the mortality estimates refer to a sixteen-year period centered eight years prior to the census. Thus, the 1900 census yields information centered by a period around 1892, and the 1910 census yields information centered by a period around 1902. We refer to these two infant mortality periods as "1900 Census mortality" (roughly 1884–1900), and "1910 Census mortality" (roughly 1894–1910), in order to keep our description as simple as possible.[9]

The procedures that we have followed are based on those described by Preston and Haines in their influential study of late nineteenth-century child mortality in the United States, *Fatal Years;* our use of these measures is described in the Appendix. The point of the analysis is to use values of the $q(x)$ parameter of a model life table to compute an expected number of dead children for every mother, based on the number of years she had been married. The expected number of dead children is the product of the total number of children that she bore, and the proportion that the model life table indicates were likely to have died by certain ages. For women married zero to four years, the analysis uses the q_2 parameter (the proportion expected to have died in

8 David Montejano. *Anglos and Mexicans in the Making of Texas, 1836–1986,* (Austin, 1987). Having one Mexican parent indicates Mexican parentage in this study. A person with one German and one Mexican parent is categorized as second-generation German. United States Census of Population and Housing, *Spanish Surname List Prepared by the Bureau of the Census* (Washington, 1980.)

9 United Nations, *Manual X. Indirect Techniques for Demographic Estimation* (New York, 1983). Preston and Haines, *Fatal Years.*

Table 3 Child Mortality Characteristics of the Population for Six Texas Counties, by Ethnic Origin

ETHNIC ORIGIN OF MOTHER	CHILDREN DEAD				MORTALITY ESTIMATES		
	WOMEN	ACTUAL	EXPECTED	RATIO	q_5	l_5	e_0
				1900			
African	656	605	525	1.152	0.226	77,418	44.9
German	498	216	387	0.558	0.109	89,057	58.4
Mexican	247	255	166	1.534	0.301	69,943	37.5
Other white	2,050	1,324	1,458	0.908	0.178	82,203	50.0
Total	3,452	2,400	2,536	0.946	0.185	81,452	49.2

ETHNIC ORIGIN OF MOTHER	CHILDREN DEAD				MORTALITY ESTIMATES		
	WOMEN	ACTUAL	EXPECTED	RATIO	q_5	l_5	e_0
				1910			
African	555	413	323	1.278	0.208	79,156	46.7
German	735	241	370	0.652	0.106	89,368	58.8
Mexican	337	292	195	1.498	0.244	75,574	42.9
Other white	2,371	1,326	1,328	0.998	0.163	83,720	51.7
Total	3,999	2,272	2,216	1.025	0.167	83,281	51.2

NOTE   Based on once-married women married fewer than twenty-five years, with spouse present and no child from a previous marriage belonging to either woman or spouse.

the first two years of life), for marriages of five to nine years, the q_3, and so on. Once we have calculated an expected number of children born, we can compare that number with the actual number who have died. The analysis of differences in mortality is based on an index that is the ratio of the actual to the expected number of births, either for each woman, or for groups of women (see Table 3). This index is the important part of the analysis, and any related life table measures—such as e_0—are less important and less precise. With that caveat, we report a few life-table estimates, in order to put rural Texas childhood mortality in context, before turning to differentials in the Texas childhood mortality experience.[10]

The mortality experience of the children of mothers enumerated in the 1900 census shows that the expectation of life for rural Texas children at birth was similar to that in a Coale-Demeny west model life table with an expectation of life of nearly forty-nine years. Ten years later, the expectation of life at birth had grown by approximately two years. Overall, life expectancy in

10   See the works cited in note 9. See the Appendix for further discussion.

Texas, as we have estimated it, was slightly lower than Glover's overall estimates for the United States in 1900–1902 and in 1909–1911, and roughly equal to the estimates produced by Preston and Haines for the United States as a whole (despite the difficulty in comparing the child mortality indexes drawn from different base populations and different model life tables). Texas is part of Preston and Haines' South-Central region, for which they report a mortality index of 1.10, which places Texas' mortality lower than their regional estimate, primarily because of lower mortality among Texas blacks than among blacks throughout a region that encompassed Kentucky, Tennessee, Alabama, Mississippi, Arkansas, Louisiana, Oklahoma Territory, and Texas.[11]

Most of the comparative data for the United States in the late nineteenth and early twentieth century separates whites from African-Americans, as we have done. However, we have gone further by differentiating, in Table 3, between African-Americans and whites of Mexican, German, and all other ethnic origins ("other white"). In both time periods, rural Texans of African and Mexican descent experienced higher levels of child mortality, and those of German descent lower levels of child mortality, than the "other white" population that constituted more than half of all women. In general, African-American rural Texans had better life chances than did African-Americans in the national samples described by Preston and Haines, and by Glover, who report expectations of life at birth for African-American children at under thirty-five years. Moreover, the life chances of African-American children in rural Texas appear to have been improving slightly in the early twentieth century. No preceding study had sufficient cases to study the mortality of the Mexican children. Our results show that the life expectation of Mexican-American children was low, as shown in the 1900 and 1910 censuses, although not as low as national estimates for blacks. The life chances of Mexican-American children were improving at the turn of the century, probably more rapidly than for any other group. Note the relatively high expectation of life (more than fifty-eight years) for rural Texans of central European origin. In both time periods, these children were less than two-thirds as likely as the model

11 James W. Glover, *United States Life Tables, 1890, 1901, 1910, and 1901–1910* (New York, 1976; reprint of United States Department of Commerce Publication, 1921), 52–55; Preston and Haines, *Fatal Years*, Table 3.5, 112.

population to have died before their mothers were enumerated, and less than half as likely as black or Mexican origin children to have died.[12]

The sharp differences between racial and ethnic groups constitutes a starting point for our analysis of the social conditions affecting child mortality in Texas at the turn of the twentieth century. Why did these groups have such varied mortality experiences? Part of the mortality difference stems from disparate economic opportunities and standards of living. These economic and social conditions were themselves a consequence of a political and social system that channeled education, wealth, and opportunity in certain directions. Yet, there were probably other fundamental reasons. One of our striking findings is that, even with other characteristics held constant, the county in which a family lived determined the likelihood of a child dying. This important finding is in keeping with the regional determination in earlier analyses of child mortality, though it reduces the unit of territorial variation to a very small scale—the individual county. This variation by county in rural Texas child mortality emphasizes the importance of studying local conditions.

Table 4 shows fundamental differences in child mortality by cross-classifying the index, as well as estimated q_5s, by ethnic and occupational group. The indexes cannot be compared across time periods because we used different basic life tables for the 1900 and 1910 data. Hence, the indexes are multiples of different starting points. The q_5s, on the other hand, can be compared across years. The columns labeled "Total" show a simple pattern in the occupational distribution of child mortality in rural Texas: The families of farmers and white collar workers had the lowest child mortality; those of tenant farmers and skilled workers (at least in the 1900 census data) fell into a middle category; and those of farm and non-farm laborers, as well as of men who had no occupation, had the highest child mortality. The child mortality indexes cross-classified by occupation and ethnic origin reveal that the story is not so simple as it may seem, partly because of the relatively small numbers of cases in some cells. The low index for other white farm laborers (and therefore all farm laborers) in 1910, for example, is the result of this group's very low mortality in Red River

12 *Ibid.;* Glover, *United States Life Tables,* 76–77, 82–83.

Table 4 Child Mortality Index and Estimated q_5 for Six Texas Counties, by Ethnic Origin and Husband's Occupation

	1900									
	AFRICAN		GERMAN		MEXICAN		OTHER WHITE		TOTAL	
OCCUPATION GROUP	INDEX	q_5	INDEX	q_5	INDEX	q_5	INDEX	q_5	INDEX	q_5
Farmer	1.12	0.220	0.54	0.105	0.81	0.159	0.86	0.168	0.79	0.156
Tenant	1.12	0.219	0.55	0.107			0.91	0.178	0.96	0.187
Farm laborer	1.13	0.221			1.48	0.290	1.20	0.235	1.24	0.243
High white collar							0.86	0.169	0.84	0.164
Low white collar	1.27	0.250			1.77	0.348	0.73	0.143	0.86	0.168
Skilled craft	1.32	0.258	0.68	0.133	1.85	0.363	0.96	0.188	1.13	0.221
Non-farm laborer	1.41	0.277			1.96	0.385	1.31	0.256	1.45	0.284
No occupation	1.44	0.283	1.09	0.213	1.58	0.310	1.01	0.199	1.21	0.236

	1910									
	AFRICAN		GERMAN		MEXICAN		OTHER WHITE		TOTAL	
OCCUPATION GROUP	INDEX	q_5	INDEX	q_5	INDEX	q_5	INDEX	q_5	INDEX	q_5
Farmer	1.22	0.199	0.65	0.106	0.96	0.157	0.92	0.150	0.86	0.140
Tenant	1.17	0.190	0.61	0.099	1.30	0.212	1.04	0.170	1.05	0.171
Farm laborer	1.59	0.260			1.11	0.180	0.69	0.112	1.09	0.177
High white collar			0.48	0.078			1.03	0.168	0.93	0.152
Low white collar					1.49	0.243	0.84	0.137	0.85	0.139
Skilled craft	1.64	0.267	0.88	0.143	2.18	0.356	0.92	0.151	1.12	0.183
Non-farm laborer	1.52	0.247			1.91	0.312	1.32	0.215	1.45	0.236
No occupation							1.48	0.241	1.53	0.250

NOTE   The 1900 and 1910 index values cannot be compared; estimated q_5s can be compared. Empty cells have fewer than ten actual child deaths. For other limitations on data inclusion, see Table 3 and text.

County. Despite the complexity, it is worthwhile to emphasize that there was little difference between farmers and tenant farmers among black families, and that the highest child mortality of all groups with significant numbers of cases afflicted the skilled workers and non-farm laborers, especially Mexicans and blacks.[13]

Table 5 reports the index of child mortality and estimated q_5s cross-classified by county and ethnic origin, in order to view those differences from another angle. The table shows a clear ranking of county mortality levels, even when ethnicity is taken into account. Gillespie County had the lowest mortality by far for every ethnic group. Jack and DeWitt counties were at an inter-

13   It is important to understand that none of these indexes can be compared with those published by Preston and Haines because they use a different baseline life table.

Table 5 Child Mortality Index and Estimated q_5 for Six Texas Counties, by Ethnic Origin and County of Residence

	AFRICAN		GERMAN		MEXICAN		OTHER WHITE		TOTAL	
					1900					
COUNTY	INDEX	q_5	INDEX	q_5	INDEX	q_5	INDEX	q_5	INDEX	q_5
Angelina	1.01	0.198					0.98	0.193	0.97	0.191
DeWitt	1.13	0.222	0.65	0.127	1.11	0.217	0.61	0.120	0.85	0.166
Gillespie	0.53	0.103	0.53	0.103			0.59	0.116	0.55	0.108
Jack			0.90	0.177			0.90	0.177	0.90	0.177
Red River	1.21	0.238					1.00	0.196	1.07	0.210
Webb					1.65	0.323	0.72	0.141	1.53	0.300

	AFRICAN		GERMAN		MEXICAN		OTHER WHITE		TOTAL	
					1910					
COUNTY	INDEX	q_5	INDEX	q_5	INDEX	q_5	INDEX	q_5	INDEX	q_5
Angelina	1.84	0.300		0.000		0.000	1.07	0.175	1.14	0.185
DeWitt	0.75	0.122	0.68	0.111	1.51	0.247	0.79	0.129	0.86	0.139
Gillespie		0.000	0.60	0.098	1.25	0.205	0.52	0.085	0.61	0.099
Jack		0.000	1.06	0.173	2.81	0.459	0.81	0.132	0.82	0.134
Red River	1.37	0.223	1.03	0.168		0.000	1.21	0.198	1.26	0.206
Webb		0.000		0.000	1.50	0.245	0.93	0.152	1.39	0.227

NOTE   The 1900 and 1910 index values cannot be compared; estimated q_5s can be compared. Empty cells have fewer than ten actual child deaths. For other limitations on data inclusion, see Table 3 and text.

mediate level, with Angelina somewhat higher. Red River and Webb counties had the highest mortality levels. County and ethnicity are not independent in this analysis, given the structure of our sample. The large concentrations of Germans in Gillespie County (and to a lesser extent DeWitt County), of African-Americans in Red River County, and of Mexicans in Webb County shape the overall level of mortality in the respective counties. But it is significant that the "other white" category shows unmistakable county differences that demand further explanation. In the 1900 census data, the other whites in DeWitt, Gillespie, and Webb counties had much lower index values than did those in Angelina, Jack, and Red River counties. In the 1910 data, those in Gillespie, DeWitt, and Jack counties had the lower child mortality, and Angelina, Red River, and Webb counties the higher.

Tables 4 and 5 demonstrate that child mortality in Texas is complicated by the interrelationships between ethnicity, occupation, and location. The families of farm owners generally had lower mortality than did those of farm tenants, except in the African-American population. Moreover, some counties had better child mortality experiences than others. These interactions demand a more complex analytic scheme that will reveal genuine patterns—namely, a multiple regression analysis in which each woman's child mortality index is the dependent variable. We must also understand the forces that shaped infant and child mortality in rural Texas.

THE DETERMINANTS OF DIFFERENTIAL CHILD MORTALITY   Reformers at the beginning of the twentieth century concentrated on three issues to lengthen the lives of children. Their first concern was medical care for mothers, before and during the process of giving birth. A mother who received competent prenatal care, and who was attended at birth by a well-trained physician or midwife, was more likely to produce a healthy child and be healthy herself, than one who was not. The second concern of children's health reformers was good infant and child nutrition. Mothers were urged to breast-feed their children and to provide a balanced diet to those who had been weaned. The third concern involved sanitation. In the rural context, representatives of reform groups and the Children's Bureau of the Department of Labor taught the need for properly protected water supplies and proper disposal of human and animal waste. They argued for deep water wells with pumps, protected from the contaminants that could foul shallow, open-topped wells. They also advocated properly designed domestic sanitation systems, consisting of, at minimum, well-constructed privies that would not foul ground water and, at maximum, modern septic systems for containing human waste.[14]

Although it would be desirable to measure the extent to which any household had access to the improved maternal, infant, and child health provisions that the reformers proposed, the available sources make it difficult to track down individual health, nutrition, and sanitation conditions. Instead of measuring the causes of good childhood health directly, we measure them indirectly. Some of the differences between mortality experiences are explained by the individual characteristics of women and their

14 Bradley and Williamson, *Rural Children*; Moore, *Maternity and Infant Care*.

Table 6 Size and Density of Texas Project Sample Counties

	ANGELINA	DEWITT	GILLESPIE	JACK	RED RIVER	WEBB	TEXAS
				1900			
Land Area (Square Miles)	940	879	1,109	962	1,039	3,219	262,398
Population	13,481	21,311	8,229	10,224	29,893	21,857	3,048,710
Density	14.3	24.2	7.4	10.6	28.8	6.8	11.6
				1910			
Land Area (Square Miles)	940	879	1,109	962	1,039	3,219	262,398
Population	9,256	23,501	9,447	11,817	28,564	22,503	3,896,542
Density	9.8	26.7	8.5	12.3	27.5	7.0	14.8

husbands. Our simplest explanations of differential child mortality come from the age and ethnic origin of the mother and the husband's occupation, from one of the eight occupational categories of Table 4. To these we add household wealth, as manifested by tax assessments, and measured in thousands of dollars.

The conclusions drawn from Table 5 suggest that the county of residence is implicated in understanding levels of mortality. However, isolating county of residence is complicated by its relationship with ethnicity. In 1910, Jack and Angelina counties were almost exclusively made up of people in our "other white" category; Webb County was more than three-fourths Mexican; and a large proportion of the Germans in our sample lived in Gillespie County (76 percent). Because these uneven distributions of ethnic origin confuse the roles of the individual counties, what gave individual counties their importance for child health? The answer comes from those very issues that health reformers raised in the early twentieth century. Child health was influenced by local sanitation conditions and by the ability of families to provide good food and medical care, which were influenced by both families' economic conditions and levels of education, and by the general degree of prosperity and knowledge in the communities. The task of measuring these conditions is beyond the scope of the present study. Instead, our multivariate analysis uses each county as a composite independent variable representing local conditions. The complexity of doing any more is evident in the population densities reported in Table 6. Webb County has the lowest density reported in the table, despite the size and density of Laredo and despite very high mortality indexes, because of its large size (see Figure 1), its aridity and ranching economy, and the relative concentration of its population in Laredo. No aggregate measure as simple as population density can reveal the characteristics of the counties' residents. County must stand as a proxy for density, poverty, standards of public health, and education and knowledge.

Our multivariate results are presented in tables 7 (for 1900 data) and 8 (for 1910 data). Each table contains four regression models, in which the dependent variable—an individual woman's child mortality index—relates to a series of independent variables. Although other variables are possible, the results with these are stable and consistent. We used Stata software, with a standard regression model, weighted by the number of children born to minimize heteroscedasticity. In their use of similar models, Preston and Haines submit that a Tobit regression might be superior, because the data are limited on one side (the index value cannot be lower than zero). We have followed their example, however, and not used the Tobit.[15]

The first two models presented in tables 7 and 8 limit information about ethnic origin to the four major categories—African, German, Mexican, and other white. They include all eight occupational groups, plus the woman's age and household wealth. One model includes a series of county dummies. All of the models are significant, although they explain relatively little of the overall variance in childhood mortality—slightly more than 10 percent in the 1900 data, and between 8 and 9 percent in the 1910 data. These results are consistent with those obtained by Preston and Haines.

The results in models 1 and 2 of tables 7 and 8 confirm much of the index-value data in tables 4 and 5. First, they demonstrate the importance of race and ethnicity. German-Americans had lower childhood mortality than other whites, followed by African-Americans and Mexican-Americans with the highest of all. Second, the demographic indicator—a woman's age—significantly raised her family's child mortality index as it increased. Third, the basic economic measure, wealth, was found to have

---

15 We have also experimented, using poisson regression, with the number of children dead as the dependent variable; the results did not suggest a different interpretation.

Table 7 Regression Models for 1900

	1	2	3	4
	COEFFICIENT	COEFFICIENT	COEFFICIENT	COEFFICIENT
R^2	0.106	0.117	0.109	0.120
Adjusted R^2	0.105	0.116	0.108	0.118
Constant	0.505****	0.208****	0.526****	0.221****
Age	0.011****	0.011****	0.010****	0.011****
Household wealth ($1,000s)	−0.041****	−0.035****	0.040****	−0.035****
Ethnic origin (without generations)				
African	0.210****	0.202****		
German	−0.324****	−0.071**		
Mexican	0.505****	0.402****		
Other white (reference group)				
Ethnic origin (with generations)				
African			0.211****	0.201****
German 1st generation			−0.326****	−0.074
German 2d generation			−0.332****	−0.057
German 3d generation			−0.281****	−0.111**
Mexican 1st generation			0.604****	0.522****
Mexican 2d generation			0.202****	0.174**
Mexican 3d generation			0.362****	0.278***
Other white (reference group)				
Husband's occupation				
Farm owner (reference group)				
Farm tenant	0.034	0.012	0.033	0.012
Farm laborers	0.213***	0.243****	0.204****	0.236****
High white collar	0.080	0.057	0.072	0.052
Low white collar	0.076	0.049	0.084*	0.058
Skilled work	0.233****	0.209****	0.233****	0.214****
Non-farm laborer	0.513****	0.457****	0.476****	0.429****
No occupation	0.359****	0.319****	0.361****	0.326****
County				
Angelina		0.292****		0.303****
DeWitt		0.073**		0.085**
Gillespie (reference group)				
Jack		0.284****		0.292****
Red River		0.393****		0.401****
Webb		0.460****		0.430****

* Significant at the .1 level.
** Significant at the .05 level.
*** Significant at the .01 level.
**** Significant at the .001 level.

an inverse relationship to the child mortality index. Finally, in comparison with the reference group, farm owners, farm tenants evinced little difference, but almost every other group had a higher mortality even if not every coefficient was significant. The biggest exception, noted earlier, were the farm laborers in 1910, who had lower child mortality because of an exceptional group of other

Table 8 Regression Models for 1910

	1	2	3	4
	COEFFICIENT	COEFFICIENT	COEFFICIENT	COEFFICIENT
R^2	0.080	0.100	0.085	0.104
Adjusted R^2	0.080	0.099	0.084	0.103
Constant	0.364****	−0.093	0.394****	−0.058
Age	0.017****	0.018****	0.016****	0.017****
Household wealth ($1,000s)	−0.019****	−0.016****	−0.018****	−0.015****
Ethnic origin (without generations)				
African	0.241****	0.156****		
German	−0.334****	0.049		
Mexican	0.517****	0.759****		
Other white (reference group)				
Ethnic origin (with generations)				
African			0.243****	0.157****
German 1st generation			−0.266****	0.077
German 2d generation			−0.364****	0.033
German 3d generation			−0.283****	0.065
Mexican 1st generation			0.662****	0.951****
Mexican 2d generation			0.214****	0.527****
Mexican 3d generation			0.252****	0.524****
Other white (reference group)				
Husband's Occupation				
Farm owner (reference group)				
Farm tenant	0.061**	0.009	0.062**	0.008
Farm laborers	−0.147***	−0.102**	−0.155***	−0.115**
High white collar	0.000	−0.019	−0.008	0.024
Low white collar	−0.055	−0.065	−0.052	−0.057
Skilled work	0.290****	0.315****	0.269****	0.301****
Non-farm laborer	0.400****	0.413****	0.371****	0.389****
No occupation	0.576****	0.581****	0.569****	0.574****
County				
Angelina		0.455****		0.457****
DeWitt		0.124***		0.134****
Gillespie (reference group)				
Jack		0.300****		0.295****
Red River		0.699****		0.695****
Webb		0.209****		0.134**

* Significant at the .1 level.
** Significant at the .05 level.
*** Significant at the .01 level.
**** Significant at the .001 level.

white farm laborers in Red River County. The greatest difference distinguished the two non-farm working-class groups—the skilled workers and the non-farm laborers—a large proportion of whom lived in Webb County. We discuss the importance of that connection below.

We expected the counties to display different child mortality experiences, and model 2 of tables 7 and 8 offer confirmation. Gillespie County, the reference, had the lowest mortality of all the counties, with age of woman, wealth, ethnicity, and husband's occupation taken into account. DeWitt's was slightly higher, Angelina and Jack Counties were intermediate, and Red River and Webb counties had the highest mortality. The models that include the counties are especially interesting because they reduce the importance of the German ethnic variable, suggesting that the advantage experienced by the Germans was a consequence of living in Gillespie and DeWitt counties, or that, because virtually all of the Germans lived in these counties, the consequences of German sanitation and cleanliness affected other groups. Put another way, there is good reason to believe that by the first decade of the twentieth century (the 1910 data reflects sixteen years centered on 1902), the child mortality experiences of German-Americans and other whites were similar in those counties where they lived in proximity. The other whites have higher mortality in the overall index values because of their residence in other counties and their different distributions of occupation and wealth. We speculate further about these relationships in the conclusion.[16]

In the third and fourth models presented in tables 7 and 8, we divide the Mexican- and German-origin populations according to generation—the foreign born (first generation) from the native born of foreign parents (second generation) and the native born with the Mexican and German surnames of native parents (third generation). Model 3 includes only ethnicity; model 4 also includes the county variables. The results for the occupation, age, wealth, and county variables, and for the models as a whole, are not too different from the simpler models in which generation was not taken into account. The results for generation raise the question of whether second- and third-generation Mexican-Americans and German-Americans were more like their immigrant parents or more like members of other ethnic groups. The answer is revealing. German-Americans were relatively consistent in all three generations. They were likely to have had lower

16 We verified the relationship between ethnicity and county of residence in another set of regression models, in which we interacted residence and ethnicity, finding that other whites had mortality that varied from county to county, but child mortality was similar to that of German Americans in DeWitt and Gillespie Counties.

childhood mortality than any of the other groups, and the differences between the generations was relatively small. The sole noticeable difference was that third-generation German-Americans were more similar to the other-white reference group than were members of the first and second generations, which might have been the result of a convergence between third-generation Germans and the other whites, or the result of a less telling choice of surnames than we had hoped. By 1910, as we saw earlier, there was no significant difference between any of the German-American groups and other whites.

Mexican-Americans were more sharply divided between generations than were German-Americans. First-generation Mexican immigrant women had the highest child mortality of any group that we examined. Their daughters and granddaughters had relatively high mortality, reflected in the 1900 and 1910 census data, but not nearly as high as for the children of immigrant women. The coefficients for second- and third-generation Mexican women were nearly the same as those for African-American women in 1900, and larger than those for African-American women in 1910, but the coefficients for first-generation Mexican women were much larger than those for African-American women in both periods.

TELLING THE STORY OF MORTALITY IN TURN OF THE CENTURY TEXAS   Based on the information thus far, childhood mortality in our sample of rural Texans was roughly comparable with that of the United States as a whole, although its components were substantially different from those of the United States, or even those of the South. The expectation of life at birth for the whole population in 1900 was approximately forty-nine years, as derived from the reports of women about the number of children to whom they had given birth, and the number that survived; the children's expectation of life at birth for the population of women reporting in 1910 had increased to c. fifty-one years. These figures are comparable with national and regional ones. The story was more complicated for the subgroups that comprised the population of Texas. Texan blacks had better life chances than blacks elsewhere in the United States, especially better than elsewhere in the South. Although their mortality levels were higher than those for whites, African-American Texans were relatively privileged c. 1900. Subdividing the white population into three groups produces two immigrant minority groups, one of central European (we call it German) origin, whose mortality experience was relatively favorable, and one of Mexican origin, whose mortality experience was not. The mix of generations in these two minority white populations meant, however, that the lot of the Mexicans was improving, whereas that of the Germans remained stable, having already improved in the late nineteenth century.[17]

The story is more about differentials than levels, because the methods available for analyzing census-based data about childhood mortality are better at revealing the differences between groups than they are at establishing an exact level of mortality or even an exactly matched model life table. The examination of differentials and multivariate combinations tells an even richer story about the social context of childhood mortality in Texas. Race and ethnicity are vital to this enhanced picture of childhood mortality differences, but there are social and economic, and even local, issues at work as well.

Wealth was crucial in determining levels of childhood mortality in rural Texas. A family's taxable wealth had a strong influence on the survival of its children. We suspect that this relationship is manifest in terms of the quality of housing and food, clean drinking water, and effective sanitary disposal. Once we factor in the role of family wealth, the means of livelihood had some impact on child mortality, but less than we might have expected. The children of farm owners had mortality experiences at least as good as any other group, probably because they were likely to live away from contaminated water on isolated farms, because they had access to good food, and because ownership gave their parents both the capital and the motivation to improve their residential situation. Every other occupational group had similar or higher mortality than farmers, although the differences were not always statistically significant in the regression analyses. The children of men employed in white-collar occupations lived as long as those of farmers, probably because of the advantages of parental education.[18]

17 Fliess, "The Historical and Genetic Demography of the Wends of Serbin, Texas, 1854 to 1920," unpub. Ph.D. diss. (University of Texas, Austin, 1986); *idem,* "Mortality Transition among the Wends of Serbin, Texas, 1854–1884: Investigation of Changes in the Pattern of Death Using Parochial Records," *Social Biology,* XXXVIII (1992), 266–276.
18 On this issue, see Preston, "Resources, Knowledge, and Child Mortality: A Comparison of the U.S. in the Late Nineteenth Century and Developing Countries Today," *Proceedings of the International Population Conference, Florence, Italy, 1985* (Florence, 1985), 373–388.

Surprisingly, the children of tenant farmers and farm laborers did not fare as poorly as we might have predicted. Tables 7 and 8 show that, for the most part, tenant farmers did not differ significantly from farmers. In the 1900 data, however, the children of farm laborers had higher mortality than farmers, although the discrepancy is not big. Remarkably, in the 1910 data, the children of farm laborers had lower mortality than the children of farmers, probably because of a dramatic improvement among white tenant farmer families in Red River County. The upshot is that, after accounting for the strong relationship between wealth and race/ethnicity as independent variables and the child mortality index as the dependent variable, the differences between farm owners, farm tenants, and farm laborers do not amount to much. Living conditions in the farm environment were determined by wealth and by the tangible attributes of race and ethnicity, more than by occupational group.

The children of skilled workers and non-farm laborers, plus the small number of children of men without occupations, were the only groups in our sample to suffer mortality notably higher than that of farmers. Leaving aside the families of men without occupations (a diverse group), these families were likely to have lived in the least satisfactory housing, and to have had access to the least adequate sanitary systems, of any in our population, as the poor mortality of their children show. That these workers were disproportionately Mexican-American and lived in Webb County may prevent our analysis from adequately disentangling the role of the more urban environment of Laredo in their high mortality count. In other words, their high mortality may have been caused by living in Laredo rather than by the material consequences of their occupational status, although the two factors are closely linked.

If occupation became less important after the inclusion of wealth, race, ethnic origin, and generation still mattered after the inclusion of wealth and occupational group. Ethnic origin had a great effect on childhood mortality, with African- and Mexican-Americans experiencing much higher mortality than German-American and other non-Mexican whites. The children of women born in Mexico had the highest mortality of all. What was it about the living conditions of Mexican-Americans and African-Americans that so diminished their life chances? Similarly, what benefited, in relative terms, the life chances of German-Americans, above and beyond their wealth and occupation? It is unlikely that genetic susceptibilities to disease were sufficient to explain the child mortality differences between these groups. Although there may have been cultural differences—that is, members of these groups may have been more likely to live in some situations than others—those cultural differences were shaped largely by social and economic opportunities.

In a recent article, Fliess shows that the Wendish population of Serbin, Texas (not included in our sample, but living in conditions similar to those in DeWitt County), reduced their levels of infant mortality between the 1850s and the 1880s, by limiting air- and waterborne contagious diseases. By the 1890s, the German-American population probably were able to do so because they lived in well-constructed farm houses and were relatively prosperous. Apparently, by 1910, other whites were making progress as well, at least where they had German-American models to follow. The higher-mortality, Mexican-American and African-American families, however, did not have the same opportunities. Studies of rural living conditions in the South suggest that the poorest whites and blacks may have been ignorant about how to improve their health and too poor to do much about it anyway. The complexity of this story is made greater by differences in mortality within each county, even for the group, "other whites."[19]

We began with the idea that differences in child mortality by county and ethnic background might have had something to do with location, in a purely geographical sense. Many of the German-Americans in our sample lived in Gillespie County. This area of the Texas "hills" has an arid climate, porous limestone soil, and relatively clean surface water. Many of the African-Americans lived in Red River County, which is at a lower elevation, has a heavy clay soil, and more surface water. DeWitt County, with its mixed population, had an intermediate geography. The greater possibility of drawing contaminated water in Red River County than in Gillespie County should have resulted in higher infant mortality. The rate in DeWitt County should have fallen between those of the other two. The presence of families in our other-

19   Fliess, "Mortality Transition."

white category in all three counties allows us to test this hypothesis. Table 5 shows that mortality for other whites was higher in DeWitt than in Gillespie County, and highest in Red River County. Terrain seems to play a role, but it is only part of the explanation.

What makes the story more complicated than just a combination of geography, wealth, and ethnic origin is that the diseases that killed the children of rural Texas were contagious. There may have been a relationship between proximity of disease and level of mortality, even for groups that were otherwise not likely to have undergone high levels of child mortality. We anticipated that in counties with dense populations of poor people living amid unsanitary conditions and using contaminated water, everyone would have had ample contact with disease, and that in counties with dense populations per se, the exposure would have been worse. These hypotheses were impossible to test with the data at hand. Nonetheless, it is noteworthy that non-Mexican and non-German whites lived in a poor, or a densely populated county, as did Germans. Living in DeWitt County, with its dense, poor population was more dangerous for children than living in Gillespie County, all other things being equal.

The reformers in the early years of this century who attempted to reduce infant mortality sought to work within the contemporary social system and to improve the health of women and children by teaching them about nutrition and sanitation. They knew that money made a difference; the children of well-to-do parents are always more able to survive childhood. However, they also argued that improvements in drinking water and sanitation would help the poorer population. The reformers of the Children's Bureau did not have our sophisticated statistical approaches, but they had a wealth of case studies that showed the importance of the measures that they advocated. Our analysis shows that they were correct. Wealth and ethnicity—along with occupational status, to some extent—were the driving forces behind differences in child mortality in rural Texas. It is just as important to note that some parts of rural Texas provided a better environment for the survival of children than others. But we wish to emphasize that the conclusions that we draw are similar to those that the reformers drew. The measurable differences in the social context of child mortality discussed in this article seem mostly to reflect the knowledge of and access to good food and the improved water and sanitation that were the goals of the reformers.

Appendix: A Rural Texas Life Table, and Constants for the Calculation of the Child Mortality Index

The methodological starting points for the foregoing estimates are United Nations *Manual X,* and Preston and Haines' *Fatal Years.* Although neither of these works is easy to follow, we have improvised an appropriate way of using them to make mortality estimates and compute the Child Mortality Index.

We begin with the average number of children ever born and the average number of children who died, per woman, categorized in five-year groups of marital durations. These averages are computable for the 1900 and 1910 censuses, because each census asked married women how long they had been married, how many children they had borne, and how many of those children still survived. We have learned from extensive analysis that these values were certain to be enumerated accurately only for once-married women of once-married husbands. In order to ensure inclusion of these women alone in our analysis, we excluded women who were said to have been married more than once (a question asked in 1910, but not always enumerated well), women who had children from a previous marriage, and women whose husbands had co-residing children from a previous marriage (often indicated by the presence of children more than one year older than the enumerated duration of marriage). We also excluded, for the same reason, all women whose number of children exceeded the number of years of the current marriage by more than one. Finally, our procedure excludes from analysis all women with an enumerated marriage duration of twenty-five years or more.

Formulas c.3 and c.4 and Table 56 of *Manual X* (p. 82) provide the means to calculate the probabilities of dying before exact age x (denoted in the life table as q_x. Each group of marital durations is associated with one point in the life table; the parity and child deaths of women married zero to four years are associated with q_2, those married five to nine years with q_3, those ten to fourteen years with q_5, those fifteen to nineteen years with q_{10}, and those twenty to twenty-four years with q_{15}. Table A 1 reflects the results of this procedure, in which the column labeled "Parameter Estimate" is the value of q_x at the appropriate ages.

Once we had estimated the values of q_x at each age, we selected an appropriate male and female Coale-Demeny West Model Life Table for each q_x, using the United Nations Mortpak Lite Match Program. We identify the life tables chosen in Table A1 by showing their expectation of life at birth. The life tables chosen are presented in the columns, "Male e_0" and "Female e_0," in Table A1. The levels of mortality implied

Table A1 Computation of Basic Life Table Values for Six Texas Counties

YEARS MARRIED	WOMEN	AVERAGE PARITY	MULTIPLIER[a]	CHILDREN DEAD		PARAMETER ESTIMATE[b]	ESTIMATED e_0^c		
				AVERAGE	PROPORTION		COMBINED	MALE	FEMALE
1900									
0–4	997	0.93	1.15886	0.15	0.15663	0.18151 q_2	45.5	45.6	45.5
5–9	830	2.59	1.01927	0.42	0.16188	0.16500 q_3	49.7	49.4	50.0
10–14	626	4.07	1.02295	0.77	0.18971	0.19406 q_5	48.3	47.8	48.7
15–19	524	5.38	1.04291	1.08	0.20121	0.20985 q_{10}	48.4	47.9	49.0
20–24	475	6.50	1.03214	1.40	0.21595	0.22289 q_{15}	48.4	47.7	49.0
Average e_0							48.1	47.7	48.5
1910									
0–4	1,211	0.91	1.16727	0.08	0.09153	0.10685 q_2	56.1	55.7	56.4
5–9	970	2.57	1.01708	0.39	0.15137	0.15396 q_3	51.0	50.7	51.4
10–14	752	3.76	1.00586	0.61	0.16361	0.16456 q_5	51.5	51.0	52.0
15–19	601	5.26	1.01703	0.98	0.18598	0.18915 q_{10}	50.5	49.9	51.1
20–24	465	5.91	1.00611	1.25	0.21205	0.21334 q_{15}	49.3	48.6	50.0
Average e_0							51.7	51.2	52.2

[a] Calculated using the formula in United Nations *Manual X*, 82.

[b] Product of the number in the "Multiplier" column and the proportion dead.

[c] Found by using the "Match" routine in the United Nations MORTPAK LITE software package, with the value in the "Parameter estimate" column as input.

Table A2 Constants Used in Calculation of Expected Child Mortality

	1900	
AGE	CONSTANT q_x	YEARS MARRIED
2	0.16344	0–4
3	0.17940	5–9
5	0.19597	10–14
10	0.21321	15–19
15	0.22618	20–24
	1910	
AGE	CONSTANT q_x	YEARS MARRIED
2	0.13669	0–4
3	0.14947	5–9
5	0.16309	10–14
10	0.17777	15–19
15	0.18892	20–24

by these life tables are fairly consistent, except for the level implied by the experience of women married zero to four years in 1900. We use the average life table from the five life tables implied by the q_xs to provide an overall estimate of mortality in rural Texas for the years preceding the 1910 census; for 1900, we use the average of the four life tables estimated for women married five to twenty-four years. Combining male and female life tables, the expectation of life at birth improved only slightly in the first decade of the twentieth century—from less than forty-nine years in 1900 to just above fifty years in 1910.[20]

The Child Mortality Index devised by Preston and Haines requires a model life table, from which the q_2, q_3, q_5, q_{10}, and q_{15} parameters are drawn. We used the average male and female life tables shown in Table A1 to choose these parameters, and then took the average of the male and female q_x parameters (weighted to represent a ratio of 1.05 male per female). The q_xs for 1900 and 1910 are reported in Table A2.

To determine the child mortality index for an individual woman, first compute her expected number of dead children—the product of her total children borne, and the appropriate q_x for her number of married years. A woman married between five and nine years, for example, would have the number of children that she bore multiplied by the q_3 of the model life table. The Child Mortality Index is computed by dividing the actual number of her children who died by the number

20   Ansley J. Coale and Paul Demeny, *Regional Model Life Tables and Stable Populations* (New York, 1983; 2d ed.). United Nations, *The United Nations Software Package for Mortality Measurement: MORTPAK LITE* (United Nations, 1988).

expected to have died. If more of her children died than expected, the index is large; if fewer died than expected, the index is small. The numbers of actual and expected children can be summed for a group of women, and an overall index computed. In the main body of this article, we used indexes computed for groups of women according to specific categories (by ethnic group, or by ethnic group and occupation or county), and we used the indexes computed for individual women in the multivariate regression analyses.

It is sometimes necessary to convert child mortality indexes back to model life tables. Preston and Haines show that it is sufficient to multiply the index by the q_5 of the reference model life tables (those we use are shown in Table A2) to determine the q_5 of the model life table that is represented by the child mortality index. The q_5 can be converted to any other parameter of the life table with the Coale-Demeny model life tables (and either the published volume or the Match program). For convenience, we usually present these life tables by showing an expectation of life at birth, sexes combined.

Irene W. D. Hecht

Kinship and Migration: The Making of an
Oregon Isolate Community

The term "isolate" is one that is familiar to the human geneticist, but not necessarily to the historian. When used in genetics the term refers to a small, closed population in which the gene frequencies are different from those found in the general population. Human geneticists have so far developed three general categories of isolates: (1) physical—in the sense of geographical—isolates, (2) ideological isolates, and (3) linguistic isolates.[1]

Geographical location has, for example, created an isolate population on the island of Tristan de Cunha. A remote continental location can cause similar isolation, as in the case of Lac St. Jean-Chicoutimi in Quebec Province. Ideological convictions have produced isolates even in circumstances where people exist in easy physical proximity to other social groups. The Old Order Amish are a good example of this phenomenon. Linguistic characteristics have contributed to the isolation of some of the Indian and Eskimo populations in Alaska, who, although they live in similar locations and circumstances, tend not to inter-marry.[2]

What is particularly significant about the isolate described here is, first, that it exists without primarily conforming to any of

Irene W. D. Hecht is Associate Professor of History and Associate Dean of the Faculty at Lewis and Clark College.

The material here was presented in part at the annual meeting of the American Society of Human Genetics, 1975. An earlier draft was read by Luca Cavalli-Sforza, Mark Skolnick, Everett Lovrien, and Frederick Hecht, each of whom provided helpful suggestions. Much of the credit for assembling the data goes to the undergraduate participants of Pacific Northwest History, a research seminar taught by the author at Lewis and Clark College.

1 A clear definition of the term "isolate" is given in L. L. Cavalli-Sforza and W. F. Bodmer, *The Genetics of Human Populations* (San Francisco, 1971), 352: "relatively small populations that have little or no exchange with other populations." Translated into vocabulary more familiar to historians an isolate is a small community whose members have little to do with those outside their group, and who above all do not marry persons outside their group. See also *ibid.*, 353, Table 7.4.
2 H. L. Bailit, St. Danon, and A. Amon, "Consanguinity on Tristan de Cunha in 1938," *Eugenics Quarterly*, XIII (1966), 30–33; James S. and Margaret W. Thompson, *Genetics in Medicine* (Philadelphia, 1973), 61; V. A. McKusick, J. A. Hostetler, J. A. Egeland, and R. Eldridge, "The Distribution of Certain Genes in the Old Order Amish," *Symposia on Quantitative Biology*, XXIX (1964), 99–114; Everett Lovrien, M.D., personal communication about research on Eskimos.

the patterns cited above, and, second, that its identification was made possible through the application of the techniques of historical demography. The linkage of sociohistorical findings with biomedical data has made it possible both to perceive the existence of the isolate and to investigate its dynamics.

Attention was first drawn to the community when a young man of Dutch extraction was referred by his physician to the University of Oregon Medical School for consultation concerning blistering of the skin upon exposure to sunshine.[3] The condition had afflicted the patient since childhood. His skin would redden easily when exposed to the sun. Small blisters would appear, become confluent, and burst, releasing clear fluid. The affected areas of skin would then heal, but as the process was repeated through further exposure to sun, areas of fissured, thickened skin marred by deposits of deeper colored pigment were left. The involved areas of skin were over the face, neck, forearms, and hands. The process could be prevented by the patient's staying in the shade or indoors or by his wearing a broad-brimmed hat and gloves. However, prevention became difficult when he began working as a heavy-equipment operator on road construction. He was seen at the Medical School and the diagnosis of sun-sensitive porphyria was made. He was given a variety of sun-screen ointments, which were partially successful in decreasing, but not eliminating his tendency to redden and blister. Because sun-sensitive porphyria is genetical, the patient was referred to the Genetics Clinic for family studies. These disclosed only two other definite cases of sun-sensitive porphyria in his family. Those involved a brother and a male cousin. Parents and other close relatives proved normal on their medical history, clinical examination, and laboratory study. Relief of symptoms was achieved by periodic removal of blood in order to decrease the red cell mass from which the skin-damaging porphyrin compounds emanate.[4]

The porphyrias are a group of hereditary biochemical disorders involving aberrations in the metabolism of porphyrin compounds which occur with the breakdown of the heme component

---

3 The case report is furnished by Drs. Lovrien and Frederick Hecht.
4 The medical practice of blood-letting is a venerable technique which is now regarded as not only outmoded, but harmful. This is one instance where purposeful bleeding of a patient—physiologically—is therapeutic.

of hemoglobin. Despite certain similarities, the various types of porphyria can be distinguished from one another by clinical, biochemical, and/or genetical criteria. Two types of porphyria have been of particular sociohistorical interest: one form, acute intermittent porphyria, involves excruciating attacks of abdominal pain and episodes of aberrant behavior. George III's madness is now thought to have been caused by acute intermittent porphyria since this disease has been diagnosed in some of his living descendants. A second form of the disease, known as porphyria variegata, is also of historic interest. An extensive genealogical study of Dutch settlers in South Africa has been done by Deane, a physician. Finding that a number of his patients had porphyria, Deane proceeded to trace the disease. He identified 1,021 affected persons, all of whom were descended from a pair of seventeenth-century migrants. Which of the two, the husband or wife, had brought the disorder to South Africa is not known, but that the gene had been carried down from one of the two original progenitors is clear. Deane's is a classic study of founder effect.[5]

The genetic mode of transmission for both of these types of porphyria is known to be autosomal dominant. "Autosomal" means that the responsible genes are carried on one of the twenty-two non-sex chromosomes (autosomes). Dominant (and fully penetrant) means that symptoms will be manifest if one porphyria gene is received by a particular offspring. (In the case of autosomal recessive disorders, both parents must carry a gene and it must be present in a double dose in the child for symptoms to be apparent.)

The type of cutaneous porphyria identified in Oregon is clinically reminiscent of the South African variety of porphyria variegata. Insofar as the Oregon patient is of Dutch descent, it seemed initially that the direction of the Oregon study would parallel that of Deane in South Africa. However, careful investigation un-

5 John B. Stanbury, James B. Wyngaarden, and Donald S. Frederickson, *The Metabolic Basis of Inherited Disease* (New York, 1960), ch. 36, classifies four types of porphyria: congenital erythropoietic, erythopoietic, intermittent acute, and variegate porphyria. *Porphyria—A Royal Malady* (London, 1968). This pamphlet includes Ida Macalpine and Richard Hunter, "The 'Insanity' of King George III: A Classic Case of Porphyria," *British Medical Journal* (8 Jan., 1966); Ida Macalpine, Richard Hunter, and C. Rimington, "Porphyria in the Royal Houses of Stuart, Hanover, and Prussia: A Follow-up Study of George III's Illness," *Ibid.* (6 Jan., 1968); John Brooke, "Historical Implications," *Ibid.* (13 Jan., 1968); Abe Goldberg, "The Porphyrias", *Ibid.* (13 Jan., 1968); Geoffrey Dean, *The Porphyrias: A Story of Inheritance and Environment* (London, 1963), ch. 12, esp. 107, 111.

earthed only two other cases of porphyria among the Oregon patient's numerous relatives. This finding was incompatible with the
dominant (fully penetrant) pattern of inheritance described in
South Africa. In turn this led the study in a new direction.

The Oregon porphyria might have a recessive pattern. Insofar
as the affected persons were biological relatives, the next logical
step was to search for possible consanguinity. That line of inquiry,
however, also broke down, for, if there were consanguinity, it
was not obvious. What did become clear was that the patient and
his relatives belonged to a very large family with a clear sense of its
ethnic identity, complex bonds of kinship with other persons of
Dutch extraction, and a strong commitment to the Roman
Catholic religion. The focus of the inquiry now turned to the possibility of the patient and his relatives being members of an isolate.

To raise the possibility that the original patient might be a
member of an isolate community invited a change in methodology, since the community bore none of the classic hallmarks of an
isolate. Located in the Willamette Valley, a fertile trough stretch-
ing 100 miles from the Columbia River to the city of Eugene, in
close proximity to the state's major metropolis, the community
can hardly be categorized as geographically isolated. Nor could
ethnocentricity be the basis of isolation for the community encompassed persons of Belgian, German, and even Irish descent, in
addition to the Dutch presumed to be so omnipresent.

Ideology offered, if anything, an even less satisfactory explanation for isolation. If religion can be defined as a form of ideology, the most one can say in this instance is that this community
has a strong sense of religious identity. Most members of the
community are devout, practicing Catholics, and as we shall see
shortly, it is the church which serves as the physical and spiritual
center of the "town." However, a distinction must be made between a strong sense of religious identity and isolation.

The importance of the group's Catholic identity is indisputa-
ble. That this identity is the basis of isolation is improbable. In the
first place the earliest sedentary European population in the
Willamette Valley was Catholic. In the 1820s and 1830s French-
Canadian fur traders began forming a small community in an area
known as French Prairie. By 1840 the community was sufficiently
numerous for a mission to be established under Father Francis
Norbet Blanchet. By 1845 Oregon became an ecclesiastical prov-

ince with Blanchet as its archbishop.[6] When the community under study began to take shape in the Willamette Valley in 1875 its Catholic character was hardly an anomaly in a state which had a well-established Catholic hierarchy, schools, and mission system. One would have expected the Catholic character of the group to have assisted in the integration of the new arrivals into the already established population of the area.

Since the community could not be assumed to be an isolate it became necessary to ask explicitly whether or not it was indeed an isolate. It was this need which led to a medicohistorical collaboration. From the medical point of view the usual manner of building a pedigree had proven insufficient to the task. It was clear that the basis for the medical problems observed would not be found within the lines of a single family. A broader study encompassing the total community was needed. Being Catholic, the community had kept careful registers of its marriages, baptisms, and burials. The historical technique of family reconstitution developed by Henry and later adapted to English registers by Wrigley held the promise of proferring an answer to the medical question.[7] As we shall see, the exercise in family reconstitution, pursued from a historical as opposed to a medical point of view, led to the conclusion that the community was in fact an isolate. Further, the same analytical technique uncovered the basis for that isolation in the system of kinship generated by certain idiosyncracies of nuptial patterns.

The start for community reconstruction was provided by the parish registers. Following the general methodology outlined by Wrigley, we transcibed the baptism, marriage, and burial records, and then proceeded to rebuild all the families.[8] It became im-

6 Dorothy O. Johansen and Charles M. Gater, *Empire of the Columbia* (New York, 1957), 219–221.

7 Michel Fleury and Louis Henry, *Noveau Manuel de depouillement et d'exploitation de l'etat civil ancien* (Paris, 1965); E. A. Wrigley, "Family Reconstitution," in D. E. C. Eversley, Peter Laslett, and E. A. Wrigley (eds.), *An Introduction to English Historical Demography* (New York, 1966), 96–159.

8 A word should be said here about research procedures. Data was collected for this project by a series of undergraduate seminar students. In three different years groups of ten to twelve students were organized into a research team. Each time the team concentrated its efforts on a particular set of records and wrote a report of its findings. Thus, the first group transcribed most of the parish register which is available on microfilm at the Oregon Historical Society. The second group completed the transcription and expanded the reconstitution process to include information from the Oregon Census of 1880 and land records. The third group utilized migration records and three Wisconsin ms. censuses for 1850, 1860, and 1870.

mediately apparent that the community had two components: those who appeared fleetingly in the parish registers, and those whose lives were traceable through multiple generations. The latter numbered approximately thirty family names, and those we refer to as the "core families."[9]

Other sources have filled in the skeletal history provided by the parish registers. We have used the Oregon manuscript census of 1880 and the Wisconsin manuscript censuses of 1840, 1850, 1860, and 1870. We have also had access to Dutch migration records, and to unofficial documentation, the most important piece being a history of the parish produced by members of the community at the time of its Diamond Jubilee in 1950.[10] Combining the data from these various sources we now have the rough outlines of the community's European history, a rudimentary understanding of the group's first North American experiences in Wisconsin, definite data on the community's establishment in Oregon, and considerable knowledge of its subsequent history in the Northwest.

The European roots of twenty-eight core families are traceable to Holland, Belgium, or Germany. In twenty-four cases we have definite national identifications. Three families were German, two Belgian, and nineteen Dutch. Of the nineteen Dutch, seventeen family names were traceable to specific towns, all of which were located in the eastern portion of the Province of North Brabant. Of four families for whom we lack definite identifications, family surnames suggest that one was Belgian, one German or Dutch, and two Dutch.

As the map indicates, the geographical origins of the core families were highly concentrated, most coming from a series of towns clustered around Uden. Three other Brabant families came from towns contiguous to the Belgian border. Insofar as that bor-

9 It is difficult to give an absolute number for the core families, for they dominate in somewhat different ways. Some families are prominently core families if one examines birth records. Others dominate land-holding. Some are demographically unimportant in a numerical and/or economic sense, but are vital as genealogical links. Depending on the focus, we found ourselves concerned with twelve to thirty family names.
10 We have had Dutch migration records furnished us through the generosity of Robert Swieringa, who provided us with the computer lists of migrants from which he is doing a study of Dutch migration to North America in the nineteenth century. We have used his lists to locate the points of origin and migration dates of our core families. Diamond Jubilee, Visitation Church, Verboort, Oregon, 1875 to 1950. Private copy.

NOORD BRABANT HOLLAND

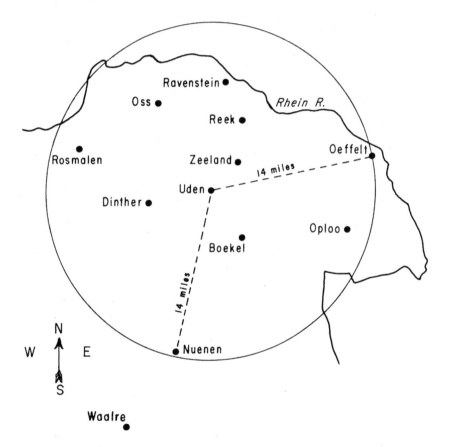

der had only been esablished in 1832, we have speculated that the kin connections between Dutch and Belgians might have preceded the imposition of the political boundary. By the same reasoning it is possible that the Germans were neighbors from across the Rhine. These possibilities are highly conjectural, but they do serve to make the point that the sharp differences one might presume to be reflected by differences in national designations may have been meaningless in the real-life world of these people.

By using the Dutch migration list we have been able to trace the arrival of the nineteen Dutch core families in North America. Their migration began in 1847 and 1848, at which time three Catholic priests sought to encourage people to move into the Fox River Valley of Wisconsin.[11] They recruited a number of North Brabanters, including two future Oregon core families. Other Dutch families arrived in the Fox River Valley in subsequent years, among them the rest of our core families. The last Wisconsin arrival date for a core family was 1870.

In tracing the Wisconsin history of the group we had as our sole source the manuscript census records, and what we have learned leaves us with important questions unanswered. The core families were somewhat scattered along the Fox River Valley, although by 1870 there was a notable concentration of thirteen of thirty-five core-family households in De Pere. Overt signs of their maintaining a separate identity are thin. The core families in all cases had other Dutch households near them. Perhaps one hint that the future Oregonians already had a sense of separate identity is the fact that Kaukana, the site of the most numerous concentration of Dutch households along the Fox in 1850, 1860, and 1870 drew a maximum of three core households, while in De Pere, which had a modest number of Dutch households, half of these were to become Oregon core families.

It is not until we come to the northwestern history of the community that we begin to have a clear understanding of the group's dynamics. A sense of identity emerges from the carefully preserved memory of the founding of the Oregon "town." According to local tradition the community's history began in 1873 when a man named John Verboort travelled from Wisconsin to the Pacific Northwest in search of a suitable location for an agrarian,

11   Henry S. Lucas, *Netherlanders in America* (Ann Arbor, 1955), 217 ff.

Catholic community. Having seen the Willamette Valley, he decided that Washington County would be the ideal geographical site. A second scouting expedition corroborated Verboort's report, and by the spring of 1875 six families made the move together to the Pacific Northwest.

The six families in question stopped initially in Portland while they arranged the cash purchase of the 550 acre Henry Black Donation Land claim. By the first week of April, 1875, the transaction had been completed, and the families took a train from Portland to the Valley station nearest their destination. For the first months the group functioned in a communal fashion, all twenty-seven in the party living together in the Black House, a ten-room, two-storied structure.[12] A large garden was laid out the produce of which was shared. Even the picking of the wild blackberries which grow so prolifically in western Oregon was carefully supervised and the crop judiciously divided. After the first harvest the land was divided into lots and individual houses were built. The community grew as new families arrived from Wisconsin, and by 1908 community expansion was sufficient to warrant the founding of a daughter parish from among the families of the original parish.

This historical overview serves to emphasize several important points about the community. First, there is no doubt about the cohesiveness of the group during the time it has lived in the Northwest. Second, the group's identity was already visible in Wisconsin. Third, circumstantial evidence suggests that community identity was already evident in Europe. Each of these observations reveals the common origins of the community and strengthens the possibility that it could be an isolate. However, we have yet to grasp the dynamics which bind the group together. These are the issues to which we must now turn.

Our concentrated analysis has so far centered on Oregon, and on the basis of what we have learned of the community's northwestern history it appears that there are three phenomena which have served to keep the group united: religion, land, and kinship.

12 There is a strong possibility that family B-4 is related to family A. The husband's widowed mother in family 4 bears the same married surname as the wife's maiden name in family 2. We have found no way to prove the linkage but suspect strongly that some relationship did exist (see fig. 1).

We suspect that the community would give greatest credit to the first element, whereas we, since the focus of our interest is on the isolate character of the group, emphasize the last. All three components are, however, interwoven, and from stray clues we think that it has been these same elements which linked the group both in the Old World and the New.

RELIGION   The importance of religion as a unifying principle is not to be belittled. Although the community may not exist insofar as the secular organization of the state of Oregon is concerned, the town being unincorporated, it definitely exists in the minds of the inhabitants. Nor is it hard for outsiders to find the community if they know for what to look. The physical center of the "town" is marked by its church, the importance of which is emphasized by its size and solidity. Although the houses of the area are generally modest in size and built of wood, the church stands out in terms of its imposing mass and its building material—red brick.

The centrality of the church, both in a physical and a spiritual sense, is nothing new to the community. According to tradition a major reason for the move from Wisconsin to Oregon was the desire to found a Catholic community. We also know that the guiding force behind the migration was Father William Verboort. His brothers, John and Albert, helped scout the Northwest for a suitable location, and fourteen members of Father Verboort's family migrated with the twenty-seven person founding group. His unexpected death at the age of forty during the summer of 1876 was a severe blow. Yet the sense of purpose and cohesiveness did not evaporate. Additional families arrived and the church continued to serve as the focal point of the community.

By 1889 the community enjoyed sufficient material comfort and its membership was large enough for a major building program to be undertaken which continued through 1894. Entries in the parish register make clear the wide and active involvement of the parishioners. It was they who provided not only funds, but also labor to erect a house for the priest, paint the church, and place a cross in the cemetery.

However, when we speak of the church as the focal point of the community, this must be understood in a wider context. The church was not just a building, but rather the basic unit of social organization. It included the parochial school—initially limited to elementary education, but later expanded to include a high school in response to changes in state educational requirements. The community orientation of the school was reinforced by teaching nuns who were frequently daughters of parish families.

Social and recreational activity also clustered around the church, and, to a degree, economic life as well. Beyond the school building stands the community hall. Once heavily used for dances and social gatherings, it is now the one "town" building which appears to be somewhat neglected. It is still used for the annual sausage festival, but the social gatherings of times past are no longer frequent.

The two centers of economic activity stand across the road from the church. These are the grocery store, today a very small enterprise catering exclusively to limited local needs, and the sausage factory. Despite its small size and necessarily limited clientele, the store is still neatly painted and carefully maintained. The sausage factory is a recent addition, and it stands in new splendor, the largest single structure in the town aside from the church. Commercial sausage-making has sprung from the annual sausage festival, a traditional Brabant celebration to which the public is invited.

LAND   The strongest physical manifestation of community identity is to be seen in what has happened to landholding in the area. To have an accurate idea of the configuration of the community requires that one take in at least one neighboring parish which was formed early in the twentieth century by the overflow from the original community. The formation of the new parish probably reflects the expansion in landholding which placed the younger generation at an increasingly inconvenient distance from the original parish church. Data about landholding in the second parish have yet to be collected. Nonetheless, within the limits of what has been done, interesting patterns are discernible.

We selected nine sections which corresponded most closely to the boundaries of the original parish, and proceeded to analyze landholding patterns for the core families from 1875 to 1972. We made three observations. The first was that once land came into the possession of community members it tended to stay there. The second discovery was that, in terms of landholding in the nine sections examined, there were two stages of development. The first stage was completed during the first decade of the twentieth century, while the second took place during World War II. Our third discovery was that within the community confines there was a lively exchange of land among members of the community.

The propensity for land to remain with members of the core families is illustrated in Table 1 which lists the total acreage held by the core families in 1907, 1937, and 1972. Total acreage remained stable from 1907 to 1937, then increased by 1972.

Close to 1,000 additional acres had been acquired in the nine sections, bringing the community holdings to 70 percent of the total land in the nine sections. The first generation had established a basic territorial claim, with minimal changes taking place during the second generation. Either late in the life of the second generation, or early in that of the third generation territorial organization did alter. The total land area held by the core families increased, possibly as a response to demographical expansion and perhaps as a response to the increased demand for agricultural products generated during World War II.

At the same time the community world was never static. Ownership changed frequently among members of the community and there was a distinct tendency for land near the church to be broken into smaller and smaller fragments. In fact, at the center of the community near the church, there is a proliferation of small parcels of land, a number of which are now utilized by the community's oldest residents who have retired from active farming. Although the macrocosm either remained static or expanded the microcosm was a kaleidoscope of change.

KINSHIP   The third and crucial element in fostering community cohesion is kinship. We first became aware of the importance of the

Table 1   Acreage Held by Core Families in First Parish, 1907, 1937, 1972.

	1907	1937	1972
Total land owned by core families	2880.82	3139.45	4070.23
Total number of acres in nine-section area	5760.00	5760.00	5760.00
% of land controlled by core families in nine-section area	50.00	54.50	70.66

kin network as we probed the history of the migrating generation. Fortunately community tradition described in minute detail the make-up of the founding group, for the patterns found among them are the same for the entire migrating generation. It is these patterns which are responsible for the development of the community as an isolate.

Figure 1 depicts the migrating group of 1875, and demonstrates that although there may have been six different households, these represented only four families. For example, families 1, 2, and 3 consisted of an elderly set of parents and their four children, two of whom were married and themselves had children. Families 4 and 5 were less complex, but they, too, were extended families. Only family 6 appears as a simple nuclear family composed of parents and young children.

The characteristics revealed by the first group deserve emphasis because, as we later discovered, the same principles affected all subsequent migrants. First, we realized the importance of the kin bonds. These bonds held the group together both vertically through the generations and horizontally among the siblings. The strength of the kin ties was such that migrants represented all stages of the life-cycle, not just the youth who are traditionally regarded as most prone to moving. Lastly, and again this is an effect of kin ties, what appear initially as six nuclear families are interconnected by family bonds which reduce the group to three major social units.

Once the process of family reconstitution was well advanced we discovered that the principles visible among the first group also shaped subsequent migrations. Without the aid of reconstitution as a technique this could not have been discovered because, after the arrival of the 1875 party, the community appears to have lost interest in the dynamics of subsequent arrivals. This may be in part because there were no further transfers from Wisconsin which were organized in the elaborate manner of the founding group. Instead subsequent immigrants trickled in, usually as nuclear families. However, once we established pedigrees for all the families who lived in the community for more than one generation we stumbled onto the underlying pattern of kinship. As Figure 2 indicates, we were able to establish that the families who migrated were linked together in a giant web. For only seven core families were we unable to establish genealogical links, but in five of these

Fig. 1   Migration of Founding Group in 1875

Dotted lines encompass households, each of which is identified by an Arabic numeral. Households are appropriately grouped into family groups, each of which is given a letter. All of the persons depicted arrived in the spring of 1875 with the exception of the male in family A who is identified as arriving in the fall.

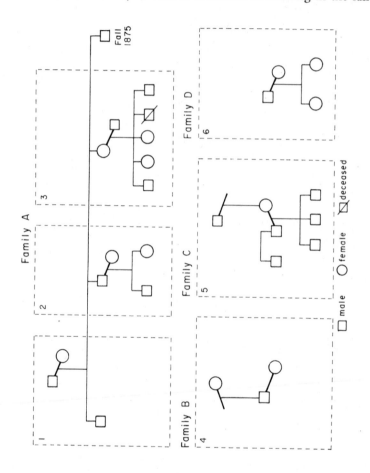

Fig. 2 Community Migration: Kinship Ring

We have placed all families whose genealogical connections could be traced on the "kinship ring." Despite the spread of arrival dates from February, 1875 to 1900, it has been possible to establish links between most of the families which arrived in the community.

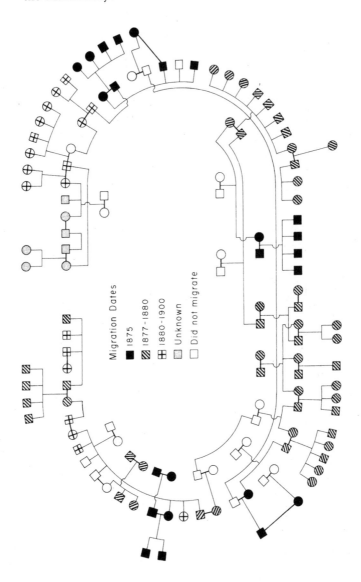

instances we are convinced that they, too, were related to the community prior to migration. We feel this to be true since these five have been traced to North Brabant. Furthermore, in examining the marriages of their Oregonian offspring we found them intertwined with families who were part of the "migration ring." Our surmise is that these five families were linked to the web through persons who remained in Wisconsin. Thus, in only two cases do we find a lack of correspondence with the general patterns for the community.

It should also be emphasized that the community migration ring reflects the same feature observed in the 1875 migration: the importance of kinship, both in terms of vertical generations, and in terms of horizontal sibling ties. It also reveals the willingness of these people to move at various stages of the life cycle, a fact which again emphasizes the importance of kin ties.

The construction of the migration ring revealed the importance of kinship in the formation of the Oregon community. It also demonstrated that the community dated its establishment to a time preceding the move to the Pacific Northwest. Furthermore, the ring gave us our first clear evidence that we were looking at an isolate. But kin ties, and with them the isolate, can evaporate quickly unless they are reinforced by each succeeding generation. Reinforcement, in turn, depends upon marital patterns.

The existence of parish records in Oregon has enabled us to examine in depth the marriage practices of the community, and we have discovered the glue which has cemented the group—certainly in Oregon, and possibly in Wisconsin and Holland as well.

There are two marriage practices which are noteworthy in this community. One is what we call "repeat alliances," defined as the creation of multiple marriage links between given families, whether in the same or in successive generations. The second is a specialized version of the above practice which anthropologists call "sibling exchange marriages." In this case sets of siblings from two families intermarry.

The marriages of twelve children from a particular family are shown in Figure 3. These children were third-generation Oregonians, their grandparents having migrated to the Northwest. One can see the sibling exchanging phenomenon in the marriages of children 2, 3, and 4 (three sisters who married three brothers from

Fig. 3 Marriages of a Third Generation Family

Marriages of twelve children, third generation ■ symbolizes a
realliance. That is to say that in either preceding, succeeding,
and/or parallel lines in this family, there were other marriages
linking the same surnames. Among the eight realliances, six different surnames are represented.

■ Re-alliance

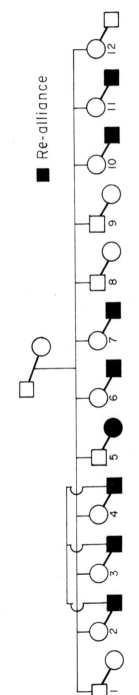

another family). In addition one can see that eight of the twelve marriages served to re-ally this family to families with which they already have established ties of kinship.

The marriages in another family over three generations illustrated in Figure 4 clarifies how the repeat alliance phenomenon operates. The central family in Generation I consisted of two brothers: I, 1 and I, 2. Brother I, 2 had three sons (Nos. II- 9, 10, 11), while brother I, 1 had five sons (Nos. II- 2, 4, 5, 7, 8) and three daughters (Nos. II- 1, 3, 6). So far as we know the wives in Generation I were unrelated. All eleven members of Generation II married, but rather than eleven new alliances there were but eight. The total number of new family alliances was less than the total number of marriages because six marriages were to pairs of siblings. Four of I, 2's children (Nos. II- 2, II- 3, II- 4, and II- 5) married pairs of siblings. I- 1's son No. II- 7 and I- 2's son No. II- 9 also married a pair of sisters. Thus, II- 7 and II- 9 were both first cousins and brothers-in-law.

When we look at the third generation we notice the effects of concentration even more strongly. We have been able to trace the marital history of fourteen of the youngsters of Generation III. Out of their fourteen alliances ties were established with only four families, and of these one was a repeat alliance. The latter occurred with the marriage of III- 4 and III- 5 who were first cousins. In this case there was legal and ecclesiastical consanguinity and, to cope with the latter, a dispensation was required.[13] It should be emphasized that such cases appear to be extremely rare. More frequent is the type of situation illustrated by the marriage of III- 6. In this case the spouses were not related genetically. However, from a social point of view their marriage served to reinforce ties between two families which were already allied both in Generation II and Generation III. The link in this case was II- 6 who was aunt to both III- 6 and to her husband. III- 6 was the child of II- 6's brother (II- 5), while III- 6's husband was the child of II- 6's brother-in-law.

As we can see from the case of this family, marriages based upon repeat alliances or sibling exchanges serve to bind a group of people into a complex biological network. If the practices are per-

13　The right to marry a relative is limited both by civil and cannon law. Exceptions to the latter can be obtained in certain cases (for example, for a first cousin marriage) through an ecclesiastical dispensation.

Fig. 4   Marriages of a Core Family: Three Generations

Three generations of marriages for a core family. ■ or ● stand for male or female members of the core family whose marriages are traced over three generations. Generations are noted with Roman numerals. Offspring in each generation are represented by Arabic numerals.

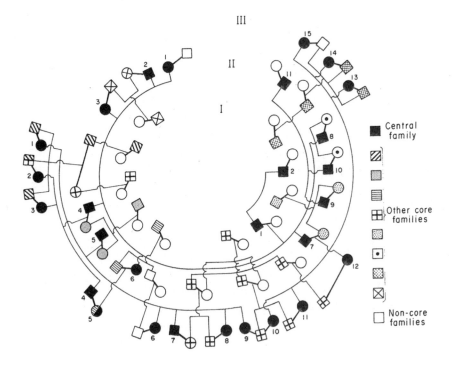

petuated over successive generations the relationships which result become so entangled that the participants cease to understand the nature of their biological relationships. It should be emphasized that this can take place without there being an elevated number of consanguinous marriages in the legal or ecclesiastical sense of the term. However, from a biological point of view these practices, if they persist, do create a gene pool which becomes concentrated. Gradually more and more genes will become unusually frequent, and, in such a situation, the chances of recessive genes pairing increases. In this way one could anticipate the emergence of an isolate population, displaying different gene frequencies from the general population, without the usual factors of geographical, ideological, or linguistic isolation found in isolates hitherto described.

The rapidity with which a biological isolate might arise out of purely social practices would depend upon three factors: the size of the founding population, the intensity with which it practiced restricted mating, and the temporal duration of the mating patterns. Thus, for a very large group of people one would need more generations for unusual genes to become fixed or frequent among the group than one would for a small founding group, assuming the same propensity for both to mate within the group.

For our group we could assume that the migration ring is the founding group. One could envisage an isolate arising from such a founding group, but would it arise within the third or fourth generation? Perhaps, but, in view of the avoidance of legal consanguinity, this is not probable. The appearance of isolate characteristics would instead suggest that the group had existed as a community for more than three to four generations. Indeed historical data tend to support that contention. Since the relationships reflected by the marriage ring were established in Wisconsin we know that there must have been a community of sorts prior to the group's establishment in Oregon. But genealogical knowledge fails to extend the relationship of the community temporally. To do that we would need some indication that the practices observed in the Northwest predate the move to Wisconsin.

Is there such evidence? At this point we move from what we have been able to unearth as "fact" into a hazier realm in which we have clues only. There is one pattern among the families practicing repeat and sibling alliances which suggests that these habits may predate the move to North America. Overwhelmingly the families indulging in these practices came from the Dutch Province of North Brabant. In analyzing Oregon marriage patterns we found fifteen families who either exhibited repeat alliances or sibling exchange marriages. Of these, nine came from North Brabant, one from Amsterdam, one from Prussia, and one from Germany. There were three cases where we could not establish a point of origin for the family, but one case at least is certainly Dutch. We traced 335 marriages for these fifteen families. Of these 216, or 66.4 percent, were repeat alliances. Among the North Brabanters 190 of 283 marriages we recorded (70 percent) were repeat alliances. This suggests that the practice may have been peculiar to the European heritage of the families in question, particularly for those from North Brabant.

At first sight this proposition may seem to be far fetched. However, it is compatible with observations made by Moroni in a study of consanguinity in northern Italy.[14] Moroni used as his source the Vatican archives on dispensations. He discovered that the rate of consanguinous marriages increased in the nineteenth century following the promulgation of the Code Napoleon. The basis for this, Moroni believes, was an effort by the northern Italians to protect family property. The Code Napoleon required the equal division of property among all offspring including the females. Applied to land, this meant that a once-handsome family plot might within one or two generations be reduced to a mosaic of useless morsels. To avoid this result, some families ingeniously arranged for intra-family marriages which enabled them to keep the overall holdings intact.

The patterns that we have seen may have been generated by a similar motive. The technique, however, was a bit different. Rather than brothers arranging that their children should marry each other, a decision which required ecclesiastical dispensation, could it be that the Brabanters utilized sibling exchanges or repeat alliances to achieve the same ends—and without the jarring need to bend the rules of their faith?

The chance detection of a case of cutaneous porphyria has led to the identification of an isolate community the existence of which has been studied over approximately 100 years in some

---

14 A. Moroni, "Andamento della consanguineità nell' Italia Settentrionale negli ultimi quattro secoli," *Atti Associazione Genetica Italiana*, XII (1966), 202-222.

depth and detail. The major findings may be cited as follows. First, the identification itself has demonstrated that isolates are not necessarily obvious. All isolates are dependent to a degree upon social behavior, but it is now clear that they are not dependent upon isolation of a geographical, ideological, or linguistic nature. They can exist purely on the basis of social practice, and they can follow those practices sufficiently unobtrusively to remain undetected. Anyone seriously interested in isolate communities needs not only to study those groups which are clearly separated from the general run of humanity, but also needs to be alert to the possibility of identifying such communities as they exist within a general population.

Second, the study has unravelled in considerable detail the social patterns and, more specifically, the nuptial patterns which have led to the formation of the isolate. Two definite patterns, realliance and sibling exchange, have been identified as the basis of biological isolation. The identification of these patterns in turn can be applied for comparative purposes to other already known isolates or to cases where one suspects, but is as yet uncertain, that an isolate does exist.

Third, the study is a demonstration that cooperative research between the fields of biomedicine and social history can be mutually productive. These two fields have appeared to stand far enough apart in terms of their concerns and methods that they have not been envisaged as a fruitful interdisciplinary area. As a result the dialogue between the two areas has been thin, particularly at the historian's end. This state of affairs does seem to be changing for, as an editorial in *The Lancet* commented, there is interplay between "gene frequencies and history."[15] In some instances historical knowledge has assisted in the understanding of genetic findings, while in others genetic data have assisted historians in interpreting the significance of archaeological data. The examples cited in *The Lancet* editorial focused on research into important problems of the past. The study reported here not only demonstrates the usefulness of interdisciplinary research linking biomedical and historical research, but also indicates that such collaboration can be utilized in what one might call current history.

15 "Gene Frequencies and History," *The Lancet*, I (May 10, 1975), 1075–1076.

In conclusion, it is appropriate to note that it is the mutual interest in social behavior which makes the cooperation of biomedical and historical researchers both possible and productive. Both disciplines are interested in tracing change over time. It is in this area that the community described here fascinates. One cannot but want to know why these particular patterns of behavior arose, why they were perpetuated, and whether in the face of modernization and urbanization the same patterns are apt to persist.